AF514723

Endoscopy of the Hip and Knee

Tun Hing Lui
Editor

Endoscopy of the Hip and Knee

Principle and Practice

Springer

Editor
Tun Hing Lui
Department of Orthopaedics and Traumatology
North District Hospital
Hong Kong
China

The Second Affiliated Hospital
Shenzhen University
Shenzhen
China

ISBN 978-981-16-3490-1 ISBN 978-981-16-3488-8 (eBook)
https://doi.org/10.1007/978-981-16-3488-8

© The Editor(s) (if applicable) and The Author(s), under exclusive license to Springer Nature Singapore Pte Ltd. 2021
This work is subject to copyright. All rights are solely and exclusively licensed by the Publisher, whether the whole or part of the material is concerned, specifically the rights of translation, reprinting, reuse of illustrations, recitation, broadcasting, reproduction on microfilms or in any other physical way, and transmission or information storage and retrieval, electronic adaptation, computer software, or by similar or dissimilar methodology now known or hereafter developed.
The use of general descriptive names, registered names, trademarks, service marks, etc. in this publication does not imply, even in the absence of a specific statement, that such names are exempt from the relevant protective laws and regulations and therefore free for general use.
The publisher, the authors, and the editors are safe to assume that the advice and information in this book are believed to be true and accurate at the date of publication. Neither the publisher nor the authors or the editors give a warranty, expressed or implied, with respect to the material contained herein or for any errors or omissions that may have been made. The publisher remains neutral with regard to jurisdictional claims in published maps and institutional affiliations.

This Springer imprint is published by the registered company Springer Nature Singapore Pte Ltd.
The registered company address is: 152 Beach Road, #21-01/04 Gateway East, Singapore 189721, Singapore

To my wife Eva and my sons Pun Lok and Pun Ho

Foreword

The interest of the Editor, Dr. T. H. Lui, in endoscopic surgery starts from the very beginning of his orthopaedic training. Throughout his career, he has been a champion for pushing and expanding the boundaries of endoscopic surgery into different parts of the human anatomy.

As a record of his footprints in various anatomical regions, he came up with a series of three books. The first one "*Arthroscopy and Endoscopy of the Foot and Ankle: Principles and Practice*" was already in print in 2019. Followed by "*Arthroscopy and Endoscopy of the Hand, Wrist and Elbow: Principles and Practice*" and then, this book on Endoscopy of the Hip and Knee.

For each region, the arrangements were similar and logical. To begin with, the anatomy as seen through the endoscope was clearly illustrated. Then, the setup and instruments for the actual practice were explained. These serve as not only essential source of information for beginners but also handy reference for those who happen to need it every now and then.

After the section on basic knowledge, are chapters on specific topics at the frontiers of endoscopic surgery of the particular region. These chapters were representative of milestones in the development of the topic under discussion. Taking the hip as an example, there were chapters addressing the use of hip arthroscopy in femoroacetabular impingement, avascular necrosis of the femoral head, developmental dysplasia of the hip and post total hip arthroplasty. In addition, chapters on endoscopies of the peritrochanteric and deep gluteal spaces were included to address the less charted areas such as Greater trochanteric pain syndrome, Piriformis syndrome, Deep gluteus syndrome, ischiofemoral impingement and anterior inferior iliac spine impingement.

For the knee, the proximal tibiofibular joint was not left out in spite of its small size. The readers will also be interested to find chapters devoted to the use of endoscopy for non-confined spaces, pathologies of bursae, ligaments, iliotibial band, sural nerve and tendoscopy of the patellar tendon. The chapter on Navigated Endoscopic Assisted Tumour Surgery for the management of benign bone tumour is particularly inspiring. Future development along this direction is expected.

In a nutshell, this book is a useful reference for those in different stages of their orthopaedic career. For posterity, it records the borders of developments of endoscopy of the hip and knee at this point in time. It is on top of this foundation that advancements will be added on in years to come.

University of Hong Kong
Hong Kong, China

Chinese University of Hong Kong
Hong Kong, China
March 2021

Sai Hung Yeung

Preface

I have had the privilege to experience firsthand the advances of hip and knee surgery during my 30 years of practice, and have witnessed technological advances in instrument design which have enabled my friends and colleagues from all over the world develop many innovative procedures to tackle hip and knee conditions. I started preparing this book 2 years ago with the aim of summarizing the current research together, and have found that as time went on, it was difficult for me to not continually expand the book's chapter index because so many new frontiers have continually been explored. Brilliant colleagues from all over the world have relentlessly pushed the boundaries of imagination in where our scope can reach.

I am optimistic about our future developments and believe that there will continually be advances in hip and knee surgery for many years to come; I anticipate that 10 years later, I might need to start rewriting this book from scratch.

Hong Kong, China
Shenzhen, China

Tun Hing Lui

Acknowledgement

I must acknowledge my good friend Prof. Xiaohua PAN of the Second Affiliated Hospital, Shenzhen University for initializing and giving life to this project.

I also like to thank the Institute of Biomedicine and Biotechnology, Shenzhen Institutes of Advanced Technology, Chinese Academy of Science and Shenzhen University for their help during preparation of this book.

My boss and mentor Dr. Ngai WK who allowed me the freedom to develop myself; you will always have my respect and gratitude.

Special thanks to Pun Ho LUI for his English editing support of this book.

Last but not least, I must take this opportunity to acknowledge my beloved wife Eva who has supported and tolerated my many late-night writing sessions, and my sons Pun Lok and Pun Ho, you boys are the joy of my life.

Contents

Part III Knee

Part I

Basic Knowledge

1 Arthroscopic Anatomy of the Hip

Marcos Del Carmen-Rodriguez, Josep Maria de Anta, Marc Tey, and Miki Dalmau-Pastor

Abstract

Hip arthroscopy is an uncommonly used surgical technique mainly due to the proximity of risk structures to the hip joint, and also to its anatomical characteristics. The coxofemoral (hip) joint is deep and narrow, features that do not facilitate arthroscopic maneuvers with surgical instruments. Recent advances in clinical diagnosis, the adaptation of young surgeons to new arthroscopic techniques, as well as the increase in training programs for surgeons, have caused a change in open surgical techniques to for minimally invasive procedures supported by arthroscopy.

The knowledge of the hip anatomy is an essential to perform this kind of surgery correctly and safely. In addition, many anatomical studies have been made in order to avoid any structural injury before entering the joint.

In this chapter, we will discuss the intraarticular and extraarticular structures that surgeons find in approaching the joint to ensure a good arthroscopic intervention of the hip.

Keywords

Hip · Anatomy · Arthroscopy · Endoscopy · Portals Compartments

1.1 Introduction

Hip arthroscopy is an uncommonly used surgical technique mainly due to the proximity of risk structures to the hip joint, and also to its anatomical characteristics. The coxofemoral (hip) joint is deep and narrow, features that do not facilitate arthroscopic maneuvers with surgical instruments. Recent advances in clinical diagnosis, the adaptation of young surgeons to new arthroscopic techniques, as well as the increase in training programs for surgeons, have caused a change in open surgical techniques to for minimally invasive procedures supported by arthroscopy.

The knowledge of the hip anatomy is an essential to perform this kind of surgery correctly and safely. In addition, many anatomical studies have been made in order to avoid any structural injury before entering the joint.

In this chapter, we will discuss the intraarticular and extraarticular structures that surgeons find in approaching the joint to ensure a good arthroscopic intervention of the hip.

M. Del Carmen-Rodriguez
Orthopedic and Traumatology Department, Hospital Universitari de Bellvitge, L'Hospitalet de Llobregat, Catalunya, Spain

J. M. de Anta
Faculty of Medicine and Health Sciences, Department of Pathology and Experimental Therapeutics, Human Anatomy and Embryology Unit, Universitat de Barcelona, Barcelona, Spain

M. Tey
Orthopedic Department, iMove Traumatologia, Barcelona, Catalunya, Spain

Orthopedic Department, Hospital del Mar, Barcelona, Catalunya, Spain

M. Dalmau-Pastor (✉)
Faculty of Medicine and Health Sciences, Department of Pathology and Experimental Therapeutics, Human Anatomy and Embryology Unit, Universitat de Barcelona, Barcelona, Spain

MIFAS by GRECMIP (Minimally Invasive Foot and Ankle Society), Merignac, France
e-mail: mikeldalmau@ub.edu

© The Author(s), under exclusive license to Springer Nature Singapore Pte Ltd. 2021
T. H. Lui (ed.), *Endoscopy of the Hip and Knee*, https://doi.org/10.1007/978-981-16-3488-8_1

1.2 Osteomusculoligamentous Anatomy of the Hip

The coxofemoral joint is a ball and socket joint formed by the union of the femoral head and the acetabulum (Fig. 1.1). It allows the following movements: flexion/extension in the sagittal plane, adduction/abduction in the coronal plane, medial/lateral rotation in the transverse plane, as well as their combination (circumduction). Active range of motion (ROM) values are approximately 115°–125° of flexion and 25°–30° of extension, 30°–45° of abduction and 25–30 of adduction, and 35° of lateral rotation and 15° of medial rotation in hip neutral flexion-extension, and 40°–60° of lateral rotation and 30°–40° of medial rotation at 90° of knee flexion. One reason of an excessive lateral or medial rotation could be compensatory of a femoral neck anteversion or retroversion angle, which is 15°. ROM values can differ according to age, population, sport type and activity, or others [1, 2].

The cervico-diaphyseal (neck-shaft) angle is normally 125° and determines the size of femoral offset. An increased angle (about 130°) produces a *coxa valga*, whereas a decreased angle (about 120°) is called *coxa vara*. Both the cervico-diaphyseal and the femoral version angles influence abductor muscles strength (less with *coxa vara* and femoral anteversion) [1] and hip contact forces (more strength with femoral anteversion) [3].

The acetabular anteversion angle is approximately 17° [4] and has a positive correlation with the femoral neck version angle [5]. Variation in acetabular morphology results in wall changes (Fig. 1.2). For example, an acetabular retroversion secondary to a posterior wall deficiency or an anterior wall

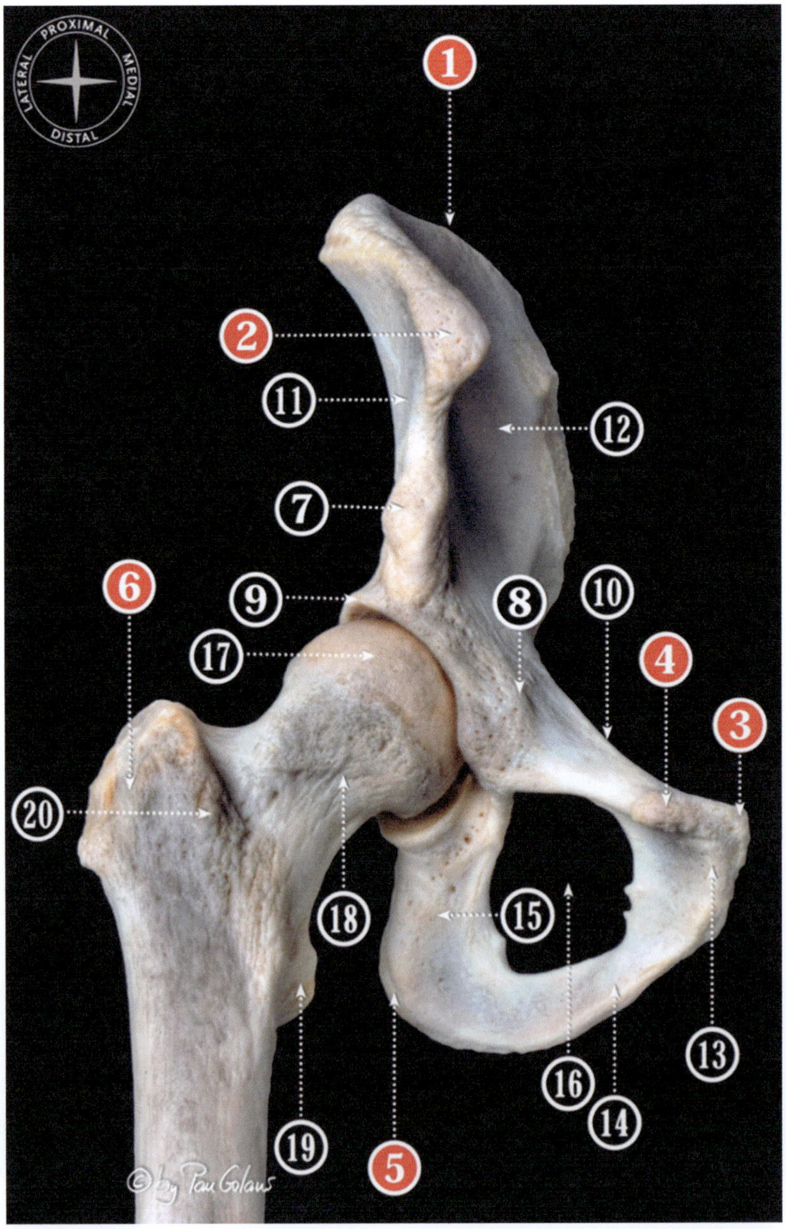

Fig. 1.1 Anterior view of the osseous components of a right hip joint (red numbers correspond to bone landmarks that can be palpated). (1) iliac crest, (2) anterior superior iliac spine, (3) pubic symphisis, (4) pubic tubercle, (5) ischial tuberosity, (6) greater trochanter, (7) anterior inferior iliac spine, (8) iliopubic eminence, (9) rim of the acetabulum, (10) pectineal line or pecten of pubis, (11) gluteal surface, (12) iliac fossa, (13) body of pubis, (14) ramus of ischium, (15) body of ischium, (16) obturator foramen, (17) head of femur, (18) neck of femur, (19) lesser trochanter, (20) intertrochanteric line. Reproduced with permission from *Dalmau-Pastor M, Vega J, Golanó P. Anatomy of the Hip Joint and how it effects groin pain. Aspetar Sports Medicine Journal 2014;3(2):418–25*

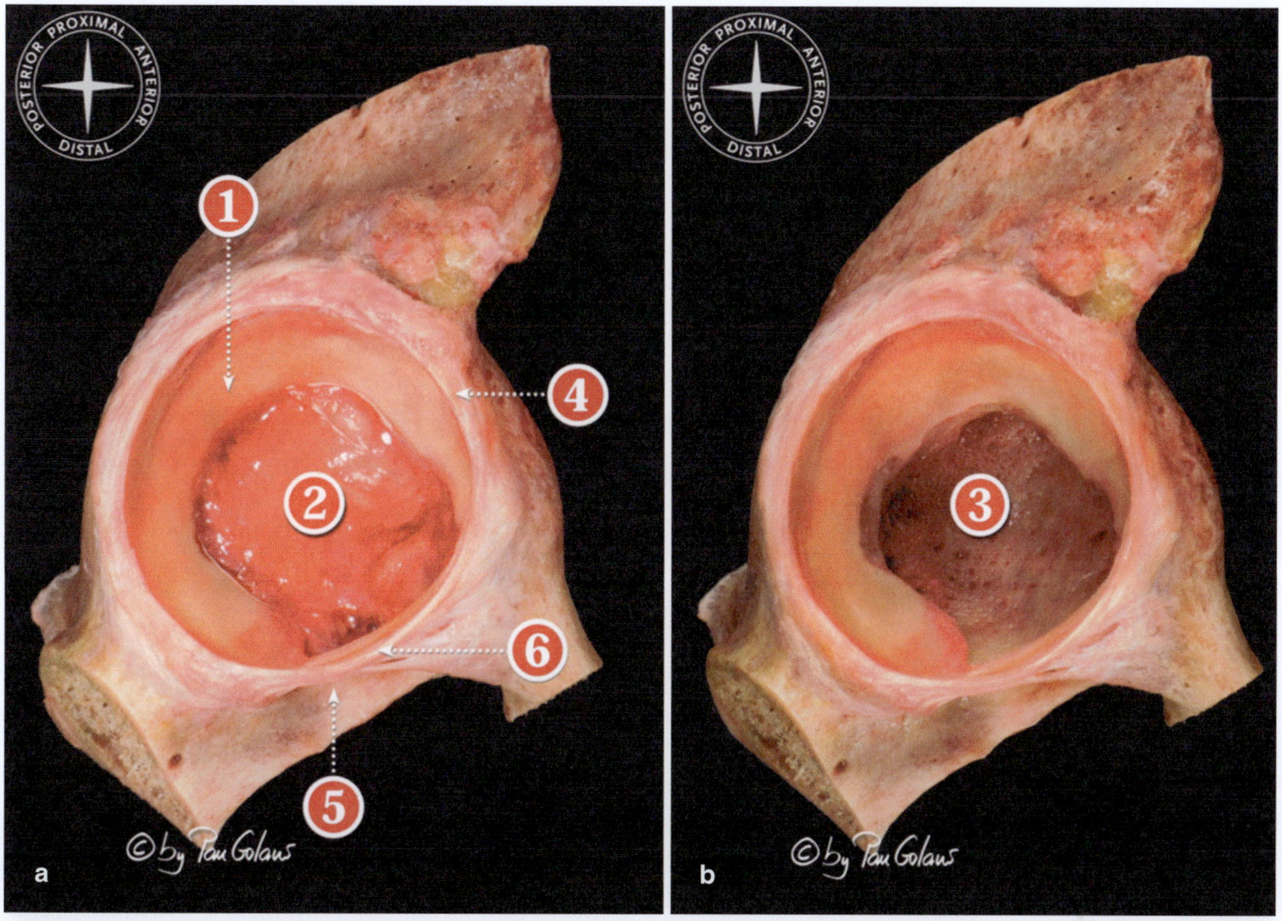

Fig. 1.2 Anterior view of an osteoarticular dissection of the acetabular area. (**a**) acetabular fossa with the pulvinar, (**b**) acetabular fossa with the pulvinar removed. (1) lunate articular surface, (2) pulvinar, (3) acetabular or cotyloid fossa, (4) acetabular labrum, (5) acetabular notch, (6) transverse ligament. Reproduced with permission from *Dalmau-Pastor M, Vega J, Golanó P. Anatomy of the Hip Joint and how it effects groin pain. Aspetar Sports Medicine Journal 2014;3(2):418–25*

overcoverage, or both, has been demonstrated to cause Pincer-type femoroacetabular impingement (FAI) [6]. It varies according to gender [7] and age, especially during skeletal maturation [8], although these variations are not pathological in many cases [9]. Because most acetabular retroversion angle changes cause pain a large study is required to improve the surgical results [10].

The coxofemoral joint capsule has a cylindrical sleeve-like shape and it travels from the periphery of the acetabulum outside the labrum to the proximal epiphysis of the femur. The capsule fibers insert distally and anteriorly along the intertrochanteric line of the femur. Posteriorly, the capsule fibers attach onto the posteromedial edge of the greater trochanter generating an arched free border that covers only the femoral neck. The orientation of the capsule fibers differs according to their location, anteriorly arranged longitudinally, and posteriorly arranged transversally, except posteriorly and inferiorly where the circular fibers of the zona orbicularis are located [11]. In the acetabular notch, the fibers are attached onto the transverse acetabular ligament [12]. The thickness of the capsular joint also varies depending on its location: it is thickest posterosuperiorly in its acetabular insertion and antero-superiorly near its femoral insertion [13]; whereas it is thinnest antero-inferiorly in its acetabular insertion and posteriorly in its femoral insertion [13].

The coxofemoral joint capsule (Fig. 1.3) is reinforced by four important ligaments: the iliofemoral ligament, the pubofemoral ligament, the ischiofemoral ligament, and the zona orbicularis.

The iliofemoral ligament (ILFL) covers the anterior, superior, and posterior part of the capsule, and comprises two distinguishable bands separated by a thinner central area. The longitudinal fibers of the superior or lateral band reinforce the capsule from its origin at the anterior inferior iliac spine (AIIS) to its insertion onto the lateral part of the intertrochanteric line, whereas the inferior or medial band originates closer to the AIIS and inserts anteriorly onto the medial part of the intertrochanteric line, and superiorly and posteriorly more transversally onto the superior border of the major trochanter. Between the two bands, a thinner area is

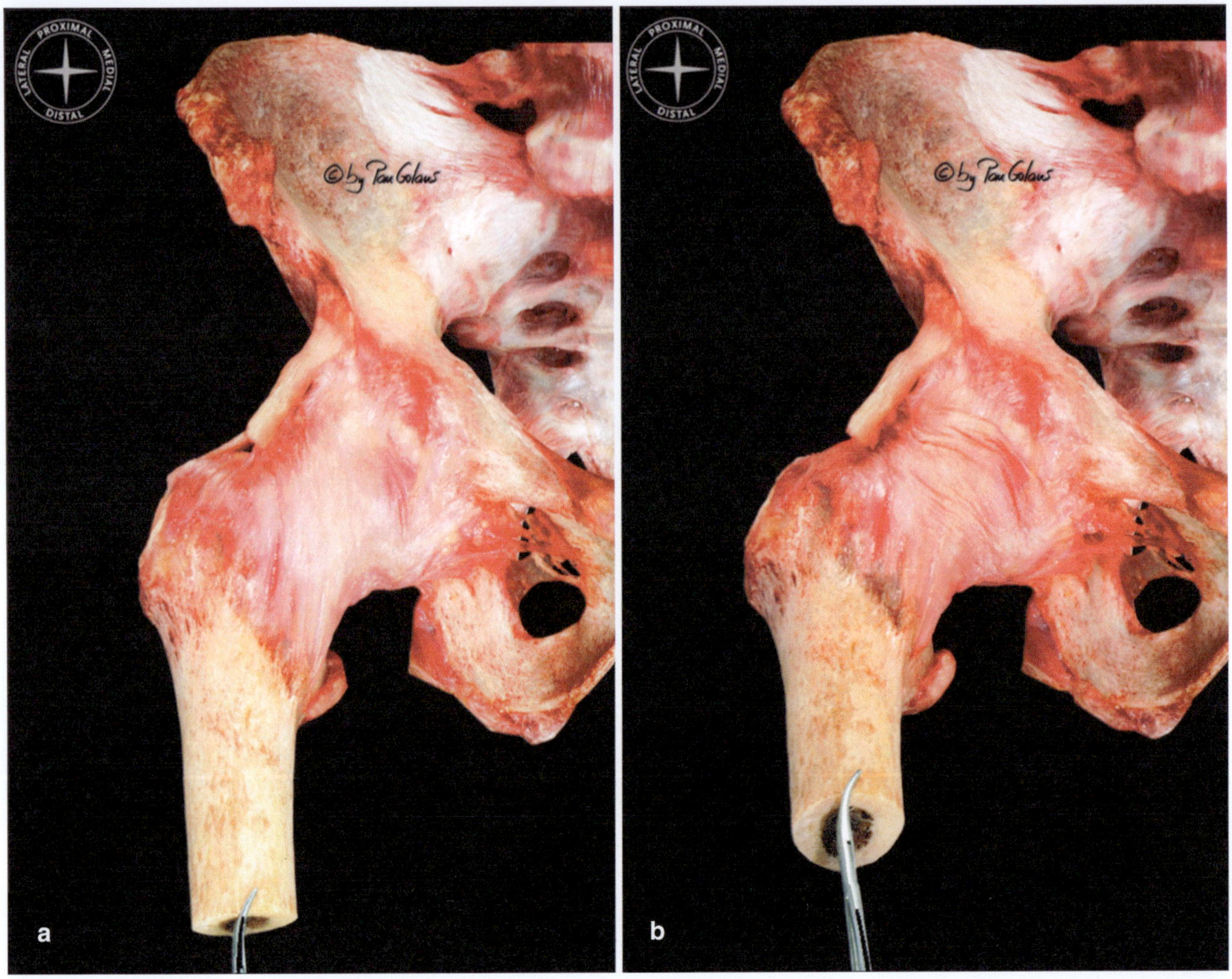

Fig. 1.3 Anterior view of an osteoarticular dissection showing osteoarticular complex of the hip joint. (**a**) Hip in anatomical position, (**b**) hip flexed. Relaxation of the anterior ligaments facilitates access to the hip joint during arthroscopy of the peripheral compartments, creating an anterior working area. Reproduced with permission from *Dalmau-Pastor M, Vega J, Golanó P. Anatomy of the Hip Joint and how it effects groin pain. Aspetar Sports Medicine Journal 2014;3(2):418–25*

described [12, 14]. The suggested functionality of this area is to balance the force of the body weight to the joint during straight position, which would explain why it is tense in extension and lax in flexion [12]. Recent studies support the importance of this ligament in rotation movements: lateral rotation is limited by both of the iliofemoral bands in extension and flexion, and medial rotation is limited by the superior arm instead of other ligaments [14].

The pubofemoral ligament (PFL) originates at the pubic portion of acetabular rim and the obturator crest and expands inferiorly blending with the inferior band of the IFL ligament to insert onto the medial part of the intertrochanteric line [12, 14]. It seems to be important limiting lateral rotation in flexion, but less than inferior band of the IFL in extension [14]. The ischiofemoral ligament (ISFL) has its origin at the ischial portion of the acetabular rim and reinforces the posterior capsule with two bands [14]. The superior band spirals superolaterally to insert medial to the anterosuperior base of the greater trochanter blending with the orbicularis fibers, while the inferior band inserts more posteriorly and also medial to the border of the greater trochanter [14]. Medial rotation is clearly impeded by the tension of this ligament [14].

The zona orbicularis is a deep annular ligament that originates superiorly at the greater trochanter, blending with the fibers of the ischiofemoral ligament [12]. It is most prominent in the posterior and inferior part of the capsule to reinforce it, suggested to act as a ring that resists femoral distraction and facilitates synovial circulation [15].

The coxofemoral joint also includes an intraarticular ligament, the ligamentum capitis femoris [(ligamentum teres (LT)]. It consists of two flat bands with origin is on the ischial and pubic aspects of the acetabulum and blends with the transverse acetabular ligament between these two attachment sites. Both bands get tubular in their transition to insert on the fovea capitis of the femoral head [16]. Its length is approximately 30–35 mm [16]. The LT fibers includes collagen types I, II, and IV [17]. It also contains small arteries (including the artery femoris capitis), veins, and nerve bundles and is surrounded by synovium [18].

LT seems to be an important stabilizer of the joint in a squatting position (flexion and external rotation) and in cross upper leg position (flexion and internal rotation) creating maximum tension on it [19]. The stability acquires more importance in patients with osseous instability, such as inferior acetabular insufficiency, borderline or frank hip dysplasia, or some forms of femoroacetabular impingement (FAI) (Fig. 1.4) [19].

The acetabular labrum (AL) is a soft tissue fibrocartilaginous structure attached along the acetabular rim. Together with the acetabular transverse ligament, both structures form a continuous ring, completing the socket of the hip joint [20]. The AL is triangular form in cross-section and includes articular and non-articular faces. The articular aspect joins the hyaline acetabular cartilage and bone through a 1–2 mm wide transition zone of calcified cartilage [21]. The non-articular surface attaches directly to bone and is characterized by presenting dense connective tissue and that allows the passage of vessels and nerves [22]. This surface is separated from the joint capsule by a capsular recess [23]. Its thickness and fiber alignment differ according to its location. The inferior and posterior AL includes the 6.4 mm widest region, with fibers attached perpendicularly, which increase resistance [22, 23]. Moreover, the 5.5 mm thickest region is located superiorly [22]. On the contrary, anterior fibers have

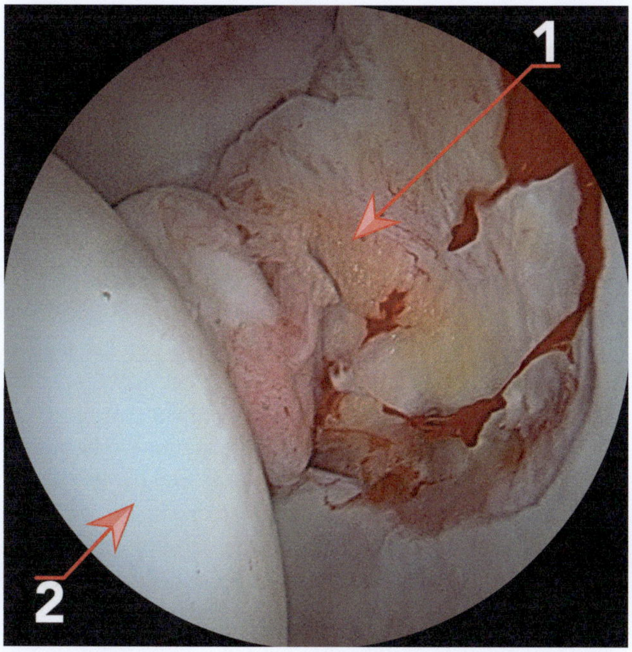

Fig. 1.4 Arthroscopic view of a pathologic ligamentum teres (1). (2) Femoral head

a parallel attachment, increasing their vulnerability to shear forces [22, 23].

Functions of AL have been studied in depth. Its mechanical role is to maintain hip stability through a suction effect between acetabulum and femoral head keeping them to resist distraction forces [24]. In this way the contact area is increased and pressure and strain to cartilage are reduced [25, 26]. Cartilage wear happens because of prolonged contact stress forces during joint movement, which may result in degenerative changes with fibrillation and delamination, something that frequently occurs in conjunction with labral tears [24, 27–29]. Different researchers have shown that joint instability is a direct contributor to cartilage degeneration and development of osteoarthritis [27, 28, 30, 31]. Another function of AL is to guarantee a pressurized layer of intraarticular synovial fluid that supports compressive loads, reducing cartilage stress and strain, and helping cartilage consolidation [32].

Seventeen muscles acting on the hip joint have been described. They are topographically divided into the posterior gluteal group (superficial and deep), the anterior iliopsoas group, and the medial adductor group.

The superficial gluteal muscles are the gluteus maximus, gluteus medius, gluteus minimus, and tensor fascia lata.

The gluteus maximus originates in the iliac gluteal region between the posterior gluteal line and the PSIS, the thoracolumbar fascia, the dorsal sacrum, coccyx, and sacrotuberous ligament. It includes a superficial (superior) and deep (inferior) part. The two superior thirds of the belly (superficial part) insert into the iliotibial tract, whereas the inferior third (deep part) inserts at gluteus tuberosity of the femur [33, 34]. This muscle is the principal extensor and lateral rotator of the hip, fully acting when the thigh is in a flexed position or climbing stairs. It is innervated by the inferior gluteal nerve.

The gluteus medius origins in the gluteal face of the iliac bone between the anterior and posterior gluteal lines. It inserts into the lateral aspect of the greater trochanter (GT) [33–35]. It is the most important hip abductor [34]. In addition, its anterior muscle fibers act as medial rotators, whereas its posterior ones act as lateral rotator. The gluteus medius is innervated by the superior gluteal nerve [33, 34].

The gluteus minor origins in the gluteal face of the iliac bone between the anterior and inferior gluteal lines and inserts onto anterior edge of the GT [35]. It also works as a weaker hip abductor. The gluteus minor is innervated by the superior gluteal nerve [33, 34]. Fibers of the gluteus medius and minimus could be in relation with branches of the superior gluteal nerve [36].

The tensor fascia lata muscle originates at the ASIS and the anterior portion of iliac crest, and runs anterior and distally to insert at the posterior edge of the iliotibial tract that extends to Gerdy's tubercle at the lateral aspect of the tibia and patella lateral retinaculum [35]. In addition, to stabilize the femoral head (adduction), it takes part, flexion and medial rotation and abduction [34]. It is innervated by the superior gluteal nerve [34].

The deep gluteal muscular group includes the piriformis, superior and inferior gemellus, obturator internus and externus, and quadratus femoris muscles, and they are located consecutively in the same plane.

The piriformis muscle origins at pelvic face of sacrum laterally to dorsal sacral foramina and at the rim of greater sciatic foramen. It crosses this foramen and inserts into the at the median edge of the GT superior to the trochanteric fossa [34, 37]. It works as abductor and lateral rotator (hip neck retroversion) at standing position [34]. It has been suggested to be a stabilizer of the posterior translation of the femoral head during hip flexion [37].

The superior gemellus originates at the ischiatic spine, the inferior gemellus at the lateral surface of the ischiatic tuberosity [33, 34], and the obturator internus originates internally to the edges of the obturator foramen and the obturator membrane and crosses the greater sciatic foramen to insert into the trochanteric fossa [33, 34]. The three muscles insert at trochanteric fossa blending in a unique tendon [34]. The obturator internus muscle originates at the inner aspect of the obturator membrane and the bone surrounding the obturator foramen. Cadaveric studies have shown a conjoined tendon conformed by piriformis and obturator internus muscles [38]. It works as a potential lateral rotator along with gluteus maximus, gemellus major and minor, and quadratus femoris muscles. When thigh is flexed the piriformis muscle works as an abductor [34]. The quadratus femoris muscle originates at the ischial tuberosity and inserts at intertrochanteric crest. It is a lateral rotator and adductor of the hip [34]. All deep gluteal muscles, except obturator externus, are innervated by the sacral plexus (nerves from fifth lumbar to second sacral spinal nerves). The obturator externus is innervated by the obturator nerve [34].

The iliopsoas muscle group includes iliacus, psoas major and psoas minor muscles. The Iliacus muscle originates from the iliac fossa, joins the psoas major to form the iliopsoas muscle, which inserts onto the lesser trochanter [33, 34]. The psoas major muscle consists of two portions: the superficial part originates onto the lateral faces of the bodies of the 12 thoracic vertebrae and lumbar vertebrae I–IV; and the deep portion originates from the transverse processes of lumbar vertebrae I–V [33, 34]. It runs over the iliopubic eminence and the anterior superior aspect of the capsulolabral complex, where its circumference is greatest, and finally attaches onto the lesser trochanter of the femur [34, 39]. Less than 50% of population has a psoas minor muscle which origin at the lateral face of 12 thoracic and first lumbar vertebrae, fuses with the iliac fascia, and finally attaches into the iliopectineus arch [34]. The psoas major muscle is innervated by direct branches of the lumbar plexus, and the iliacus muscle by the second to fourth branches of the lumbar plexus through the femoral nerve [34].

The sartorius muscle is not included in this group because it is superficial location. It runs from ASIS to the pes anserinus at antero-medial surface of the tibia [33, 34].

The iliopsoas group muscles are the most important flexors of the hip, being the sartorius muscle a weak flexor and lateral rotator due to its oblique trajectory to the knee [34]. The second stronger hip flexor is the rectus femoris muscle, a part of the quadriceps femoris muscle. The rectus femoris includes two heads: the direct head arising from the anterior inferior iliac spine (AIIS), and the reflected head emerging from the posterolateral margin of the acetabular rim. Both heads insert as a common tendon with the rest of quadricipital muscles at the patella and indirectly as a reflected tendon at the anterior tibial tuberosity [33, 34]. The quadriceps femoris is innervated by the femoral nerve [34].

The hip adductors group includes the pectineus, adductor brevis and longus, adductor magnus and gracilis. The pectineus muscle originates at the pecten of the pubis between the iliopubic eminence and the pubic tubercle and inserts at the pectineal line of the femur [33, 34]. The adductor brevis and longus muscles originate onto the inferior branch of the pubis. The adductor brevis inserts at the superior third of linea aspera, whereas the adductor longus inserts at the middle third of linea aspera. Both muscles are innervated by the anterior branch of the obturator nerve [34]. The adductor magnus muscle originates at the anteroinferior margins of the inferior branch of the pubis and the ischiatic tuberosity. Two parts are distinguished: the adductor and the ischiocondylar portions. The first arises from the lower pubic ramus and inserts onto the distal third of linea aspera, and is innervated by the posterior branch of the obturator nerve. The second part originates from the ischiatic tuberosity, inserts to the adductor tubercle of the medial epicondyle of the femur through a visible tendon [33, 34], and is innervated by the tibial nerve as other hamstring muscles [34]. The gracilis muscle originates at inferior branch of the pubis and inserts along with the semitendinosus and sartorius muscles at the anterior and medial face of proximal tibia. Sartorius, gracilis, and semitendinosus muscles constitute the pes anserinus. The gracilis muscle is innervated by the obturator nerve [34]. All these muscles are hip adductors, whereas adductor magnus also acts as a hip extensor (ischiocondylar portion) [34].

Finally, the hamstring muscles also act on the hip joint. They are the biceps femoris, semitendinosus, and semimembranosus muscles. They originate from the ischiatic tuberosity (and also from the linea aspera in the case of the short head of biceps femoris muscle) and insert below the knee joint. All these muscles are extensors of the hip, mainly at stand position [34]. They are innervated by the tibial nerve, with the exception of the short head of biceps femoris muscle.

1.3 Neurovascular Structures

The knowledge of the surrounding neurovascular hip structures is vital importance for the safety of hip arthroscopy procedures.

Before surgery, it is important to find these hidden structures in relation to anatomical visible edges. Marking these points will let to know their location and injury of vessels and nerves. In decubitus patient position, two bone structures are distinguished with palpation: the anterior superior iliac spine (ASIS) and the greater trochanter (GT).

First, the ASIS must be identified and marked, and a line distal to the patella line must be drawn. The workspace will be lateral to this line to protect sensitive structures. The anterior and posterior edges as well as GT tuberosity must be also marked.

- *Femoral vein, artery, and nerve*: these structures are located medial to the drawn line. Therefore, beyond this line in medial direction, the risk of injuries is very high. The femoral nerve (L2–L4), artery, and vein are placed from lateral to medial at this point. Palpation of the femoral artery pulse is always recommended to ensure location of the structures.
- Veins exhibit a great deal of anatomical variability at the saphenous opening [40], although infrequently some accessory veins may appear lateral to the femoral nerve. The femoral nerve may also present some ramifications that exceed the safety line, usually the sartorius and anterior cutaneous branches, but these usually do not go beyond 1 cm lateral to it [41].
- *Circumflex femoral arteries*: at a deep plane, the femoral artery is located medial and anterior to the anterior wall of the acetabulum, running above the muscle fibers of iliopsoas until it divides into the superficial and deep femoral arteries approximately at the level of the femoral neck [42]. The deep femoral artery runs toward the distal portion of the iliopsoas muscle and its tendon which is inserted onto the lesser trochanter of the femur. Before reaching this point, the deep femoral artery gives rise to the medial and lateral circumflex branches that will form a peri-cervical anastomotic ring [42, 43].
  - The lateral circumflex artery (LCFA) gives rise to three branches (ascending, transverse, and descending) that supplies blood to the head and neck of the femur and also part of the GT [44]. The medial circumflex branch (MCFA) is the most important blood supplier of femoral neck and head [42, 45], being observed posteriorly between the inferior gemellus and quadratus femoris muscles. It runs posteriorly from the profunda femoris artery, goes around the lesser trochanter, and provides a trochanteric branch before running anterior to the conjoint tendon of the superior gemellus, obturator internus, and inferior gemellus muscles, and posterior to the obturator externus tendon [42]. Here, it perforates the coxofemoral joint capsule and anastomoses with LCFA forming an arch around the neck that provides from two to four posterior retinacular vessels [43]. Lesion of these vessels could cause avascular necrosis of the femoral head. Veins vessels with the same track as arteries are also present.

    Based on the vascularization of the head provided by retinacular vessels, safe vascular zones for hip arthroscopy have been described [46].The "femoral neck safe zone" represents the anterior half of the femoral neck. The "psoas tendon release safe zone" is divided in two zones. The first one is located adjacent to the lesser trochanter. The second is located at the inferior border of coxofemoral junction, avoiding the MCFA which is medial to this point [47].
- *Gluteal arteries*: they arise from the internal iliac artery and include the superior and inferior gluteal arteries. The superior gluteal artery exits the pelvic cavity through the suprapiriformis foramen [33, 34] and divides in superficial and deep branches in the gluteal region. The superficial branch emerges between gluteus maximus and medius muscles, and finishes anastomosing with the inferior gluteal artery. The deeper branch runs laterally between gluteus minimus and medius to provide blood to these muscles and also to tensor fascia lata muscle. It also gives an anastomotic branch to LCFA [33, 48]. On the other hand, the inferior gluteal artery exits the pelvic cavity through the infrapiriformis foramen of the greater sciatic foramen [33, 34]. In the gluteal region, it runs under the gluteus maximus muscle supplying several branches to it and other lateral rotators muscles. Anastomoses of the inferior gluteal artery with the obturator, gluteal superior, and MCFA are common [42]. Some authors indicate the importance of the inferior gluteal artery, along with MCFA, in the blood supply of the femoral head and neck. Therefore it is essential that surgeons should know their exact locations to avoid hip injury during arthroscopic approaches, to prevent femoral head avascular necrosis [42, 45, 49].
- *Lateral femoral cutaneous nerve* (*LFCN*): this nerve has a constant path. It passes medial to ASIS and crosses the muscular space behind the inguinal ligament. At this point, it divides usually in 2–5 branches, superficially to the sartorius muscle. The two most lateral branches, superior and posterior, provide sensation to the lateral

thigh and may be injured during arthroscopic approaches [50]. The superior lateral branches exit the fascia lata distally and provide sensation from the anterolateral thigh to the knee. The posterior division provides sensation to the skin covering the GT halfway up the thigh [51].

- *Sciatic nerve*: this nerve usually exits the pelvic cavity through the infra-piriform foramen and covered by the gluteus maximus muscle, runs distally [52] superficial to the superior gemelli, internal obturator, inferior gemelli, and quadratus femoris muscles. Four different morphologic patterns of the sciatic nerve have been described [53]:
  - Pattern 1: Most of individuals (>80%) shows a unique nerve emerging under the piriformis muscle.
  - Pattern 2: In 10–15% of cases there is an accessory piriformis belly and between both parts of the sciatic nerve. The common peroneal nerve (L4, L5, S1, S2) crosses superiorly to piriformis muscle, and the tibial nerve emerges inferior to it.
  - Pattern 3: 3–5% of individuals show a non-divided piriformis muscle and a sciatic nerve divided in common peroneal nerve emerging superior to the muscle and the tibial nerve inferior to it.
  - Pattern 4: The less common pattern (0.5–1%) is characterized by a bi-headed piriformis with the sciatic nerve emerging between both bellies.
  - The sciatic nerve is 29 mm medial to the posterior GT rim [54], so all maneuvers to access inside the articular cavity should be performed close to the GT rim to avoid injuring this nerve.

1.4 Arthroscopic Portals

1.4.1 Positioning and Marking

In process to obtain enough data to accomplish a safe surgical approach, up to 18 arthroscopic portals have been described, being only 9 safe and reproducible [55]. The correct placement of the portals supposes the success of the surgery, and small errors in the location of the portals may make the surgical intervention very difficult and affect their success. In this context, specific arthroscopic portal complications of 0.5–0.6% have been described [56].

Supine or lateral decubitus positions are used for hip arthroscopy depending on surgeon's preferences. Each surgeon should feel comfortable with one of them and develop it use.

General anesthesia producing muscular paralysis, with concomitant use of spinal anesthesia or regional anesthesia to help postoperative pain, is the most frequently used method. In this context, it is essential to get complete muscular relaxation to perform a successful procedure. A standard fluoroscope is also necessary to perform distraction and arthroscopic portal placement. Independent to the position selected, skin marks may be drawn after joint distraction. Neurovascular femoral structures must be identified by palpation and marked. Bone structures, ASIS and GT, and a rectangular line directed from the ASIS to the patella should be marked to avoid injury of femoral neurovascular structures. In relation with these, the portal location (see later) should also be marked.

During surgery, the mean blood pressure should be less or equal to the arthroscopic pump pressure (around 65 mmHg) to allow an adequate visualization of the joint [57]. It is known that low pressures can lead to poor visualization, and high pressures can lead to fluid extravasation, and sometimes fatal complications [58, 59]. Joint-calibrated systems seem to be more accurate showing the real joint pressure, reducing the risk of related complications [60].

In supine decubitus position, a traction fracture table is used. To avoid pudendal neuropraxia, a well-padded perineal post is required to provide a transverse force vector against the patient's thigh [57, 61]. This position allows to lateralize femur and stops traction. The post size is important. Oversized post (9–12 cm) has been associated with less pudendal neuropraxia [61, 62]. It is necessary to pay attention to the scrotum position, as an excessive pressure may result in edema, hematoma, or scrotal necrosis [63]. A fluoroscope C-arm is situated at contralateral side for dynamic fluoroscope evaluation of the hip. It is recommended before surgery to recognize possible undiagnosed lesions. Traction of the hip is applied with 15° of hip flexion, 0° of adduction, and 10° of medial rotation to give parallelism to the femoral neck with the horizontal floor reference [61]. An excess of flexion may injure sciatic nerve.

Glick and Sampson, in lateral decubitus position, use marks and portals similar than those used in supine decubitus position [64]. Traction is done by elastic bandage and taping, traction booties with belt buckles or Velcro straps like shoulder lateral position, or with an external lateral hip distractor. Fracture traction table with special accessories could be used too. A padded perineal post is necessary as in supine decubitus position. Fluoroscopic C-arm is brought under the table centered at the level of the greater trochanter. Flexion at 15°–20° is recommended, no exceeding it to avoid sciatic neurapraxia. 3°–5° of adduction is applied to take mechanical advantage of the perineal post.

Traction should be carefully performed under fluoroscopic guidance. The force required depends on the patient and the pathologic condition, but it is often required from 25 to 50 lb (11–23 kg) to achieve adequate joint distraction [57, 61]. An adequate traction is confirmed with the presence of a vacuum crescent sign under fluoroscopy. In case of not appearing, the use of a spinal needle to introduce air into the joint is an alternative [65] to assure that the hip is correctly distracted and reduce the force necessary to distract the joint [66]. A distraction of 10–12 mm of the joint is also a sign of correct traction [66]. Sometimes this sign is not present because of presence of specific pathologic conditions like hemarthrosis, synovial chondromatosis, and pigmented villonodular synovitis [61]. Duration of traction and extremity manipulation should be controlled during the surgery to avoid possible injuries. Total duration of traction may be less than 2 h and continuous traction should be limited by 1 h with intermittent release of traction to minimize risks [61, 67].

1.4.2 Main Arthroscopic Portals

Portal placement in hip arthroscopy is difficult because of the presence of large amount of muscular and other soft tissues around the joint, as well as the significant thickness of capsule that provides a high resistance to trocar introduction hindering the joint access.

The authors prefer to talk about a "hip arthroscopy safe zone," what refers to the skin area where multiples portals can be performed without risk of deep structures injuries. The knowledge of this area facilitates the placement depending on the locations of the pathologies. Anyway, the classical portals described in this chapter are all located in this area.

Five portals have been described for most hip arthroscopy procedures involving central and peripheral compartments. In this chapter we will deal with the correct portal position, the structures on which instruments cross to get into the joint, and the neurovascular structures related with.

1.4.2.1 Anterolateral Portal (AL)

This is the preferred portal used to introduce the arthroscopic instruments because of its low injury risk of adjacent structures. Due to the characteristics of muscular layers and the hip joint capsule, it is easier to get into the joint at this level. Once this portal is done and the camera is placed into the joint, the rest of portals are easier to perform.

It is located 1 cm anterior and 1 cm lateral to the tip of GT. For accessing the joint a spinal needle is needed. By touching the bone rims, seeing the marks and always under fluoroscope guidance, the needle is introduced into the anterosuperior space [68] before introducing the trocar into the joint. During this process, the structures crossed from superficial to deep are the major gluteal fascia in its union with the fascia lata muscle, the gluteus medius muscle, and finally the joint capsule. A minimum resistance is provided by the gluteus medius muscle, but the hip joint capsule is hardest and provides more resistance to needle introduction. After passing the capsule, its resistance disappears. To avoid injuring the labrum, the whole process should be performed with a good prior training and under fluoroscopy guidance. Feeling resistance into the joint means that the needle is hindered by the labrum or the chondral surface [66]. The inferior branches of the deep branch of superior gluteal artery and nerve are 45 mm proximal to the portal [54, 65].

This classical technique has reported a 20% of complications such as iatrogenic labral tears or chondral lesions [69]. In another technique [70], the needle is located more anterior and distal (above the femoral head as observed by fluoroscopy) to avoid this kind of lesions during trocar introduction.

To confirm the correct position of the AL, a 70° arthroscope is introduced by a second portal previously established.

1.4.2.2 Posterolateral Portal (PL)

It is not a routinely performed portal. It is located 1-cm posterior and 1-cm lateral to the tip of GT. It crosses the gluteus medius and minimus, anterosuperior to the piriformis muscle tendon, crossing the coxofemoral capsule at this level. The sciatic nerve is 29 mm medial to this portal [54]. Medial rotation of the hip during creation of the PL has been recommended to avoid injury of the nerve, but it is known that this movement increases the contact between the nerve and the posterior capsule, so some authors do not endorse its utility and recommend avoiding it [65]. The deep branch of the MCFA is located 10 mm to the portal and protected by the piriformis muscle, assuming a normal trochanteric anatomy [71], for what a normal GT shape and a skin penetration close to the bone rim will decrease the risk of injury. Light secondary bleedings of the anastomotic branch between the MCFA and the superior gluteal artery situated above the piriformis have been observed [42].

1.4.2.3 Anterior Portal (AP)

It is located at the intersection between a line drawn from the ASIS to superior pole of the patella, and a perpendicular line from the AL and PL portals, approximately 6 cm below the ASIS. It crosses the sartorius and rectus femoris muscle, and finally the iliofemoral ligament before entering the joint.

The LFCN nerve is at risk, because it is located only 3 mm medial to the portal [50, 54]. For that reason, only skin is incised at the portal site, and non-piercing instruments must be used to access the joint. Common injuries may cause hypoesthesia or anesthesia of the superior lateral skin of the thigh or painful neuroma formation [50]. High number of lesions has been reported, and currently this portal is not in use.

A more lateral AP portal position, 10 mm to the original, has been described [55] to avoid LFCN injury. The structures crossed are the fascia lata muscle, the soft interval between gluteus minimus and rectus femoris muscles, and finally the articular capsule. Small bleedings may appear due to injuries of the superior branch of the LCFA [50] situated 14 mm from the portal [55]. At the capsular level the portal passes 39 mm lateral to the femoral nerve [50].

1.4.3 Secondary Portals

Diverse accessory portals used in hip arthroscopy have been described. They are the following:

- *Mid-Anterior Portal* (*MAP*): it is located at the distal apex of an equilateral triangle with a union base line between AL and AP (about 5 cm in 45° angle distal to AL). It crosses the rectus femoris muscle and the IFL before entering the joint. This portal is selected instead of AP due to a lesser risk of LFCN injury and a better angle for Pincer's cases or placement of anterolateral acetabular anchors [55]. As with the AP, it is recommended not to use sharping material to perform the portal. The ascending branch of the LCFA is located at 19 mm from the portal [55].
- *Proximal Mid-Anterior Portal* (*PMAP*): it is placed in line with the MAP but in this case proximal to AL and AP portals (about 5 cm in 45° proximal to AL). It goes through the tensor fascia lata and rectus femoris muscles before crossing the IFL. Due to its anterior situation, the branches of LFCN are at risk [55].
- *Distal Accessory Anterolateral Portal* (*DALA*): it is located 3–6 cm distal to the AL portal. It goes through vastus lateralis muscle and the IFL. It lets a better working angle of the anterolateral acetabular rim in the central compartment and a good view of the peripheral compartment. It is also used to perform lesser trochanter pathology or to place percutaneous implants [55, 65, 72]. 5–8 mm anteriorly, the LFCN and the terminal branches of LCFA are at risk [72].
- *Proximal Accessory Anterolateral Portal* (*PALA*): it is located 2–4 cm proximal to the AL portal. It goes through the junction of gluteus maximus and tensor fascia lata muscles. It is useful to get a direct view of superior and anterior central compartment and provides a good angle to attack CAM lesions [65].
- *Peritrochanteric Space Portal* (*PSP*): it is located in line 2 cm distal to the AL portal or at the same distance of the MAP from the AL, immediately anterior to the intertrochanteric line. It goes through the interval between the tensor fascia lata muscle and the iliotibial tract. This portal is used for proximal and distal peritrochanteric work [55, 65].

Portal	Muscle pathway	Neurovascular structures at risk
Anterolateral Portal (ALP)	Gluteal fascia, gluteus medius	Superior gluteal nerve (45 mm) Terminal branches of the superior gluteal artery
Posterolateral Portal (PLP)	Gluteus medius, gluteus minimus	Sciatic nerve (29 mm)
Anterior Portal (AP)	Sartorius, rectus femoris	LFCN (25 mm) Terminal branches of LCFA (14 mm) Femoral nerve at capsule level (39 mm)
Mid-Anterior Portal (MAP)	Rectus femoris	LFCN Ascending branch of LCFA (19 mm)
Proximal Mid-Anterior Portal (PMAP)	Tensor fascia lata, rectus femoris	LFCN
Distal Accessory Anterolateral Portal (DALAP)	Vastus lateralis	LFCN (5–8 mm) Terminal branches of LCFA (8 mm)
Proximal Accessory anterolateral Portal (PALAP)	Junction of gluteus maximus and tensor fascia lata	Superior gluteal nerve Terminal branches of superior gluteal artery
Peritrochanteric Space Portal (PSP)	Interval between tensor fascia lata muscle and the iliotibial tract	

1.5 Compartments

Hip joint arthroscopy surgeons classically divide the joint into two compartments: central and peripheral [55, 57, 64–66, 68–70, 73, 74]. Technical advances in arthroscopy have provided a better diagnosis of the hip pain, and the knowledge of other compartments around the hip: the peritrochanteric compartment and the deep gluteal space [65, 75–78]. Knowledge of normal landmarks is essential to procedure a routine and safety arthroscopy. In this chapter the normal anatomy viewed from a camera will be described in each one.

1.5.1 Central Compartment

The central compartment contains the femoral head and acetabulum covered by hyaline cartilage, the acetabular labrum and the acetabular bone rim, the ligamentum teres, and the articular face of joint capsule.

The clock face method is used for a better understanding of the location of the different structures in the acetabular cavity from the ALP, PLP, and AP/MAP [50]. The transverse ligament is the reference for the inferior border or the 6 o'clock, and the acetabular roof with the superior labrum (Fig. 1.5) for the superior border or the 12 o'clock. For the anterior border or the 3 o'clock our reference is the anterior labrum (Fig. 1.6), and for posterior border or the 9 o'clock the posterior labrum.

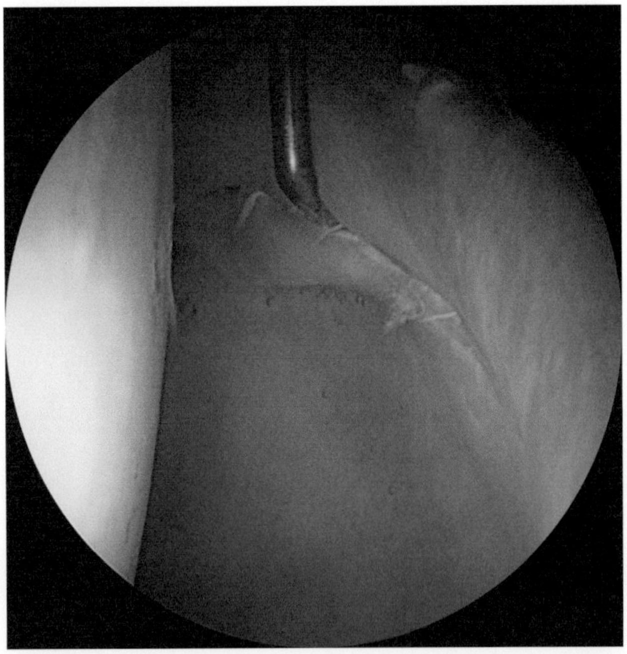

Fig. 1.5 Arthroscopic view of a superior labrum rupture

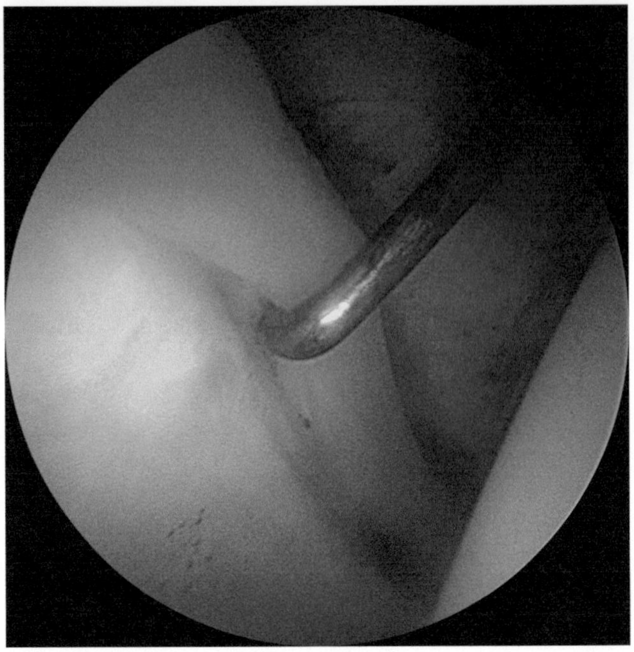

Fig. 1.6 Arthroscopic view of an anterior labrum rupture

To distinguish a right to a left hip, the 3 o'clock will be at our camera right or at our left, respectively.

The structures seen, depending on the portal of view used, are described using the clock face method:

- ALP: the camera shows from 4 to 9 o'clock. The ligamentum teres is seen in the acetabular fossa at 6. It usually measures 30–35 mm of length and 10 mm of thickness, covered by synovial membrane, inserting medially at the cotyloid fossa. The labrum attachment to the acetabular rim, on both sides (capsular and acetabulum), is identified from 4 to 9. The hyaline cartilage covers the lunate surface of acetabulum except the cotyloid fossa, where pulvinar fat tissue is visualized. The anterior and superior aspect of the view, the anterior triangle is seen. Its landmarks are the anterior labrum, the femoral head, and the anterior capsule, and it allows a direct view to perform the AP/MAP. Normal anatomy structures used as landmarks have been described. Its knowledge is important to not confuse with pathological changes. The traces of fused triradiate cartilage are frequently observed as grooves on the articular surface crossing horizontal from 3 to 11, and vertical through the cotyloid fossa. A fibrous cartilage area of 10 mm wide, corresponding to the iliac cartilage fusion, named "stellate crease," locates at 12:30–1 o'clock on acetabular roof, good acetabular mark to locate the top of the cartilage into the camera view. Labral sulcus is often seen at 8 o'clock, but other locations at 9 and 11 have been described. Other less normal frequently variants are the supra-acetabular fossa and the supra-acetabular notch. An identification of these structures in magnetic resonance prior to surgery can help us not to confuse them with pathology. The femoral head surface can be examined. The articular space between the femoral head and the acetabulum can be determined and monitored with traction and movement changes.

- PLP: the camera shows from 6 to 2 o'clock. The inferior gutter of the hip joint with the transverse ligament, the anterolateral labrum, the posterosuperior femoral head, and the bearing dome of the acetabulum are visualized. Loose bodies are usually found at the inferior gutter.
- AP/MAP: the camera shows from 6 to 10 o'clock, being possible to visualize the posterior, superior, and anterior labrum, the anterior and posterior transverse ligament, the posterior and superior capsule, the acetabular and antero-superior femoral head, the acetabular fossa, and the ligamentum teres.

1.5.2 Peripheral Compartment

The peripheral compartment is lateral to the labrum and contains the femoral neck including the femoral head–neck junction [73]. Even after the portals are established, a limited capsulotomy is performed to facilitate maneuverability of the instruments. To access to it, traction of the hip is performed and 20°–30° of flexion required. The ALP and AP allow good diagnoses and to perform most of the techniques. In case of posterior disorder, PLP is then used. 10° of lateral rotation of the hip should give additional visualization. Two approach techniques: intracapsular and extracapsular, have been described. The intracapsular approach avoids extended capsulotomies [79]. Central compartment portals are commonly used, changing the direction of the camera and instruments. The camera is placed in MAP and the instruments in ALP, placing the camera against the orbicularis area [79, 80]. The extraarticular approach, as the "T" patter or those performed from ALP and DALAP [72], allows better visualization of the peripheral compartment from 9 to 7:30 o'clock and is useful in deep overcovered cases [75]. Complications related to extensive capsulotomy and instability of the hip in association with hyperlaxity have been described [76, 77]. To prevent these complications, more superior and anterior capsulotomies have been proposed in an anterior capsule relaxed position [68]. From ALP, lateral and inferior synovial shaving is performed when loosing traction and changing to lateral rotation with flexion hip position, technique really useful to manage posterosuperior peripheral compartment pathology [50, 68].

With the camera inside the joint, the first structures viewed are the medial aspects of the neck, femoral head, acetabular labrum, and antero-medial capsule with the zona orbicularis and the medial synovial fold [80]. Introducing the camera toward the bottom of the circular limit or the zona orbicularis, allows to visualize the medial gutter space with the capsular recess. Other medial structures observed are the edge of medial neck and the medial synovial fold, good landmarks to assess correct peripheral space location and as a limit to osteochondroplasty [50, 61]. Introducing the camera beyond the anterior border of the neck allows to visualize in the anterior region the anterolateral neck and the anterior femoral head with anterior labrum. Anterior synovial fold can be identified here. The congruence between the femoral head and the labrum is evaluated in this point when traction is released. Importantly, impingement disorders have to been evaluated with dynamic test in this region [50]. Anterior synovial fold can be identified here. The access to the lateral region is facilitated with a partial reduction of the hip in flexion changing to medial rotation. The lateral aspect of the femoral neck with lateral synovial folds is the limits of work in order to preserve retinacular vessels and arteries from injuries and prevent avascular necrosis of the head of the femur [50].

Portal	Compartment	Structure identified
Anterolateral (AL)	Central	Anterior acetabular wall Posterior acetabular wall Acetabular fossa (Ligamentum capitis femoris/Ligamentum teres and fat pad) Anterior superior labrum Anterior capsule
	Peripheral	Anterior, superior, and posterior femoral head—neck junction Antero-medial capsule Zona Orbicularis
Posterolateral (PL)	Central	Bearing dome of the acetabulum Posterosuperior femoral head Anterolateral labrum Transverse ligament
Anterior (AP) and Mid-Anterior (MAP)	Central	Acetabular fossa Anterosuperior femoral head Ligamentum capitis femoris/ Ligamentum teres Transverse ligament Anterior, superior, and posterior labrum Posterior and superior capsule
	Peripheral	Anterolateral neck Anterior femoral head (anterior and inferior head–neck junction) Anterior labrum Medial synovial fold Transverse ligament MFCA and retinacular vessels Zona Orbicularis Capsular recess

1.5.3 Peritrochanteric Compartment

The peritrochanteric compartment lies between the iliotibial tract and the proximal femur. Hip arthroscopy of this compartment requires two specific portals.

The *anterior portal for peritrochanteric compartment* (APPC) is placed 1 cm lateral to ASIS in neutral flexion-extension and slight medial rotation of the thigh, going through the tensor fascia lata and sartorius muscles, and allowing visualization of the peritrochanteric space [65]. Proximally, the GT with the insertion of gluteus medius and minimus tendons, the iliotibial tract and the vastus lateralis muscle are viewed.

The distal posterior portal for peritrochanteric compartment (DPPC) is placed at the posterior third of the GT halfway between the tip of the GT and the vastus tubercle, not trespassing any muscular structure [65]. It allows the visualization of the working area for the proximal iliotibial tract, the greater trochanter and its bursa, and the gluteal medius and minimus muscles under the tensor fascia lata muscle.

1.5.4 Deep Gluteal Space

The Deep Gluteal Space (DGS) comprises the space and structures located under the gluteus maximus muscle [78, 81, 82]. Its proximal border is the origin of gluteus maximus near the iliac crest, whereas its inferior border corresponds to the insertion onto the linea aspera. Anteriorly, from medial to lateral, the sacrotuberous ligament and the falciform fascia, the ischium, the greater sciatic foramen, the hamstring origin, and the inferior border of sciatic notch are observed. The lateral border corresponds to the linea aspera and the posterior margin the femoral neck. This space includes the ischium, the sacrotuberous and sacrospinous ligaments, the origin of the ischiofemoral ligament, the piriformis muscle, the obturator internus/externus muscles, the gemelli muscles, the quadratus femoris muscle, the hamstrings muscles, the lateral ascending vessels of the MFCA, the superior and inferior gluteal nerves, and the sciatic nerve [52, 78, 81, 82].

A 30° camera is inserted from the MAP portal crossing the peritrochanteric compartment in 30° of abduction and slightly medial rotation of the hip. It is important to identify the gluteus maximus insertion onto the linea aspera by placing the camera parallel to the patient body [78]. From here, the sciatic nerve is identified leaving the subgluteal space above the piriform muscle. It lies between the ischial tuberosity, 12 ± 2 mm proximal to the hamstring muscles origin [83]. Different auxiliary posterolateral portals around the GT can be performed to facilitate work in this space [78].

References

1. Heller MO, Bergmann G, Deuretzbacher G, Claes L, Haas NP, Duda GN. Influence of femoral anteversion on proximal femoral loading: measurement and simulation in four patients. Clin Biomech. 2001;16:644–9.
2. Mc RR. The hip. In: 3rd, editor. Orthopaedic examination. New York: Churchill Livingstone; 1994. p. 142–70.
3. Lenaerts G, De Groote F, Demeulenaere B, et al. Subject-specific hip geometry affects predicted hip joint contact forces during gait. J Biomech. 2008;41:1243–52.
4. Reikerås O, Bjerkreim I, Kolbenstvedt A. Anteversion of the acetabulum and femoral neck in normals and in patients with osteoarthritis of the hip. Acta Orthop Scand. 1983;54(1):18–23.
5. Buller LT, Rosneck J, Monaco FM, Butler R, Smith T, Barsoum WK. Relationship between proximal femoral and acetabular alignment in normal hip joints using 3-dimensional computed tomography. Am J Sports Med. 2012;40:367–75.
6. Ganz R, Parvizi J, Beck M, Leunig M, Nötzli H, Siebenrock KA. Femoroacetabular impingement: a cause for osteoarthritis of the hip. Clin Orthop Relat Res. 2003;(417):112–20. https://doi.org/10.1097/01.blo.0000096804.78689.c2.
7. Kang AC, Gooding AJ, Coates MH, Goh TD, Armour P. Computed tomography assessment of hip joints in asymptomatic individuals in relation to femoroacetabular impingement. Rietveld J Am J Sports Med. 2010;38(6):1160–5.
8. Grammatopoulos G, Jamieson P, Dobransky J, Rakhra K, Carsen S, Beaulé PE. Acetabular version increases during adolescence secondary to reduced anterior femoral head coverage. Clin Orthop Relat Res. 2019;477(11):2470–8.
9. Hingsammer AM, Bixby S, Zurakowski D, Yen YM, Kim YJ. How do acetabular version and femoral head coverage change with skeletal maturity? Clin Orthop Relat Res. 2015;473(4):1224–33.
10. Direito-Santos B, França G, Nunes J, et al. Acetabular retroversion: Diagnosis and treatment. EFORT Open Rev. 2018;3(11):595–603.
11. Wasielewski RC. The hip. In: Callaghan JJ, editor. The adult hip. Philadelphia: Lippincott-Raven. 1998. p. 57–74. Stewart KJ, Edmonds-Wilson RH, Brand RA, Brown TD. Spatial distribution of hip capsule structural and material properties. J Biomech 2002;35:1491–98.
12. Wagner FV, Negrao JR, Campos J, et al. Capsular ligaments of the hip: anatomic, histologic, and positional study in cadaveric specimens with MR arthrography. Radiology. 2012;263:189–98.
13. Cooper HJ, Walters BL, Rodriguez JA. Anatomy of the hip capsule and pericapsular structures: a cadaveric study. Clin Anat. 2015;28(5):665–71.
14. Martin HD, et al. The function of the hip capsular ligaments: a quantitative report. Arthroscopy. 2008;24(2):188–95.
15. Malagelada F, Tayar R, Barke S, Stafford G, Field RE. Anatomy of the zona orbicularis of the hip: a magnetic resonance study. Surg Radiol Anat. 2015;37(1):11–8.
16. Bardakos NV, Villar RN. The ligamentum teres of the adult hip. J Bone Joint Surg Br. 2009;91(1):8–15.
17. O'Donnell JM, Pritchard M, Salas AP, Singh PJ. The ligamentum teres-its increasing importance. J Hip Preserv Surg. 2014;1(1):3–11.
18. Dehao BW, Bing TK, Young JL. Understanding the ligamentum teres of the hip: a histological study. Acta Ortop Bras. 2015;23(1):29–33.
19. Martin RL, Palmer I, Martin HD. Ligamentum teres: a functional description and potential clinical relevance. Knee Surg Sports Traumatol Arthrosc. 2012;20(6):1209–14.
20. Blankenbaker DG, Tuite MJ. Acetabular labrum. Magn Reson Imaging Clin N Am. 2013;21:21–33.
21. Ishiko T, Naito M, Moriyama S. Tensile properties of the human acetabular labrum-the first report. J Orthop Res. 2005;23:1448–53.
22. Seldes RM, Tan V, Hunt J, et al. Anatomy, histologic features, and vascularity of the adult acetabular labrum. Clin Orthop Relat Res. 2001;382:232–40.
23. Grant AD, Sala DA, Davidovitch RI. The labrum: structure, function, and injury with femoro-acetabular impingement. J Child Orthop. 2012;6:357–72.
24. Smith MV, Panchal HB, Ruberte Thiele RA, Sekiya JK. Effect of acetabular labrum tears on hip stability and labral strain in a joint compression model. Am J Sports Med. 2011;39(Suppl):103S–10S.
25. Lee S, Wuerz TH, Shewman E, et al. Labral reconstruction with iliotibial band autografts and semitendinosus allografts improves hip joint contact area and contact pressure: an in vitro analysis. Am J Sports Med. 2015;43:98–104.
26. Greaves LL, Gilbart MK, Yung AC, Kozlowski P, Wilson DR. Effect of acetabular labral tears, repair and resection on hip cartilage strain: a 7T MR study. J Biomech. 2010;43:858–63.
27. Katta J, Jin Z, Ingham E, Fisher J. Effect of nominal stress on the long term friction, deformation and wear of native and glycosaminoglycan deficient articular cartilage. Osteoarthr Cartil. 2009;17:662–8.
28. Forster H, Fisher J. The influence of loading time and lubricant on the friction of articular cartilage. Proc Inst Mech Eng H. 1996;210:109–19.
29. Wilson W, van Burken C, van Donkelaar C, et al. Causes of mechanically induced collagen damage in articular cartilage. J Orthop Res. 2006;24:220–8.
30. Setton LA, Elliott DM, Mow VC. Altered mechanics of cartilage with osteoarthritis: human osteoarthritis and an experimental model of joint degeneration. Osteoarthr Cartil. 1999;7:2–14.
31. Mavcic B, Iglic A, Kralj-Iglic V, Brand RA, Vengust R. Cumulative hip contact stress predicts osteoarthritis in DDH. Clin Orthop Relat Res. 2008;466:884–91.
32. Ferguson SJ, Bryant JT, Ganz R, Ito K. An in vitro investigation of the acetabular labral seal in hip joint mechanics. J Biomech. 2003;36:171–8.
33. Netter FH. ATLAS DE ANATOMÍA HUMANA. 7° ed. Barcelona: Elsevier; 2019.
34. Platzer W, Fritsch H, Kahle W. ATLAS DE ANATOMÍA con Correlación Clínica. 11° ed. Madrid: Médica Panamericana; 2018.
35. Flack NA, Nicholson HD, Woodley SJ. A review of the anatomy of the hip abductor muscles, gluteus medius, gluteus minimus, and tensor fascia lata. Clin Anat. 2012;25:697–708.
36. Flack NA, Nicholson HD, Woodley SJ. The anatomy of the hip abductor muscles. Clin Anat. 2014;27(2):241–53.
37. Roche JJ, Jones CD, Khan RJ, Yates PJ. The surgical anatomy of the piriformis tendon, with particular reference to total hip replacement: a cadaver study. Bone Joint J. 2013;95-B:764–9.
38. Solomon LB, Lee YC, Callary SA, Beck M, Howie DW. Anatomy of piriformis, obturator internus and obturator externus: implications for the posterior surgical approach to the hip. J Bone Joint Surg Br. 2010;92:1317–24.
39. Alpert JM, Kozanek M, Li G, Kelly BT, Asnis PD. Cross-sectional analysis of the iliopsoas tendon and its relationship to the acetabular labrum: an anatomic study. Am J Sports Med. 2009;37:1594–8.
40. Ricci S, Caggiati A. Echoanatomical patterns of the long saphenous vein in patients with primary varices and in healthy subjects. Phlebology. 1999;14:54–8.
41. Gustafson KJ, Pinault GC, Neville JJ, et al. Fascicular anatomy of human femoral nerve: implications for neural prostheses using nerve cuff electrodes. J Rehabil Res Dev. 2009;46(7):973–84. https://doi.org/10.1682/jrrd.2008.08.0097.
42. Gautier E, Ganz K, Krugel N, Gill T, Ganz R. Anatomy of the medial femoral circumflex artery and its surgical implications. J Bone Joint Surg Br. 2000;82:679–83.
43. Zlotorowicz M, Czubak-Wrzosek M, Wrzosek P, Czubak J. The origin of the medial femoral circumflex artery, lateral femo-

ral circumflex artery and obturator artery. Surg Radiol Anat. 2018;40(5):515–20.
44. Prough H, Alsayouri K. Anatomy, bony pelvis and lower limb, lateral circumflex femoral artery. [Updated 2019 Sept 14]. In: StatPearls. Treasure Island, FL: StatPearls Publishing. 2020. Available from: https://www.ncbi.nlm.nih.gov/books/NBK546684/
45. Beaule PE, Campbell P, Lu Z, et al. Vascularity of the arthritic femoral head and hip resurfacing. J Bone Joint Surg Am. 2006;88(Suppl 4):85–96.
46. McCormick F, Kleweno CP, Kim YJ, Martin SD. Vascular safe zones in hip arthroscopy. Am J Sports Med. 2011;39(Suppl):64S–71S. https://doi.org/10.1177/0363546511414016.
47. Dora C, Leunig M, Beck M, Rothenfluh D, Ganz R. Entry point soft tissue damage in antegrade femoral nailing: a cadaver study. J Orthop Trauma. 2001;15(7):488–93.
48. Ebraheim NA, Olexa TA, Xu R, Georgiadis G, Yeasting RA. The quantitative anatomy of the superior gluteal artery and its location. Am J Orthop (Belle Mead NJ). 1998;27(6):427–31.
49. Grose AW, Gardner MJ, Sussmann PS, Helfet DL, Lorich DG. The surgical anatomy of the blood supply to the femoral head: description of the anastomosis between the medial femoral circumflex and inferior gluteal arteries at the hip. J Bone Joint Surg Br. 2008;90(10):1298–303.
50. Aprato A, Giachino M, Masse A. Arthroscopic approach and anatomy of the hip. Muscles Ligaments Tendons J. 2016;6(3):309–16.
51. Carai A, Fenu G, Sechi E, Crotti FM, Montella A. Anatomical variability of the lateral femoral cutaneous nerve: findings from a surgical series. Clin Anat. 2009;22(3):365–70.
52. Barone Papaianni I, Di Paolo M, Chilo JJ, Alonso H, Enriquez R, Cancelliere Fritzler R. Variaciones anatómicas del nervio ciático: Su relación con el músculo piriforme Revista Argentina Anatomía. Online. 2016;7(3):125–9.
53. Beaton L, Anson B. The relationship of the sciatic nerve and its subdivisions to the piriform muscle. Anat Rec. 1937;70(1):1–5.
54. Byrd JW, Pappas JN, Pedley MJ. Hip arthroscopy: an anatomic study of portal placement and relationship to the extra-articular structures. Arthroscopy. 1995;11:418–23.
55. Robertson WJ, Kelly BT. The safe zone for hip arthroscopy: a cadaveric assessment of central, peripheral, and lateral compartment portal placement. Arthroscopy. 2008;24(9):1019–26.
56. Clarke MT, Arora A, Villar RN. Hip arthroscopy: complications in 1054 cases. Clin Orthop Relat Res. 2003;406:84–8.
57. Stubbs AJ, Stone AV. Position and distraction options. In: Byrd JWT, editor. Operative hip arthroscopy. 3rd ed. New York: Springer; 2013. p. 121–9.
58. Kocher MS, Frank JS, Nasreddine AY, et al. Intraabdominal fluid extravasation during hip arthroscopy: a survey of the MAHORN group. Arthroscopy. 2012;28:1654–1660.e2.
59. Gupta A, Redmond JM, Hammarstedt JE, Schwindel L, Domb BG. Safety measures in hip arthroscopy and their efficacy in minimizing complications: a systematic review of the evidence. Arthroscopy. 2014;30:1342–8.
60. Ross JA, Marland J, Whiting DR, Payne B, West HS. Do arthroscopic fluid pumps display true surgical site pressure during hip arthroscopy? Arthroscopy. 2018;34:126–32.
61. Mannava S, Howse EA, Stone AV, Stubbs AJ. Basic hip arthroscopy: supine patient positioning and dynamic fluoroscopic evaluation. Arthrosc Tech. 2015;4(4):e391–6. https://doi.org/10.1016/j.eats.2015.05.005.
62. Kong KF, Chien P, Wong JW, Yip DK. Peroneal padding: an alternative to a peroneal post in hip arthroscopy. Arthroscopy. 2003;19:1027–9.
63. McCarthy JC, Day B, Busconi B. Hip arthroscopy: applications and technique. J Am Acad Orthop Surg. 1995;3:115–22.
64. Glick JM, Sampson TG, Gordon RB, Behr JT, Schmidt E. Hip arthroscopy by the lateral approach. Arthroscopy. 1987;3(1):4–12.
65. Abrams GD, Harris JD, Safran MR. Hip arthroscopy: portal placement. In: Nho S, Leunig M, Larson C, Bedi A, Kelly B, editors. Hip arthroscopy and hip joint preservation surgery. New York, NY: Springer; 2015.
66. Byrd JW. Avoiding the labrum in hip arthroscopy. Arthroscopy. 2000;16:770–3.
67. Byrd JWT. Complications associated with hip arthroscopy. In: Byrd JWT, editor. Operative hip arthroscopy. 2nd ed. New York: Thieme; 2005. p. 229–35.
68. Simpson J, Sadri H, Villar R. Hip arthroscopy technique and complications. Orthop Traumatol Surg Res. 2010;96:S68–76.
69. Badylak JS, Keene JS. Do iatrogenic punctures of the labrum affect the clinical results of hip arthroscopy? Arthroscopy. 2011;27:761–7.
70. Aoki SK, Beckmann JT, Wylie JD. Hip arthroscopy and the anterolateral portal: avoiding labral penetration and femoral articular injuries. Arthrosc Tech. 2012;1(2):e155–60. https://doi.org/10.1016/j.eats.2012.05.007.
71. Sussmann PS, Zumstein M, Hahn F, Dora C. The risk of vascular injury to the femoral head when using the posterolateral arthroscopy portal: cadaveric investigation. Arthroscopy. 2007;23(10):1112–5.
72. Thorey F, Ezechieli M, Ettinger M, Albrecht UV, Budde S. Access to the hip joint from standard arthroscopic portals: a cadaveric study. Arthroscopy. 2013;29(8):1297–307.
73. Dienst M, Seil R, Kohn DM. Safe arthroscopic access to the central compartment of the hip. Arthroscopy. 2005;21:1510–4.
74. Studler U, Kalberer F, Leunig M, Zanetti M, Hodler J, Dora C, Pfirrmann CWA. MR arthrography of the hip: differentiation between an anterior sublabral recess as a normal variant and a labral tear. Radiology. 2008;249(3):947–54.
75. Sampson TG. Arthroscopic treatment of femoroacetabular impingement. Am J Orthop (Belle Mead NJ). 2008;37(12):608–12.
76. Domb BG, Philippon MJ, Giordano BD. Arthroscopic capsulotomy, capsular repair, and capsular plication of the hip: relation to atraumatic instability. Arthroscopy. 2013;29(1):162–73.
77. Nakano N, Khanduja V. Complications in hip arthroscopy. Muscles Ligaments Tendons J. 2016;6(3):402–9.
78. Guanche C. Hip arthroscopy techniques: deep gluteal space access. 2015. p. 351–60.
79. Gutierrez RC, Iban MA, Ayestaran AC, Sobrino AS, Oteo-Alvaro A. Peripheral compartment as the initial access for hip arthroscopy in complex cases: technical note. Orthopedics. 2013;36(6):456–62.
80. Stone AV, Howse EA, Mannava S, Miller BA, Botros D, Stubbs AJ. Basic hip arthroscopy: diagnostic hip arthroscopy. Arthrosc Tech. 2017;6(3):e699–704.
81. Carro LP, Hernando MF, Cerezal L, Navarro IS, Fernandez AA, Castillo AO. Deep gluteal space problems: piriformis syndrome, ischiofemoral impingement and sciatic nerve release. Muscles Ligaments Tendons J. 2016;6(3):384–96.
82. Martin HD, Palmer IJ, Hatem MA. Deep gluteal syndrome. In: Nho S, Leunig M, Kelly B, Bedi A, Larson C, editors. Hip arthroscopy and hip joint preservation surgery. New York: Springer; 2014. p. 1–17.
83. Miller SL, Gill J, Webb GR. The proximal origin of the hamstrings and surrounding anatomy encountered during repair. A cadaveric study. J Bone Joint Surg Am. 2007;89(1):44–8.

Endoscopic Anatomy of the Knee

2

Guillermo Cortés, Josep Maria De Anta, Francesc Malagelada, and Miki Dalmau-Pastor

Abstract

Knee arthroscopy is one of the most common arthroscopic procedures performed in the orthopedic surgery.

Professor Kenji Takagi in Tokyo has been considered as the first surgeon who performed an arthroscopic examination of a knee joint in 1919 (Takagi, J Jpn Orthop Assoc 8:132, 1933). In 1920 the Swiss Eugen Bircher published several papers describing his experiences regarding knee arthroscopy with diagnostic purposes. He was the first surgeon to introduce the term arthroscopy (Bircher, Beitr Klin Chir 127:239–50, 1922).

The first interventional arthroscopy was conducted by the Japanese surgeon Masaki Watanabe and his student and consisted of the removal of an intraarticular pigmented villonodular synovitis (Watanabe et al. Atlas of arthroscopy, Springer, 1969).

Arthroscopy techniques developed significantly during the 1970 and 80 decades due to the improvement of the optical and imaging technologies.

Keywords

Knee · Arthroscopy · Endoscopy · Anatomy Extra-articular

2.1 Knee Anatomy

The knee joint consists of several structures including the distal epiphyses of the femur, the proximal epiphysis of tibia and fibula, the patellar bone, the surrounding and the internal soft tissues.

G. Cortés
Orthopedic and Traumatology Department, Knee Unit, Hospital Universitari de Bellvitge, L'Hospitalet de Llobregat, Catalunya, Spain

J. M. De Anta
Faculty of Medicine and Health Sciences, Department of Pathology and Experimental Therapeutics, Human Anatomy and Embryology Unit, Universitat de Barcelona, Barcelona, Spain

F. Malagelada
Department of Trauma and Orthopaedic Surgery, Royal London Hospital, Barts Health NHS Trust, London, UK

MIFAS by GRECMIP (Minimally Invasive Foot and Ankle Society), Merignac, France

M. Dalmau-Pastor (✉)
Faculty of Medicine and Health Sciences, Department of Pathology and Experimental Therapeutics, Human Anatomy and Embryology Unit, Universitat de Barcelona, Barcelona, Spain

MIFAS by GRECMIP (Minimally Invasive Foot and Ankle Society), Merignac, France
e-mail: mikeldalmau@ub.edu

© The Author(s), under exclusive license to Springer Nature Singapore Pte Ltd. 2021
T. H. Lui (ed.), *Endoscopy of the Hip and Knee*, https://doi.org/10.1007/978-981-16-3488-8_2

It is helpful to divide the knee joint into a medial compartment, a lateral compartment, a central pivot, and the patellofemoral joint (Fig. 2.1).

2.1.1 The Medial Compartment

The medial compartment of the knee consists of the medial femoral condyle, the medial tibial plateau, the medial meniscus, and the medial part of the joint capsule and its ligaments (Fig. 2.2).

2.1.1.1 The Anterior Third

The anterior third of the medial compartment is mainly capsular. Superficial to the capsule, the part of the vastus medialis muscle attached to the patella, the vastus medialis obliquus (VMO), is found. The VMO is the most distal segment of the vastus medialis muscle and it is not clearly delineated. The

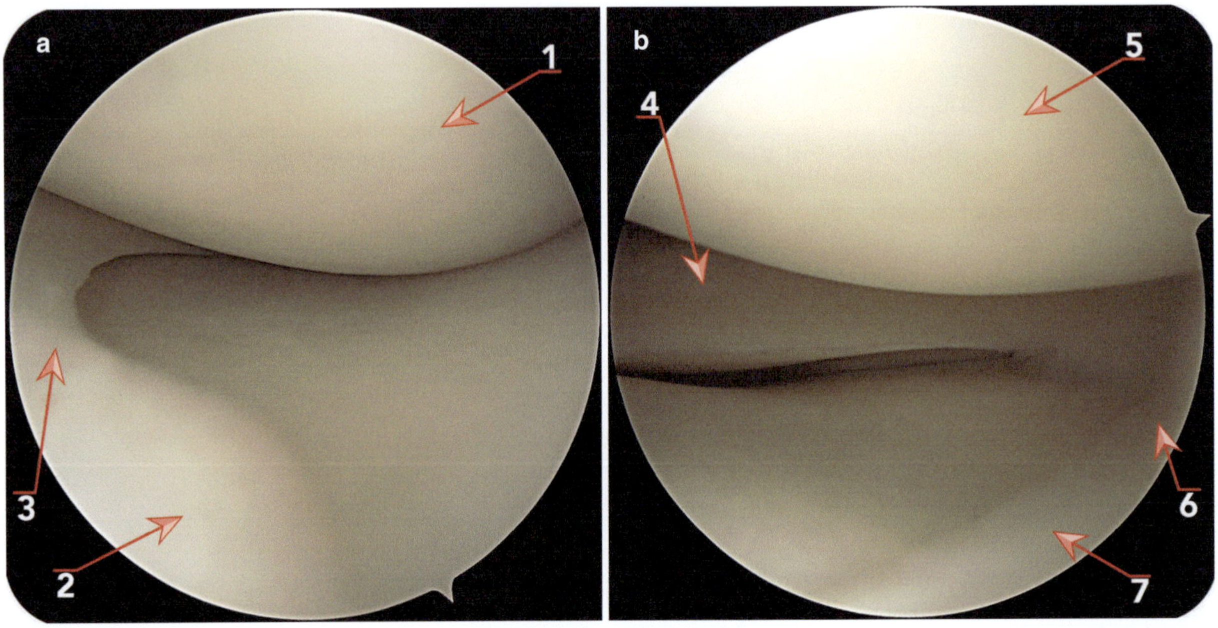

Fig. 2.1 Arthroscopic view of the medial (**a**) and lateral (**b**) compartments of the knee. (1) Medial femoral condyle. (2) Anterior horn of the medial meniscus. (3) Medial meniscus. (4) Posterior horn of the lateral meniscus. (5) Lateral femoral condyle. (6) Lateral meniscus. (7) Anterior horn of the lateral meniscus

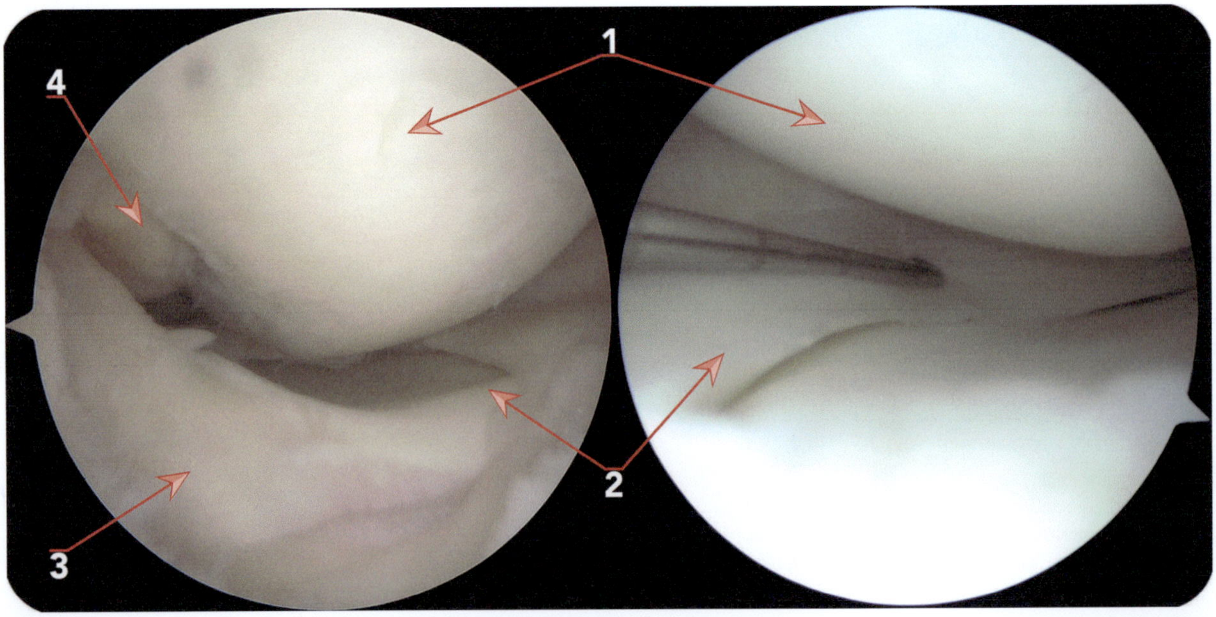

Fig. 2.2 Arthroscopic view of the medial compartment of the knee. (1) Medial femoral condyle. (2) Medial meniscus. (3) Tibial insertion of ACL. (4) Femoral insertion of ACL

distal border of the VMO is attached along the proximal edge of the medial patellofemoral ligament. It has an important role in maintaining patellar stability.

The medial patellofemoral ligament (MPFL) is found superficially to the anterior joint capsule. The distal border of the vastus medialis obliquus is attached to this ligament. It is inserted on the superomedial aspect of the medial border of the patella. The ligament coursed medially, and it is attached just distal and anterior to the adductor tubercle and 10 mm proximal and 8 mm posterior to the medial epicondyle [1]. The MPFL is the main static medial restraint of the patella and the VMO the main dynamic stabilizer, with obliquely oriented fibers [2]. The MPFL is frequently damaged in patients with patellar instability with recurrent lateral patellar dislocation. Many techniques are described for MPFL reconstruction with minimally invasive-arthroscopically assisted surgery.

At the anterior medial distal knee, the pes anserinus tendon attachment is found. It consists of the sartorius, gracilis, and the semitendinosus muscle attachments at the anteromedial aspect of the proximal tibia. The sartorius tendon is attached to the superficial fascial layer and the gracilis and semitendinosus are located deep to the fascial layer. The sartorius tendon is located superiorly to the gracilis and semitendinosus tendons, which follow inferiorly. The pes anserinus attachment is located anteriorly and superficial to the distal insertion of the superficial medial collateral ligament [3]. The pes anserinus helps knee stability to valgus stress. The semitendinosus and/or the gracilis tendons are frequently harvested for ACL reconstruction and other ligament reconstruction surgeries.

2.1.1.2 The Middle Third

The middle third of the medial aspect of the knee includes the medial collateral ligament of the knee as the main structure (Fig. 2.3). It consists of a superficial and a deep part.

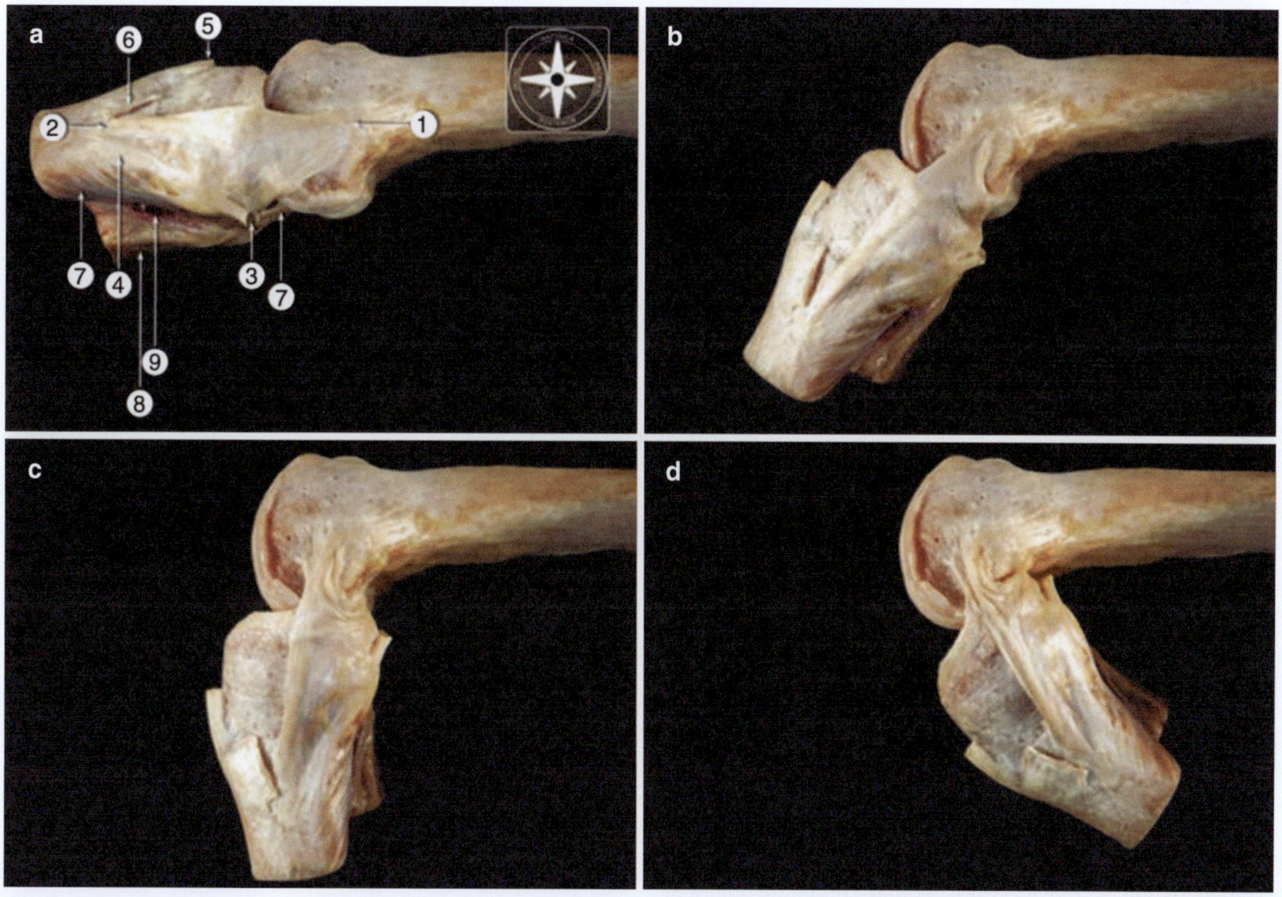

Fig. 2.3 Osteoarticular anatomic dissection of the medial collateral ligament during the range of motion of the knee joint (**a**, extension to **d**, maximal flexion). (1) Medial epicondyle. (2) Tibial insertion of medial collateral ligament. (3) Semimembranosus tendon (cut). (4). Inferior or popliteal expansion of the semimembranosus tendon. (5) Patellar tendon (cut). (6) Pes anserinus (cut). (7) Popliteus muscle. (8) Soleus muscle (cut). (9) Neurovascular bundle (popliteal artery, veins, and tibial nerve). Figure reproduced with permission from: Malagelada F, Vega J, Golanó P. Chapter 91: Knee Anatomy and Biomechanics of the Knee. In Miller MD, Thompson SR (Eds.). De Lee & Drez's Orthopaedic Sports Medicine: Principles and Practice. 4th ed. Elsevier, 2015

The superficial part of the Medial Collateral Ligament (sMCL) is the largest structure over the medial knee. Its proximal insertion is on the femur, in a depression found proximal and posterior to the medial epicondyle and distal to the adductor and gastrocnemius tubercles. As the superficial part of the medial collateral ligament travels distally it presents two different attachments at the tibia. A superior attachment is found on the bone insertion of the anterior part of the semimembranosus tendon, just distal to the joint line. Its inferior attachment is anterior to the posteromedial crest of the tibia and runs deeply to the pes anserinus tendons attachments. Between these two tibial attachments of the superficial medial collateral ligament the inferior medial genicular artery and vein along with their nerve branch from the tibial nerve can be found. The proximal division of the sMCL serves as the primary static stabilizer to valgus stress and rotational forces. The distal division of the sMCL stabilizes the knee against rotational forces specially with the knee in flexion [3, 4].

The deep part of the medial collateral ligament (dMCL) is considered as a thickening of the medial joint capsule. The anterior rim runs parallel to the superficial medial collateral ligament. The posterior rim is inseparable from the posterior oblique ligament. The dMCL consists of meniscofemoral and meniscotibial ligament at the middle third of the medial compartment. The dMCL acts as a stabilizer against valgus and internal rotation forces [3, 4].

2.1.1.3 The Posterior Third

The medial posterior knee includes the following structures: the posterior oblique ligament, the semimembranosus tendon, the adductor magnus tendon, and the medial gastrocnemius tendon.

The posterior oblique ligament (POL): the POL was considered part of the superficial medial collateral ligament, but it is considered to be an independent structure. The POL is a primary restraint to internal rotation and is a secondary restraint to valgus translation and external rotation of the knee specially with the knee in extension. It is attached at the femur proximal and posterior to the insertion of the superficial medial collateral ligament and just anterior to the gastrocnemius tubercle. As it runs distally it has three arms: the superficial, central, and capsular arms. The superficial arm coursed parallel to the anterior arm of the semimembranosus muscle. The central arm is the thickest arm of the POL and it is distally inserted direct to the medial meniscus, the meniscotibial ligament and the deep medial collateral ligament, and the posteromedial side of the tibia. The capsular arm is attached to soft tissue, the medial gastrocnemius tendon and the adductor magnus tendon femoral attachment.

Semimembranosus tendon: The main tendon of the semimembranosus muscle is divided in two arms in its tibial course, the anterior and the direct arms. The anterior arm attaches to the tibia deeply and distally to the proximal attachment of the proximal sMCL. The direct arm attaches posterior to the medial tibial crest at an osseous prominence, the *tuberculum tendinis*, and distally to the joint line. Before its final attachment the direct arm attached to the posterior aspect of the coronary ligament and the posterior horn of the medial meniscus (Fig. 2.4).

Adductor magnus tendon: it is inserted on the femur just proximal and posterior to the adductor tubercle. The distal aspect of the adductor magnus tendon is attached to the gastrocnemius tendon and the capsular arm of the posterior oblique ligament and the posterior capsule.

The medial gastrocnemius tendon: it is attached onto the femur, just proximal and posterior to the gastrocnemius tubercle. The tendon has fascial attachments to the adductor magnus tendon and the capsular arm of the posterior oblique ligament and capsule [3, 4].

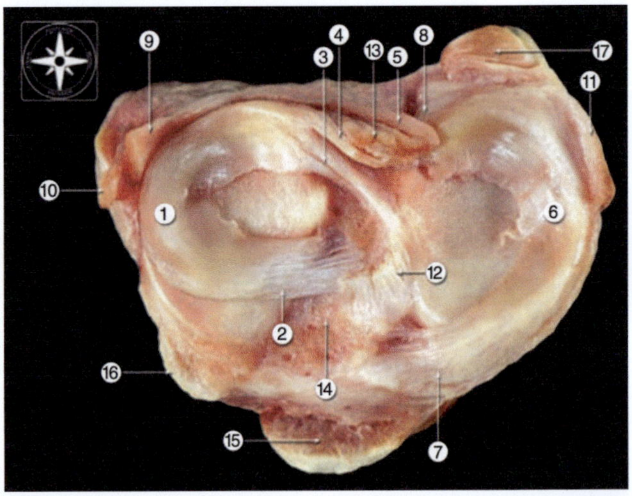

Fig. 2.4 Osteoarticular dissection showing the morphology and relationship of the proximal epiphysis of the tibia in a superior view. (1) Lateral meniscus. (2) Anterior horn of the lateral meniscus. (3) Posterior horn of the lateral meniscus. (4) Anterior meniscofemoral ligament. (5) Posterior meniscofemoral ligament. (6) Medial meniscus. (7) Anterior horn of the medial meniscus. (8) Posterior horn of the medial meniscus. (9) Popliteus tendon (cut). (10) Lateral collateral ligament (cut). (11) Medial collateral ligament (cut). (12) Tibial footprint of the anterior cruciate ligament. (13) Posterior cruciate ligament (cut). (14) Anterior intercondylar area. (15) Patellar tendon (cut). (16) Iliotibial tract insertion in the anterior tubercle or Gerdy's tubercle (cut). (17) Semimembranosus tendon (cut). Figure reproduced with permission from: Malagelada F, Vega J, Golanó P. Chapter 91: Knee Anatomy and Biomechanics of the Knee. In Miller MD, Thompson SR (Eds.). De Lee & Drez's Orthopaedic Sports Medicine: Principles and Practice. 4th ed. Elsevier, 2015

2.1.2 The Lateral Compartment

The lateral compartment of the knee consists of the lateral femoral condyle, the lateral tibial plateau, the lateral meniscus, and the lateral part of the capsule and its ligaments (Fig. 2.5).

2.1.2.1 The Anterior Third

At the anterior third of the lateral compartment of the knee the following structures are present: the lateral patellofemoral retinaculum, the iliotibial tract, and the anterolateral ligament.

The lateral patellofemoral retinaculum consists of a condensation of tissue that braces the patella from its lateral side. This tissue comes from the deep fascia, the vastus lateralis aponeurosis, and the iliotibial tract.

The Iliotibial tract is a broad fascial structure that originates at the anterolateral external crest and inserts at the Gerdy's tubercle. It has an anterior extension to the patella that is called the iliopatellar band or the superficial oblique retinaculum of the patella. The deep layer of the iliotibial tract that attaches to the distal femur is known as Kaplan fibers. It also has attachment to the lateral head of the gastrocnemius and the biceps femoris tendon. Due to its attachments, the iliotibial tract acts as a lateral femorotibial collateral ligament.

The anterolateral ligament (ALL) has been previously known as the mid-third lateral capsular ligament or the capsule-osseus latter of the iliotibial tract. The ligament originates from the prominence of the lateral femoral epicondyle and runs distally to the proximal tibia between Gerdy's tubercle and the fibular head. During it course it also attaches to the lateral meniscus. The anterolateral ligament provides rotary stability and the distal avulsion, have been its fracture correlated with the Segond Fracture characteristic of the anterior cruciate ligament injuries [5, 6]. The ALL reconstruction associated with ACL reconstruction surgery could be performed in patients with complete ACL tears with major rotational instability.

2.1.2.2 The Posterolateral Corner of the Knee

The following structures are located in this area: the fibular collateral ligament, the popliteal tendon, the popliteofibular ligament, the biceps femoris tendon, the lateral gastrocne-

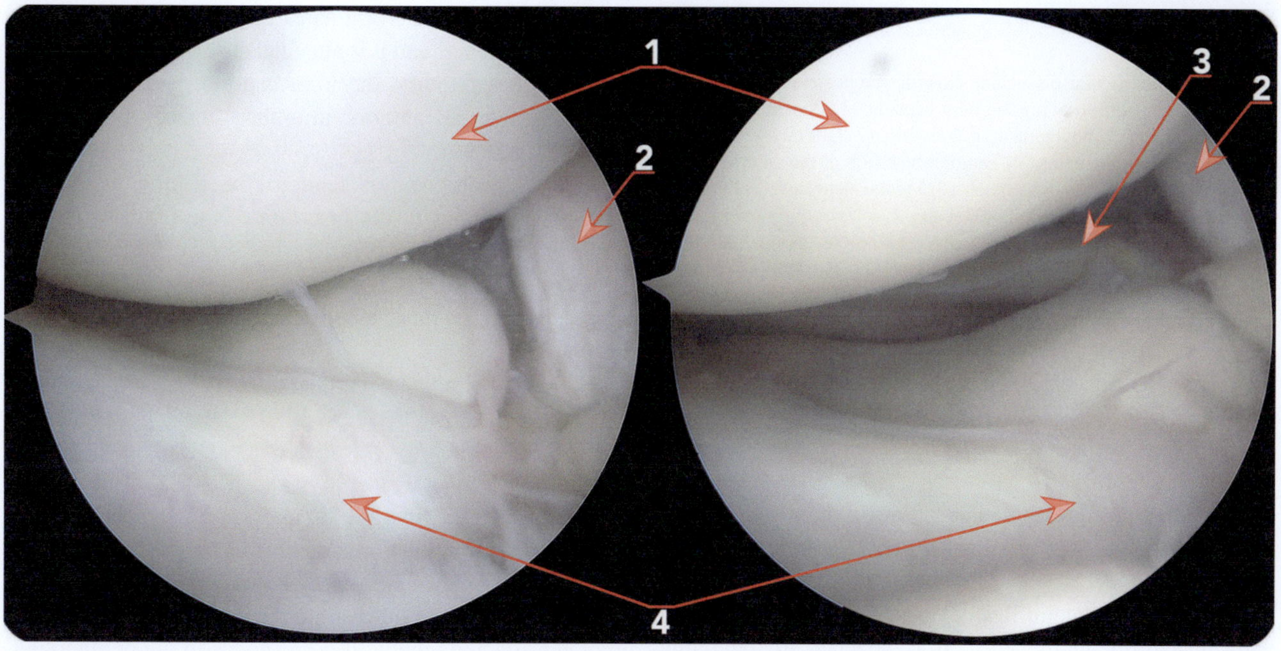

Fig. 2.5 Arthroscopic view of the lateral compartment of the knee. (1) Lateral femoral condyle. (2) ACL. (3) Posterior horn of the lateral meniscus. (4) Anterior horn of the lateral meniscus

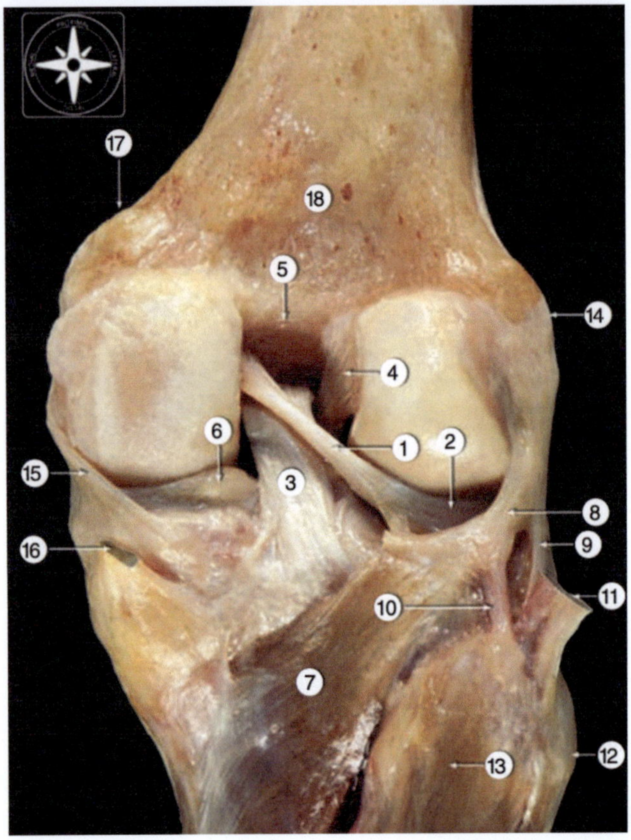

Fig. 2.6 Osteoarticular dissection showing the posterior structures of the knee joint after removing the joint capsule. (1) Posterior meniscofemoral ligament or the ligament of Wrisberg. (2) Lateral meniscus. (3) Posterior cruciate ligament. (4) Femoral insertion of the anterior cruciate ligament. (5) Intercondylar notch. (6) Medial meniscus. (7) Popliteus muscle. (8) Popliteus tendon. (9) Lateral collateral ligament. (10) Popliteus capsular extension. (11) Biceps femoris tendon (cut). (12) Head of the fibula. (13) Soleus fibular insertion muscle. (14) Lateral epicondyle. (15) Medial collateral ligament. (16) Semimembranosus (cut). (17) Adductor tubercle. (18) Popliteal surface. Figure reproduced with permission from: Malagelada F, Vega J, Golanó P. Chapter 91: Knee Anatomy and Biomechanics of the Knee. In Miller MD, Thompson SR (Eds.). De Lee & Drez's Orthopaedic Sports Medicine: Principles and Practice. fourth ed. Elsevier, 2015

mius tendon, the fabello-fibular ligament, the arcuate popliteal ligament, and the proximal tibiofibular joint ligaments (Fig. 2.6).

The fibular collateral ligament is the primary restraint to varus instability in the knee. It is attached to the femur 1.4 mm proximal and 3.1 mm posterior to the lateral epicondyle in a small bony depression and 18.5 mm proximal and posterior to the popliteal tendon attachment. It runs distally to the anterior and lateral aspect of the fibular head and attaches in a small depression 8 mm posterior to the anterior margin of the fibular head and 28.4 mm distal to the apex of the fibular styloid.

Popliteus muscle tendon: it is attached just posterior to the limit of the cartilage of the femoral condyle at the anterior end of the popliteal sulcus. The tendon runs obliquely in posterior and inferior direction, passes the popliteal hiatus, and attaches at the posterior aspect of the tibia. The tendon is attached to the lateral meniscus at the popliteal hiatus with three popliteomeniscal fascicles. It can be explored arthroscopically as it is an intraarticular structure. The popliteus tendon is loose in extension and tight in flexion, it is a stabilizer against varus and rotational stresses during flexion. With its attachment to the lateral meniscus helps to keep it in place as the knee flexes.

Popliteofibular ligament: it is attached to the popliteus musculotendinous junction and runs distally to the tip of the fibular head. It is a primary stabilizer during external rotation specially around 60° of flexion [6, 7].

Biceps femoris muscle has two heads. The long head originates from the ischial tuberosity and runs through the posterior and lateral aspect of the thigh. It is attached lateral to the fibular apex at the fibular head. The short head of the biceps femoris muscle originates medial to the linea aspera on the distal femur and it is attached distally to the long head of the biceps femoris, the joint capsule, and the iliotibial tract. There is an anterior arm that attaches posterior to Gerdy's tubercle.

Lateral gastrocnemius tendon: the tendon is attached 13.8 mm posterior to the insertion of the fibular collateral ligament. It has also fibers attached to the fabella and the supracondylar process. It is connected to the meniscofemoral joint capsule. The muscle belly runs superficial to the popliteus muscle.

Fabello-fibular ligament: the fabella is a sesamoid bone or cartilage located at the head of the lateral gastrocnemius muscle. This structure is presented in most but not all people. The fabello-fibular ligament is attached at the fabella and runs distally to the tip of the fibula.

The arcuate popliteal ligament is a classic dissection that involves an Y-shape extraarticular structure that connects the fibular head to the popliteus tendon and the posterolateral joint capsule and fabella. It corresponds to the popliteofibular ligament, fabello-fibular ligament, popliteo meniscal fascicles, and the capsular arm of the short head of the biceps femoris.

Proximal tibiofibular joint ligaments: the anterior and posterior ligaments connect the medial side of the head of the fibula to the lateral sides of the lateral condyle of the tibia [6, 7].

2.1.3 The Posterior Knee

The posterior knee includes two major structures: the posterior semimembranosus complex and the posterior popliteus complex. These major complexes have been already described in this chapter. These complexes are connected by the oblique popliteal ligament (OPL). The OPL is a structure that originates together with the tendon of the semimembranosus muscle. It arises in the semimembranosus tendon proximal to the tibial plateau, runs superolaterally, and then is attached to the fabella or to the tendon of the lateral head of the gastrocnemius and blended with the posterolateral joint capsule. However, it has a broad anatomical variability. It is the primary ligamentous restrain to knee hyperextension [8–11].

2.1.4 The Menisci

Menisci play an important role in the distribution of loads, shock absorption, joint stability, and lubrication of joint surfaces (Fig. 2.4). Arthroscopic surgery for the treatment of meniscal injuries is one of the most common orthopedic procedures worldwide. The operative treatment for meniscal injuries is continuously evolving as a result of the better understanding of its anatomy, histology, and function. Nowadays the meniscal preservation surgery is emerging in front of the classic meniscectomy procedures. Specific arthroscopic techniques for different locations and patterns of meniscal tears are developed. The meniscal allograft transplantation is also an option for those young patients with, apart from the meniscus, a healthy knee who have lost meniscal tissue.

2.1.5 The Medial Menisci

The medial meniscus is C-shaped. It has a wedge section with the free edge facing to the joint and the rim attached to the capsule. Its radius of curvature varies so it is larger anteroposterior than mediolateral. The meniscus is narrower anteriorly than posteriorly. The anterior horn is attached to the tibial plateau at the intercondylar fossae anteriorly to the ACL insertion. Berlet et al. have described four different insertion patterns for the anterior horn of the medial meniscus [12]. The anterior horns of the lateral and medial meniscus are connected by the transverse ligament of the knee. The medial meniscus is attached to the joint capsule along the entire periphery. The inferior or tibial portion of this peripheric capsular attachment is the coronary ligament. At the region of the tibial collateral ligament, a superior (femoral) attachment is present, the medial meniscus is firmly attached to the femur and tibia through a robust thickening in the capsule, the deep tibial collateral ligament. The POL and the semimembranosus complex have insertions at the posterior horn of the medial meniscus. These attachments explain the generation of some special meniscal tears at the posterior horn of the medial meniscus in knees affected by rotational instability. The posterior root is attached to the tibia at the intercondylar fossae between the posterior cruciate ligament and the posterior horn of the lateral meniscus insertion [13].

2.1.6 The Lateral Menisci

The lateral meniscus covers a wider area of the plateau of the lateral tibial condyle. Its radius of curvature is constant resulting in an O-shaped structure. The anterior horn is attached anterior to the intercondylar eminence, just posterior and lateral to the ACL insertion. The anterior and posterior horns of the lateral meniscus are inserted close to each other, both are visible during the ACL reconstruction surgery and can be used as a reference for ACL tibial positioning [14].

The lateral meniscus has fewer attachment to the periphery than the medial meniscus. It is only attached to the capsule through the coronary ligament, which is absent at the area of the hiatus popliteus, so the lateral meniscus is more mobile than the medial one.

The posterior root of the lateral meniscus is attached posterior to the lateral tibial eminence at the intercondylar notch and just posterior to the insertion of the anterior horn. The anterior fibers of the posterior root of the lateral meniscus extend to the lateral aspect of the medial femoral condyle, forming the anterior meniscofemoral ligament (ligament of Humphrey) which can be found in 50% of the population. The posterior fibers of the posterior root of the lateral meniscus can cross the PCL posteriorly and attach to the intercondylar fossa of the medial femoral condyle, forming the posterior meniscofemoral ligament (ligament of Wrisberg) which can be found in 75% of the population.

2.1.7 The Central Pivot

The central pivot includes the cruciate ligaments, which are the central stabilizers of the knee joint. They are the anterior cruciate ligament of the knee (ACL) and the posterior cruciate ligament of the knee (PCL).

The anterior cruciate ligament of the knee (ACL) is the most surgically reconstructed ligament of the body [15]. The ACL is inserted anteromedially onto the anterior intercondylar area of the tibia in front of the medial tibial spine, between the anterior roots of the lateral and medial meniscus. It ascends through the intercondylar fossa to insert at the posteromedial aspect of the lateral femoral condyle.

The ACL is divided into two different bundles, the anteromedial bundle (AM) and the posterolateral bundle (PL) according to their insertion on the tibia. In full extension, both bundles run parallel being the AM bundle relaxed while the PL bundle is tightened. During the knee flexion the bundles wrapped together, the AM becomes tight while the PL bundle is relaxed [16].

The ACL stabilizes the tibia when it is anteriorly displaced relative to the femur. The posteromedial angle, the semimembranosus complex, and the anterolateral ligament also act as anterior translation stabilizers. Due to its orientation, it is also a powerful restraint against internal rotation forces.

The ACL has poor healing capacity, so the techniques for ACL repair are limited. Therefore, most of the ACL procedures consist of autograft ligament reconstruction using hamstring tendons, bone-patellar tendon bone, or quadricipital tendon.

The posterior cruciate ligament (PCL) is inserted on the lateral side of the medial femoral condyle and runs to the posterior intercondylar area of the tibia. It also has two bundles, the anterolateral and posteromedial. Posteromedial fibers are tighten during extension and thus limit hyperextension. The anterolateral bundle is also tight during semi and full flexion. Due to its fiber orientation, the PCL mostly prevents posterior displacement of the tibia when the knee is flexed.

2.1.8 The Patellofemoral Compartment

The patella is the largest sesamoid bone of the body. The articular surface of the patella is divided into two surfaces by a median ridge. The lateral surface is longer and more sloped than the medial articular surface. The Wiberg classification of patella size includes four different types based on the location of the median ridge.

The quadriceps tendon is inserted at the base of the patella. This tendon is formed by the confluence of four muscle bellies, the rectus femoris, the vastus medialis, the vastus lateralis, and the vastus intermedius. An intraarticular space extends from the tip of the patella to the quadriceps tendon, along the front side of the femur, the suprapatellar recess.

The medial patellofemoral ligament, which runs from the femoral medial epicondyle, is inserted on the proximal two thirds of the medial edge of the patella. The distal part of the vastus medialis obliquus is overlaid the proximal side of the MPFL. From the inferior border of the medial patellar edge, the medial patellomeniscal ligament connects the patella to the anterior horn of the medial meniscus.

On the lateral side of the patella, the lateral patellofemoral retinaculum is identified. It is frequently divided into a superficial and deep layer. The superficial layer is composed of the oblique lateral retinaculum. The deep layer is composed of oblique fibers running distally (the patellotibial band) and transverse fibers to the lateral epicondyle and Iliotibial tract (the epicondylopatellar band).

The patellar tendon is inserted onto the vertex of the patella. It courses distally to the tibial tubercle. The infrapatellar fat separates the posterior side of the patellar tendon from the synovial membrane of the joint, and distally a bursa separates the tendon from the tibia [17–19].

2.1.9 The Neurovascular Structures of the Knee

Saphenous nerve (SN): it is a sensory nerve, being the longest cutaneous branch of the femoral nerve. It descends along with femoral vessels and crosses the adductor canal anterolateral to the femoral artery. After piercing the anteromedial septum along with the saphenous branch of descendent genicular artery, it passes through the fascia between the sartorius and the gracilis muscles and gives rise to the infrapatellar branch. It runs anteriorly on the medial side of the capsule and carries the sensitivity of the anterior and medial knee. The saphenous nerve continues travelling distally and provides sensitivity to the skin of the medial side of the leg and the dorsomedial ankle and midfoot.

The SN is particularly vulnerable during arthroscopic surgical procedures. It is at risk in meniscal repair procedures, when the posteromedial portal is established, or the meniscal repair needles are passed for the medial meniscus repair. It can also be damaged during the hamstring harvest as for ACL reconstruction [20]. The saphenous nerve injury is the most frequent neurovascular complication in knee arthroscopy procedures [21].

The sciatic nerve is divided at the superior edge of the popliteal fossae into the tibial nerve and the common peroneal nerve. The tibial nerve passes between the two heads of the gastrocnemius muscle, crosses the tendinous arch of the soleus muscle, and lies in the deep posterior compartment of the lower leg. In the popliteal fossa, it receives sensitive branches: the medial sural cutaneous nerve and the genicular posterior articular branch, and gives motor branches to the popliteus, plantar, and gastrocnemius muscles.

The common peroneal nerve runs distally along with the biceps femoris muscle. Then, it, passes medial to the head of the fibula, and courses laterally then anteriorly around the neck of the fibula. The common peroneal nerve is at risk during lateral meniscus repair surgery. The use of a posterior incision and a deflecting retractor is the most important factor in avoiding neurovascular injury during meniscal repair. The common peroneal nerve is also at risk when posterolateral corner ligament reconstruction procedures are performed.

The femoral artery travels anterodistally through the adductor canal, crosses the adductor hiatus, and enters to the popliteal fossa to become the popliteal artery. The genicular arteries arise from it and supply the structures around the knee. In the adductor canal, the femoral artery gives the descending genicular artery (supreme genicular artery) which divides into an articular branch (and also a saphenous branch) to supply the superior and anterior regions of the knee.

From the popliteal artery the medial and lateral superior genicular arteries branch off, running anteriorly and supplying the patella. There is also a small artery, the medial superior genicular artery, that pierces the capsule and supplies the cruciate ligaments and posterior structures. It may emerge from the popliteal superior or inferior genicular arteries (Int. J. Morphol. vol.35 no.3 Temuco set. 2017 https://doi.org/10.4067/S0717-95022017000300019). At the joint line, the lateral and medial inferior genicular emerge. At the lower end of the popliteal fossa, the popliteal artery passes between the two heads of the gastrocnemius muscle and gives rise to two muscular branches to each head. After crossing the tendinous arch of the soleus muscle, it branches into the anterior and posterior tibial arteries. Major vascular complications involving the popliteal artery are very uncommon during knee arthroscopy. Probably the most common vascular injury during knee arthroscopy is the damage of the lateral inferior genicular artery when an anterolateral portal is performed [22].

2.2 Arthroscopy Portals

The anterolateral and the anteromedial portals are the main portals used for routine knee arthroscopic procedures.

The anterolateral portal is the standard viewing portal. It is placed on a soft spot located on a triangle bounded by the lateral border of the patellar tendon, the lateral femoral condyle, and the anterolateral rim of the tibia plateau. The patellar distal apex is the key landmark to determine the height of the portal. The anterolateral portal is performed slightly distal to the vertex of the patella.

The anteromedial portal is the main working and instrumentation portal. It is performed under direct arthroscopic visualization with the camera placed through the anterolateral portal. The entry point should be close to the patellar tendon on the medial soft spot.

In addition, several accessory portals may be used depending on the specific surgical procedure requirements.

The superomedial and superolateral portals give good access to the suprapatellar recess with the knee in extension and are located, medial and lateral, respectively, at the height of the proximal patellar vertex. Both can be used for irrigation or aspiration and during surgical procedures involving the patellofemoral compartment.

The accessory medial portal is more medial and inferior to the standard medial portal and is used in meniscal repair and ACL repair.

The accessory lateral portal is more lateral and inferior to the standard portal and could be useful as a visualization portal or for certain meniscal repair procedures.

The posterior portals are used for posterior horn repair and posterior cruciate ligament reconstruction. Making the posterior portals could be challenging because of the proximity of the neurovascular structures, not just the popliteal artery but the common peroneal nerve at the lateral side and the saphenous nerve at the medial side. The knee should be flexed over 90° so the posterior structures relax and move backwards. The portals are made under direct visualization with the arthroscope placed on an anterior portal.

The posteromedial portal is located 1 cm above the joint line posterior to the tibial collateral ligament. The posterolateral portal is made 1 cm above the joint line between the peroneal collateral ligament and the biceps femoris tendon.

Finally, the transpatellar tendon portal is located 1 cm distal to the patella splitting the tendon longitudinally. It can be helpful during some complex meniscal surgeries and for reduction of tibial spine fractures but can led to side effects as anterior knee pain due to tendon scarring [23].

References

1. Amis AA, Firer P, Mountney J, Senavongse W, Thomas NP. Anatomy and biomechanics of the medial patellofemoral ligament. Knee. 2003;10(3):215–20.
2. Warren LF, Marshall JL, Girgis F. The prime static stabilizer of the medial side of the knee. JBJS. 1974;56(4):665–74.
3. LaPrade RF, Engebretsen AH, Ly TV, Johansen S, Wentorf FA, Engebretsen L. The anatomy of the medial part of the knee. JBJS. 2007;89(9):2000–10.
4. LaPrade MD, Kennedy MI, Wijdicks CA, LaPrade RF. Anatomy and biomechanics of the medial side of the knee and their surgical implications. Sports Med Arthrosc Rev. 2015;23(2):63–70.
5. Sanchez AR, Sugalski MT, LaPrade RF. Anatomy and biomechanics of the lateral side of the knee. Sports Med Arthrosc Rev. 2006;14(1):2–11.
6. James EW, LaPrade CM, LaPrade RF. Anatomy and biomechanics of the lateral side of the knee and surgical implications. Sports Med Arthrosc Rev. 2015;23(1):2–9.
7. LaPrade RF, Resig S, Wentorf F, Lewis JL. The effects of grade III posterolateral knee complex injuries on anterior cruciate ligament graft force. Am J Sports Med. 1999;27(4):469–75.
8. LaPrade RF, Morgan PM, Wentorf FA, Johansen S, Engebretsen L. The anatomy of the posterior aspect of the knee: an anatomic study. JBJS. 2007;89(4):758–64.
9. Wu X-D, et al. Anatomical characteristics and biomechanical properties of the oblique popliteal ligament. Sci Rep. 2017;7:42698.
10. Fam LP, Fruheling VM, Pupim B, Ramos CH, de Moura MF, Namba M, da Silva JL, da Cunha LA, de Oliveira Franco AP, Stieven FE. Oblique popliteal ligament—an anatomical study. Rev Bras Ortop (English Edition). 2013;48(5):402–5.
11. Morgan PM, LaPrade RF, Wentorf FA, Cook JW, Bianco A. The role of the oblique popliteal ligament and other structures in preventing knee hyperextension. Am J Sports Med. 2010;38(3):550–7.
12. Berlet GC, Fowler PJ. The anterior horn of the medial meniscus. Am J Sports Med. 1998;26(4):540–3.
13. Śmigielski R, Becker R, Zdanowicz U, Ciszek B. Medial meniscus anatomy—from basic science to treatment. Knee Surg Sports Traumatol Arthrosc. 2015;23(1):8–14.
14. Prejbeanu R, Crisan D. Arthroscopic treatment of intraarticular fractures around the knee. In: Atlas of knee arthroscopy. London: Springer; 2015. p. 141–8.
15. Granan LP, Forssblad M, Lind M, Engebretsen L. The Scandinavian ACL registries 2004–2007: baseline epidemiology. Acta Orthop. 2009;80(5):563–7.
16. Markatos K, Kaseta MK, Lallos SN, Korres DS, Efstathopoulos N. The anatomy of the ACL and its importance in ACL reconstruction. Eur J Orthop Surg Traumatol. 2013;23(7):747–52.
17. Andrikoula S, Tokis A, Vasiliadis HS, Georgoulis A. The extensor mechanism of the knee joint: an anatomical study. Knee Surg Sports Traumatol Arthrosc. 2006;14(3):214–20.
18. Zaffagnini S, Dejour D, Grassi A, Bonanzinga T, Muccioli GM, Colle F, Raggi F, Benzi A, Marcacci M. Patellofemoral anatomy and biomechanics: current concepts. Joints. 2013;1(2):15.
19. Sherman SL, Plackis AC, Nuelle CW. Patellofemoral anatomy and biomechanics. Clin Sports Med. 2014;33(3):389–401.
20. Sanders B, Rolf R, McClelland W, Xerogeanes J. Prevalence of saphenous nerve injury after autogenous hamstring harvest: an anatomic and clinical study of sartorial branch injury. Arthroscopy. 2007;23(9):956–63.
21. Small NC. Complications in arthroscopic meniscal surgery. Clin Sports Med. 1990;9(3):609–17.
22. Kim TK, Savino RM, McFarland EG, Cosgarea AJ. Neurovascular complications of knee arthroscopy. Am J Sports Med. 2002;30(4):619–29.
23. Pujol N, Beaufils P. Knee arthroscopy: general setup, portal options, and how to manage a complete arthroscopic investigation. In: Arthroscopy. Berlin: Springer; 2016. p. 69–78.

3 Setup and Instruments

Chong Yin Mak and Tun Hing Lui

Abstract

With advancement in arthroscopic and endoscopic technique and instruments, arthroscopy has become feasible in most human joints and extra-articular potential spaces. With the introduction of this minimal invasive technique, a wide variety of treatment can be performed without the need of traditional open surgery. Arthroscopic and endoscopic approaches have the advantages of better visualization by magnified arthroscopic views, minimal trauma to the surrounding soft tissues, and less post-operative pain. In this chapter, the operative room setup, patient positioning, and instruments for hip and knee endoscopy are described.

Keywords

Hip · Knee · Endoscopy · Portals · Position · Setup Instruments

3.1 Patient Position

Most endoscopic knee and hip procedures can be performed in supine and lateral positions. Floppy lateral position can be employed for knee endoscopy for flexibility when both anterior and lateral access are important. The knee can be flexed by using leg holder and dropping the foot of the bed, or by

C. Y. Mak
Department of Orthopaedics and Traumatology, North District Hospital, Hong Kong, China

T. H. Lui (✉)
Department of Orthopaedics and Traumatology, North District Hospital, Hong Kong, China

The Second Affiliated Hospital, Shenzhen University, Shenzhen, China

© The Author(s), under exclusive license to Springer Nature Singapore Pte Ltd. 2021
T. H. Lui (ed.), *Endoscopy of the Hip and Knee*, https://doi.org/10.1007/978-981-16-3488-8_3

using foot rest or posterior wedge with a full table (Fig. 3.1). Mechanical positioners, some motorized, are available for versatile and dynamic positioning for specific procedures. Precautions should be employed for the pressure-sensitive areas during lateral positioning. Pelvic holders can ensure the stability of lateral positioning. Whilst traction is necessary in certain endoscopic procedures of the hip (Fig. 3.2), care should be taken to avoid distraction injury and compression injury to the perineum by countertraction [1]. Post-less distraction options are being developed.

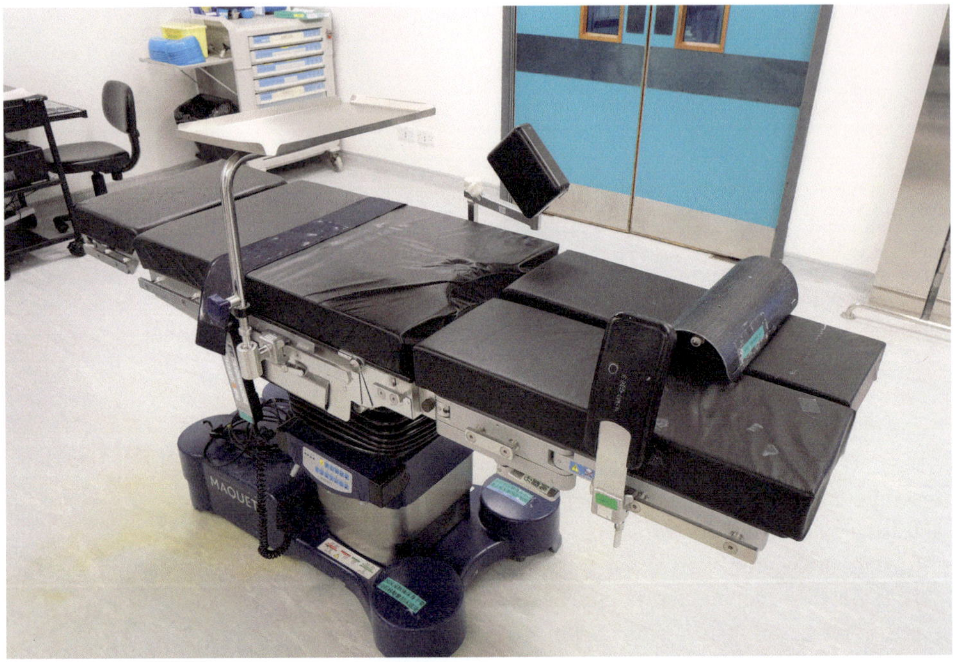

Fig. 3.1 Operation table

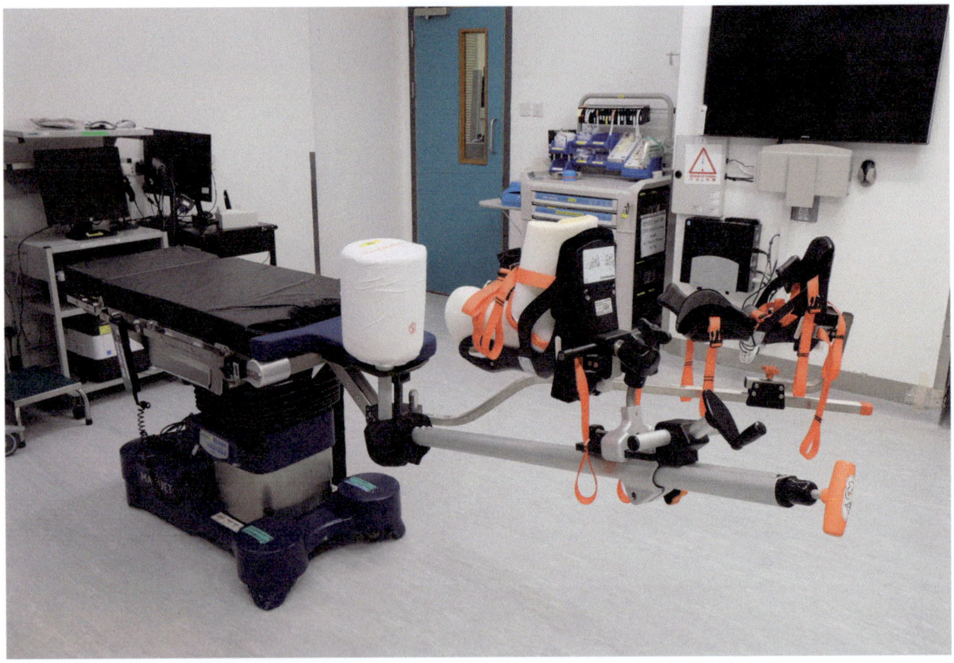

Fig. 3.2 Traction table for hip endoscopy

3.2 Theatre Arrangement

Factors to be taken into consideration for theatre arrangement include anaesthetic arrangement, surgical instruments and equipment, fluoroscopy requirement, overall theatre flow, and surgeon ergonomics. The theatre setup should be tailored to the specific procedure. In general, for endoscopic procedures, the chief surgeon and the assistants should be positioned on the ipsilateral side of the operative site whilst the endoscopy tower and fluid management devices should be positioned on the contralateral side. The scrub nurse and the back sterile instrument table are usually placed behind the surgical team. Mayo trays are used to place the frequently used instruments, such as the camera and scope assembly, trocar and cannula, motorized shaver, radiofrequency probe, and switching sticks, close to the operative site for efficient access.

3.2.1 Instruments

3.2.1.1 Scopes

Standard arthroscopes with 30°or 70° inclination (Fig. 3.3) can be used for hip and knee endoscopic procedures. 4 mm arthroscopes have optical field of view of 115°. By rotating a 30° scope along its axis, a scanning field of view of 175° can be achieved. While most procedures can be performed using 30° scopes, 70° scopes can provide better view round corners. This is especially useful when the manoeuvring of the scope is limited by the bony anatomy, tight fascial layers, and deep tissue tract. Orientation with a 70° scope can be difficult especially for beginners. Whilst 70° 4 mm scopes can achieve a scanning field of view of 255°, surgeons must be aware of the 25° of blind field in the middle to avoid missed pathologies.

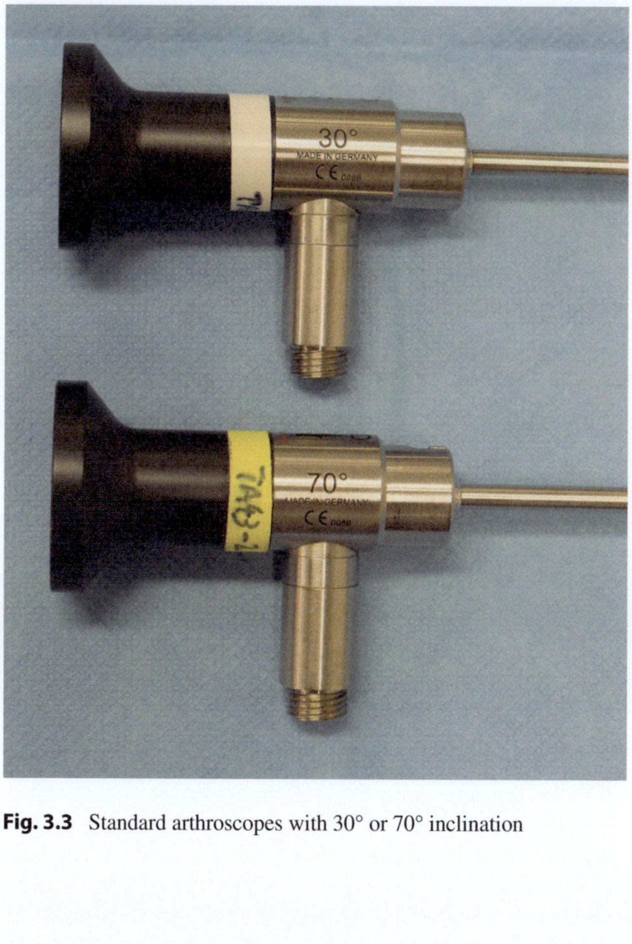

Fig. 3.3 Standard arthroscopes with 30° or 70° inclination

3.2.1.2 Fluid Management System

Fluid management system is important for the optimization of visualization and distension of working space. When application of tourniquet is not desirable or possible, achieving tamponade effect on bleeding with adequate fluid pressure is important. Consistent flow can constantly refresh the visualization medium. Automated peristaltic fluid pump systems with pressure and flow regulation (Fig. 3.4) can generate consistent flows with greater degree of joint distension. Real-time regulation of fluid flow can compensate for the rapid volume loss during the use of motorized instruments with suction. Whilst inadequate pressure and flow can limit visualization, high pressure can lead to inadvertent fluid extravasation. Apart from local complications, intra-abdominal fluid extravasation during hip arthroscopy or endoscopy can cause intra-abdominal compartment syndrome which is potentially life-threatening. The prevalence of symptomatic intra-abdominal fluid extravasation has been reported to be 0.16% in a multicentre study [2]. Intra-thoracic fluid extravasation after hip arthroscopy has also been reported [3]. Low-cost gravity flow systems were first described and are still commonly used. Although the flow rate is controlled by the flow resistance of the system, which is relatively fixed, desired pressure can be reliably achieved by elevating the fluid bag above the infusion site by specific distances. 1 m of elevation corresponds to approximately 70 mmHg of pressure. In a cadaveric study, gravity feed was proven to be accurate with minimal pressure overshoot and

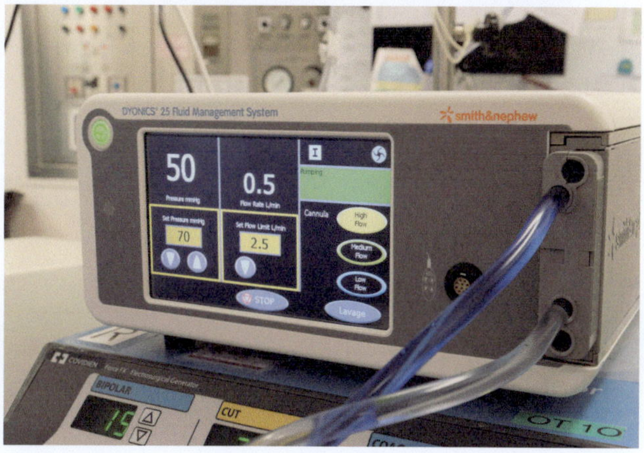

Fig. 3.4 Automated peristaltic fluid pump systems with pressure and flow regulation

lower intra-articular pressure ranges [4]. With the understanding of the different properties, the choice of irrigation system should be made based on the individual scenario.

3.2.1.3 Cannulas

Whilst most rigid scopes have accompanying cannulas, working portal access cannulas are optional depending on the portal location, depth, and application. They are often utilized for locations where maintenance of soft tissue tract is difficult. They can also assist suture management. Spigots are usually available for fluid delivery or drainage. Metallic reusable and plastic disposable cannulas are available on the market. Hard cannulas are pierce resistant but its rigidity may limit manoeuvrability. Soft cannulas are more flexible but they are not suitable for sharp-tipped instruments. Most disposable cannulas are held in place during procedure by threads or lips. Some soft cannulas have wide internal flanges to increase fall-out resistance and to assist internal soft tissue retraction. Open, or half-pipe, cannulas are commonly used for hip arthroscopic instruments exchange.

3.2.1.4 Hand Instruments

The probe is an important diagnostic instrument. It provides tactile feedback so that the consistency and continuity of deep structures can be better evaluated in addition to the visual information provided by the scope. Most probes have 90° bend at their ends which form hooks of 3–4 mm long with rounded blunt tips. The knowledge of the hook size can be used to estimate the size of lesions. The probe is also useful for suture manipulation and soft tissue handling. Cutting instruments comes in the form of cutting blades, straight scissors, hooked scissors, retrograde hooked knife, and punches of various attack angles (Fig. 3.5). Whilst straight cutting blades and scissors can precisely separate structures in tension, loose soft tissue often "escape" the cutting jaws. Hooked scissors and punches are more suitable for separation of loose tissue. With the development of motorized instruments and radiofrequency devices, the roles of many traditional cutting instruments are gradually being replaced. Antegrade and retrograde suture passing devices with various attack angles are available (Fig. 3.6). Caution should be taken when choosing instrument for suture handling. Whilst graspers are suitable for loose bodies retrieval, their sharp grasping teeth can inadvertently abrade suture fibres and jeopardize the security of tissue repair. Suture retrievers and probes should be used for the purpose.

3.2.1.5 Motorized Instruments

Motorized instruments deliver their action by either rotatory or reciprocating motion. The most commonly used motorized instrument is the shaver. Used in conjunction with controlled suction, the shaver can efficiently clear the path for visualization and excise pathological structures. The oscillating mode can prevent tissue tangling caused by unidirectional rotation. Burr with protection sleeve is suitable for endoscopic osseous excision and preparation. Reciprocating file can generate flat bony surfaces which are difficult to achieve with burr. With reciprocating saw, endoscopic osteotomy can be performed with minimal bone loss.

3.2.1.6 Radiofrequency Devices

Radiofrequency probes are electrical devices which employ high frequency alternating electrical current for heat genera-

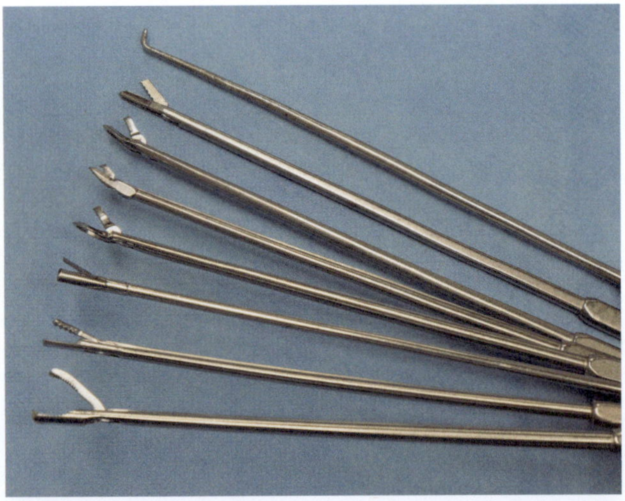

Fig. 3.5 Cutting instruments comes in the form of cutting blades, straight scissors, hooked scissors, retrograde hooked knife, and punches of various attack angles

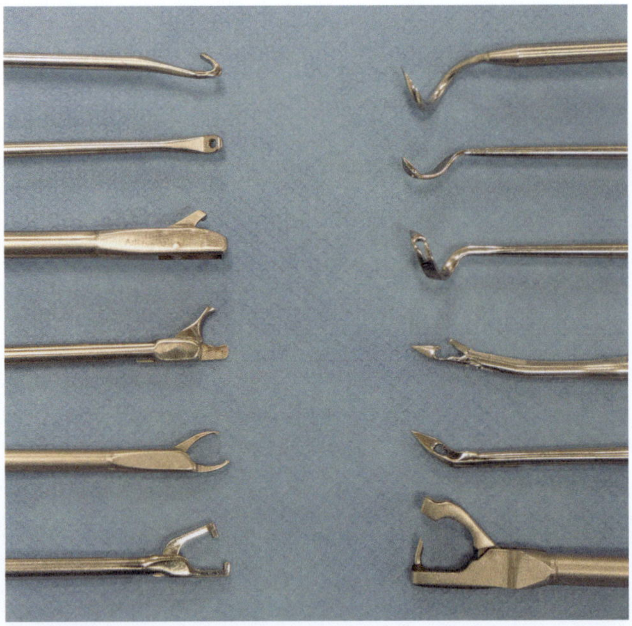

Fig. 3.6 Antegrade and retrograde suture passing devices with various attack angles

tion to achieve tissue coagulation or ablation. With conventional monopolar radiofrequency devices, the current oscillates between the active electrode and the patient return electrode. Heat is electrically induced close to the tip of the active electrode, where the current density is the highest. Instead of passing electrical current through tissue, modern radiofrequency instruments, such as Coblation-based devices (Fig. 3.7) use bipolar electrodes to generate a focused plasma layer which coagulate or ablate soft tissue at lower temperatures (25–35 °C) with lower thermal penetration and thus more targeted energy delivery [5]. Some systems have built-in suction pump with variable suction pressure for different energy delivery modes. Bipolar radiofrequency devices have been proven to be time and cost saving compared with monopolar devices.

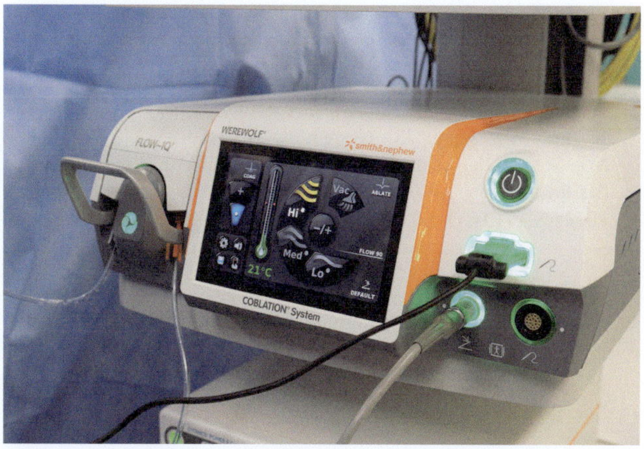

Fig. 3.7 Radiofrequency system

References

1. Papavasiliou AV, Bardakos NV. Complications of arthroscopic surgery of the hip. Bone Joint Res. 2012;1(7):131–44.
2. Kocher MS, Frank JS, Nasreddine AY, Safran MR, Philippon MJ, Sekiya JK, et al. Intra-abdominal fluid extravasation during hip arthroscopy: a survey of the MAHORN group. Arthroscopy. 2012;28(11):1654–60.e2.
3. Verma M, Sekiya JK. Intrathoracic fluid extravasation after hip arthroscopy. Arthroscopy. 2010;26(9 Suppl):S90–4.
4. Mayo M, Wolsky R, Baldini T, Vezeridis PS, Bravman JT. Gravity fluid flow more accurately reflects joint fluid pressure compared with commercial peristaltic pump systems in a cadaveric model. Arthroscopy. 2018;34(12):3132–8.
5. Anderson SR, Faucett SC, Flanigan DC, Gmabardella RA, Amin NH. The history of radiofrequency energy and Coblation in arthroscopy: a current concepts review of its application in chondroplasty of the knee. J Exp Orthop. 2019;6(1):1.

Part II

Hip

Endoscopy of Peritrochanteric Space for Greater Trochanteric Pain Syndrome (GTPS)

4

Tun Hing Lui, Chunbao Li, Xiangyu Tang, Lilei He, Kan Ouyang, Jian Xu, Xintao Zhang, Zuru Liang, and Yan Xu

Abstract

Snapping hip is a condition characterized by an audible and/or palpable snapping during hip movement and can be associated with pain around the hip. It can be classified into two types by various causes of this condition. The most common type is the external extra-articular, where the snapping is due to encumbered passage of the iliotibial band or gluteus maximus over the greater trochanter. This can be resulted from inflammatory thickening of iliotibial band, great trochanteric bursitis and degeneration, necrosis, and fibrosis of the gluteal muscles and fascia resulting in gluteal muscle contracture. Surgery is needed if conservative treatment is ineffective. Endoscopic iliotibial band release has the advantages of minimally invasive surgery. Under endoscopy, trochanteric bursectomy, release of the iliotibial band with or without release of the gluteus maximus insertion is performed. Special attention should be paid to the anatomical position of the sciatic nerve and superior gluteal nerve to prevent injury during operation. Besides external snapping hip, tendinopathy or tear of gluteus medius and minimus muscles can also present with lateral hip pain. Surgery is indicated if conservative treatment fails to relieve symptoms. The safety and efficacy of endoscopic repair of gluteal tendons is supported by the literature. In this chapter, the endoscopic techniques are outlined.

Keywords

External snapping hip · Iliotibial band · Endoscopic release · Radiofrequency · Gluteal muscle contracture Gluteus maximus · Trochanteric bursitis · Bursectomy Gluteus medius tears · Gluteal muscles · Hip abductors Hip arthroscopy · Greater Trochanteric pain syndrome

The corresponding author of section 4.1 is Chunbao Li, Email: lichunbao301@163.com
The corresponding author of section 4.2 is Lilei He, Email: helilei@fshtcm.com.cn
The corresponding author of section 4.3 is Kan Ouyang, Email: 2019310687@stu.gzhmu.edu.cn
The corresponding author of section 4.4 is Xintao Zhang, Email: zhangxintao@sina.com
The corresponding author of section 4.5 is Yan Xu, Email: yanxu@139.com

T. H. Lui (✉)
Department of Orthopaedics and Traumatology, North District Hospital, Hong Kong, China

The Second Affiliated Hospital, Shenzhen University, Shenzhen, China

C. Li
The PLA General Hospital, Beijing, China

X. Tang
The 985th Hospital of PLA Joint Logistic Support Force, Yingze, Taiyuan, China

L. He
Foshan Hospital Affiliated to Guangzhou University of Chinese Medicine, Guangzhou, Guangdong, China
e-mail: helilei@fshtcm.com.cn

K. Ouyang
The First Affiliated Hospital of Shenzhen University (Shenzhen Second People's Hospital), Shenzhen, Guangdong, China
e-mail: 2019310687@stu.gzhmu.edu.cn

J. Xu
The Fourth Affiliated Hospital of Guangxi Medical University, Guangxi, China

X. Zhang · Z. Liang
Peking University Shenzhen Hospital, Shenzhen, Guangdong Province, China

Y. Xu
Institute of Sports Medicine, Peking University Third Hospital, Beijing, China

© The Author(s), under exclusive license to Springer Nature Singapore Pte Ltd. 2021
T. H. Lui (ed.), *Endoscopy of the Hip and Knee*, https://doi.org/10.1007/978-981-16-3488-8_4

4.1 Endoscopic Iliotibial Band Release for External Snapping Hip

Chunbao Li and Xiangyu Tang

4.1.1 Introduction

- External snapping hip (ESH) is caused by an enlarged or tight posterior portion of the iliotibial band (IT band) and tight anterior border of the tendinous insertion of the gluteus maximus muscle. The mechanism of snapping is that IT band slides over and catches of the superior border of the greater trochanter of the femur as the flexion and extension of the hip during exercise or simply ordinary daily activities. Continuously presenting of external snapping always causes pain due to inflammatory thickening of IT band and great trochanteric bursitis [1–4].
- ESH can be occurred separately, or combined with gluteal muscle contracture and femoroacetabular impingement (FAI). Patients with both FAI and ESH will get optimistic outcome if underwent hip arthroscopy combined with IT band release in primary surgery [5, 6].
- Conservative treatment of ESH, including anti-inflammatory drugs, stretching, and avoidance of inciting activities, usually could successfully make patients get pain relief but has poor effect on conquering hip snapping. Therefore, for the refractory patients who do not respond well to the nonsurgical treatments, surgical intervention such as open or endoscopic IT band release is an excellent alternative [7, 8].
- Yujie Liu et al. firstly reported their research work about arthroscopic release for ESH in 2003 in Chinese and 2009 in English [9, 10]. It had obvious advantages over traditional open surgery and had been widely accepted as one of the main minimally invasive treatment methods, which will be introduced in this chapter

4.1.2 Indications

- External snapping hip with or without greater trochanteric bursitis
- External snapping hip combined with femoroacetabular impingement
- External snapping hip combined with IT band contracture

4.1.3 Contra-Indications

- Infection
- Severe external snapping hip
- Hip deformities: developmental dysplasia of the hip, ankylosis of the hip
- Abduction weakness of hip

4.1.4 Author's Preferred Technique

4.1.4.1 Pre-operative Planning

- Careful pre-operative planning is required to ensure surgical quality and safety, which includes the material preparation, portals location, and patient positioning.
- Required instruments: 4 mm, 30° arthroscope, lightweight camera, joint shaver system, probes, injector needle, periosteal strippers, and an arthroscopic radiofrequency system.
- Before surgery, outline the greater trochanter, anterior and posterior borders of the contracted gluteal muscle, portals, and the sciatic nerve.

4.1.4.2 Patient and Medical Team Positioning

- Lateral position is selected for the patients. Before surgery, the most tense posture of affected IT band of lower limb is founded by performing Ober's test, then keep this posture, which is usually at appropriate flexion, slight adduction, and internal rotation of hip.
- To make the operational procedure smooth, the surgeon could select the most convenient side which could be at the anterior or posterior side of the patient. The first assistant is positioned at the opposite side and is responsible for keeping the position of the operated lower limb (Fig. 4.1).

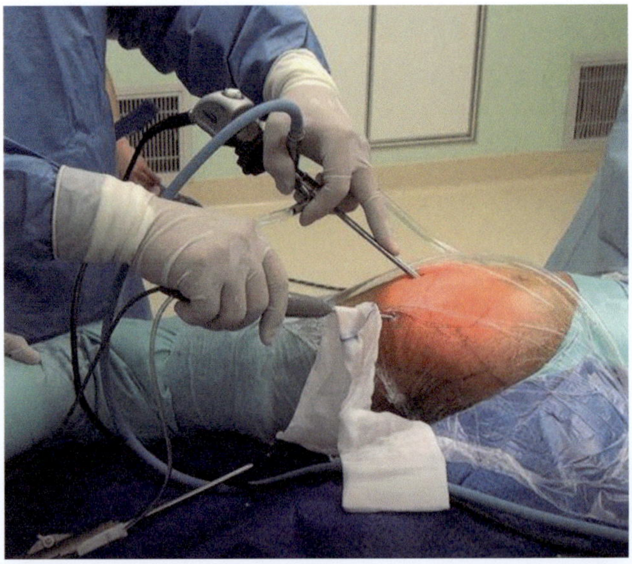

Fig. 4.1 Positioning of the patient and surgeon for the endoscopy of external snapping hip

- The arthroscope is connected with a video screen and all the other electronic equipment and arthroscopic accessories are positioned in front of the surgeon. An extra video screen is installed to help the first assistant following the arthroscopic procedure for his/her appropriate understanding and assistance of the surgical procedure.
- Surgery can be performed under epidural anesthesia and sedation.

4.1.4.3 Portal Design

- Two arthroscopic portals are used to access the IT band (anterior and posterior portals). Both of these portals are placed at 5–6 cm distal of the greater trochanter. The distance of the two portals is about 1–7 cm (Fig. 4.2).
- Care must be taken when preparing the posterior portal because the sciatic nerve runs the dorsal of the portal. Thus, the course of sciatic nerve should be marked on the skin to remind the surgeon.

4.1.4.4 Step-by-Step Description of the Technique

- Saline is locally injected to the surface of IT band (Fig. 4.3).
- Then a 5 × 5 cm operation zone is created above the surface of IT band (in the technique, surgeons developed and enlarged a potential space between the IT band and the subcutaneous fat using blunt dissection via the portal site).

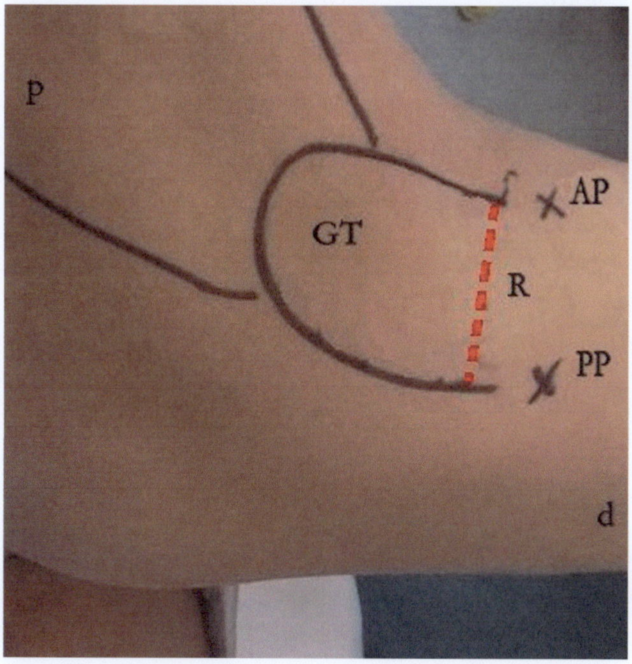

Fig. 4.2 Two arthroscopic portals are used to access the IT band. *AP* anterior portal, *PP* posterior portal, *R* pathway of release, *GT* greater trochanter; *p* proximal, *d* distal

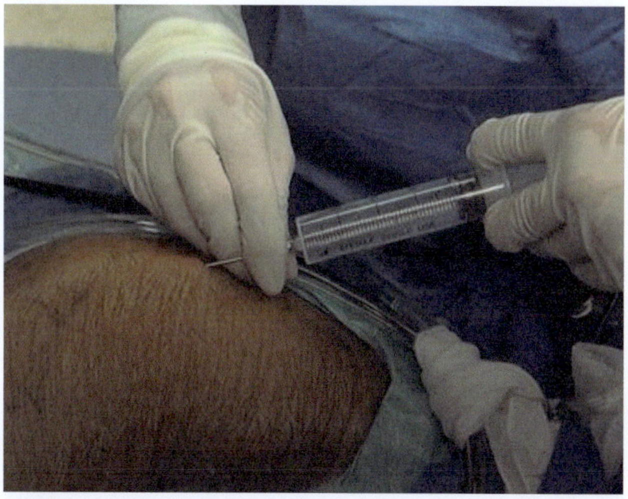

Fig. 4.3 Saline is locally injected to create an operation space for endoscopy

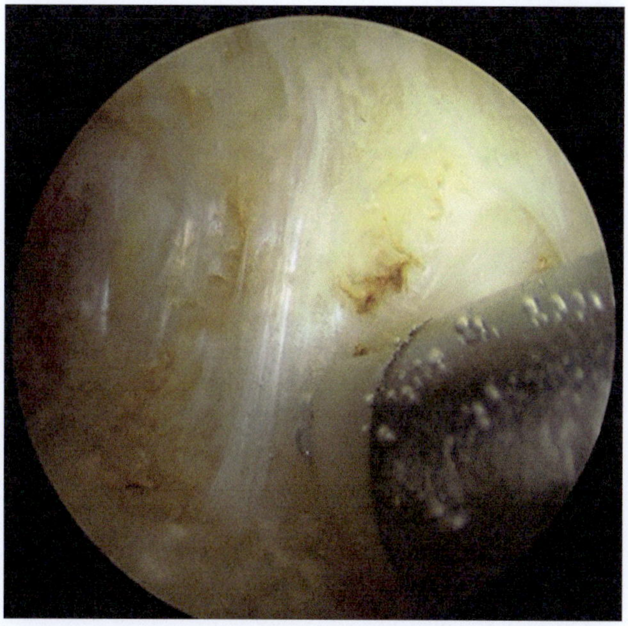

Fig. 4.4 The IT band is transversely released from superficial to deep

- Then insert the arthroscope to the operation space, fat and fibrous tissues are cleared by shaver and electrocautery device over the surface of the IT band.
- Arthroscopic evaluation of the IT band is performed through the two portals, and the anterior and posterior borders of the IT band are confirmed.
- The IT band is then transversely released from superficial to deep at the level 5–7 cm distal to the proximal end of greater trochanter (Fig. 4.4).
- For patients with gluteal muscle contracture, the contracted tissue connecting to the posterior border of the IT band should be released.

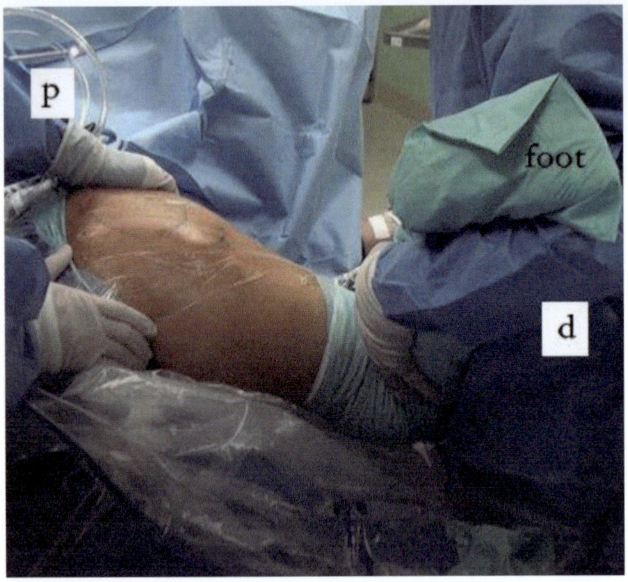

Fig. 4.5 After release, passive gentle flexion, adduction, internal rotation and abduction of hip is performed until there is no movement restriction. *p* proximal, *d* distal

- For the patients with severe bursitis, the inflammatory tissue around the greater trochanter is debrided with radiofrequency blade after the IT band is transversal released.
- After release, the hip joint is moved in different directions until the hip joint gets full ROM without snapping and has a negative Ober's sign (Fig. 4.5).
- During the endoscopic procedure, meticulous hemostasis will be very important as the inflammatory tissue is likely to bleed and influent the view.
- Special attention should be paid to the anatomical position of the sciatic nerve and superior gluteal nerve to prevent injury during operation.
- If the patient has bilateral symptoms, the IT band of contralateral limb will be released in the same way after turning over the patient.
- For FAI patients, the procedure is performed in supine position. The IT band will be released after the procedure for treatment of FAI.

4.1.4.5 Complications and Management

- Sciatic nerve impairment
- Subcutaneous hematoma
- Infection
- Hemorrhage

4.1.4.6 Postoperative Care

- Postoperative analgesia and treatment for preventing myositis ossificans are given.
- The day after operation, functional exercise is employed, including: squatting while closing knees together, hip abduction, and crossing leg after the recovery of anesthesia.

4.1.4.7 Outcomes

- Endoscopic IT band release for external snapping hip is a safe and reproducible technique. The snapping phenomenon can disappear with no muscle weakness in nearly all of the patients [11–14].
- Pain VAS score and Harris Hip Score will reflect a statistically significant improvement in patient's satisfaction after operation.
- About 40% of patients complain of very light pain after strenuous sporting activities [11–14].

4.1.5 Summary

- Endoscopic release of IT band is an effective method for ESH.
- Endoscopic IT band release is a quite simple and safe method, but regional anatomy knowledge is crucial for avoiding complication and improving outcomes.
- Greater trochanteric bursitis, gluteal muscle contracture, femoroacetabular impingement may co-exist, which can be managed at the same times to insure the clinical outcomes.

4.2 Endoscopic Iliotibial Band Release for External Snapping Hip: Two Posterior Portals Approach

Lilei He

4.2.1 Introduction

- With the increasing sport population, the number of patients with external snapping hip (ESH) has also increased. Owing to the distinct anatomical location of the lesion and often visible snapping, ESH is usually easily diagnosed without turning to imaging modalities [15–17].
- An external snapping hip (ESH) is characterized by encumbered passage of the iliotibial band (ITB) or gluteus maximus (GM) over the greater trochanter (GT), typically at some angle of flexion of the hip [18, 19].
- ESH is not always successfully treated with conservative management, and the clinical course is not the same in all cases [20].
- There are several operative techniques that may be considered for external snapping hip refractory to non-operative management. Some of these techniques involve an open lengthening or release of the ITB while others make use of endoscopic lengthening. While each has their own advantages and disadvantages, they have been reported to have positive outcomes in the short-term in small case series [16, 21–23].
- Recently, endoscopic technique to release the ITB in patients with ESH is introduced with excellent contracture release and fast recovery [24].

4.2.2 Indications

- The indication for this endoscopic technique is a painful external snapping hip not relieved by at least 3 months of non-operative treatment (physical therapy and local corticosteroid bursal injection).

4.2.3 Contra-Indications

- Patients with systemic or local infectious diseases;
- Patients with severe hypertension, heart disease, diabetes, and other diseases;
- Patients cannot tolerate anesthesia and surgery.

4.2.4 Author Preferred Technique

4.2.4.1 Pre-operative Planning

- The pre-operative evaluation includes physical examination and AP pelvis radiographs.
- The snap is identified by palpation of the trochanteric region with flexion-extension of the hip.

4.2.4.2 Patient Positioning

- The patient is placed in the lateral decubitus position on a standard operating table.
- The leg is draped so that a full range of motion of the hip can be achieved during the surgery (Fig. 4.6).

4.2.4.3 Portal Design

- With the surgical site prepared, the GT is outlined and two portal sites are marked on the skin: the posterosuperior trochanteric portal (PSTP) is placed at the 2 cm

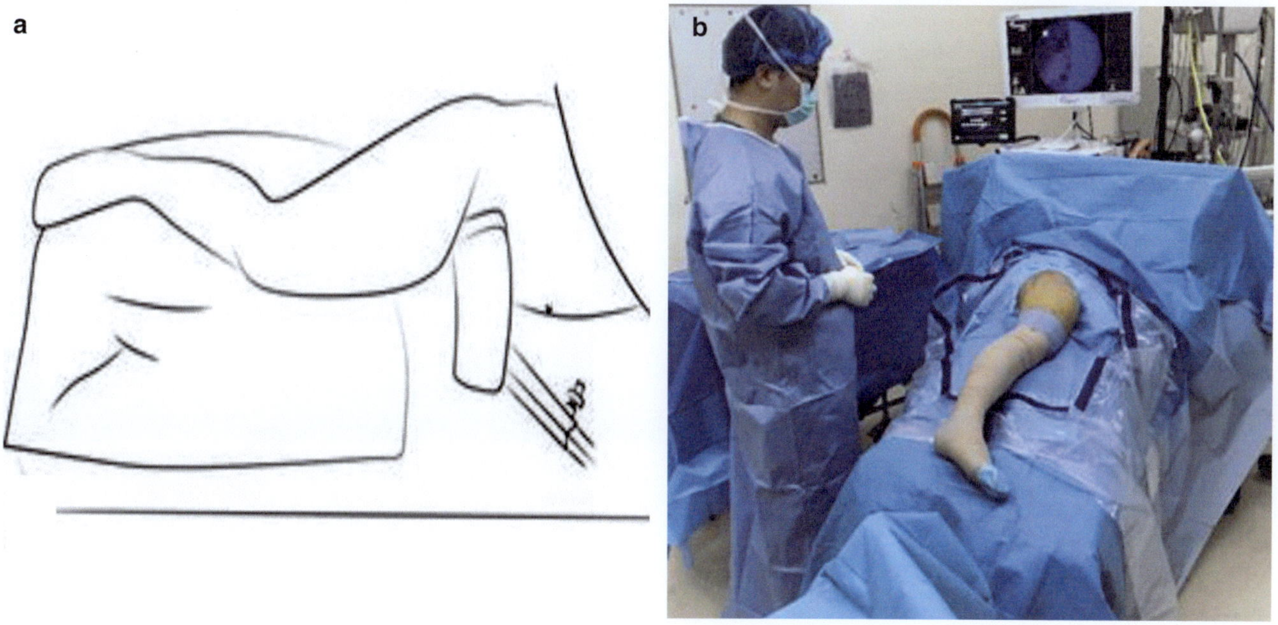

Fig. 4.6 Positioning of the patient, equipment for the arthroscopy of the external snapping hip

behind the intersection of the anteroposterior line at the tip of the GT and the line along the posterior edge of the femur and the posteroinferior trochanteric portal (PITP) is placed approximately 10 cm below the posterosuperior trochanteric portal (Fig. 4.7).

- For portals, oblique incision of 5 mm in size is made on the skin and subcutaneous tissue.

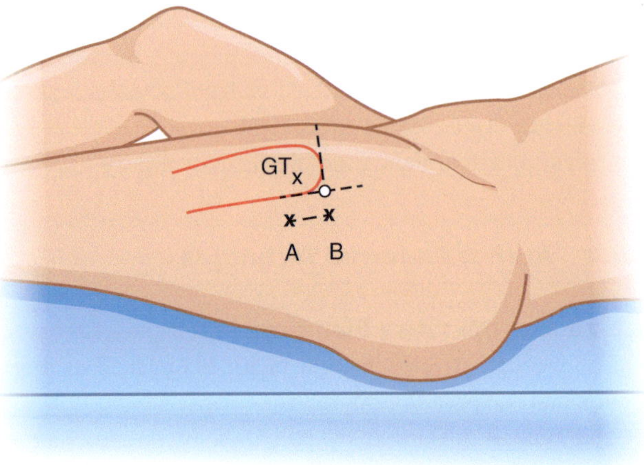

Fig. 4.7 Arthroscopic portals. (**a**) posteroinferior trochanteric portal (PITP). (**b**) posterosuperior trochanteric portal (PSTP)

4.2.4.4 Step-by-Step Description of the Technique

- The posteroinferior trochanteric portal (PITP) is created first. This follows by inserting a hand stripper directly over the prominence of the GT to develop a space between the subcutaneous tissue and the ITB (Fig. 4.8).
- The arthroscopic cannula with the blunt obturator is introduced, directed toward the tip of the GT, positioned above the ITB.
- The 30° 4-mm arthroscope is then introduced and fluid inflow with an arthro-pump at low pressure (80 mmHg) is started to develop a space between the subcutaneous tissue and the ITB.
- A needle is introduced at the site of the posterosuperior trochanteric portal (PSTP) and located under direct endoscopic vision. The skin incision is then made and a shaver blade is introduced through the portal to the ITB. The fat and fibrous tissues in the operating space are cleaned and

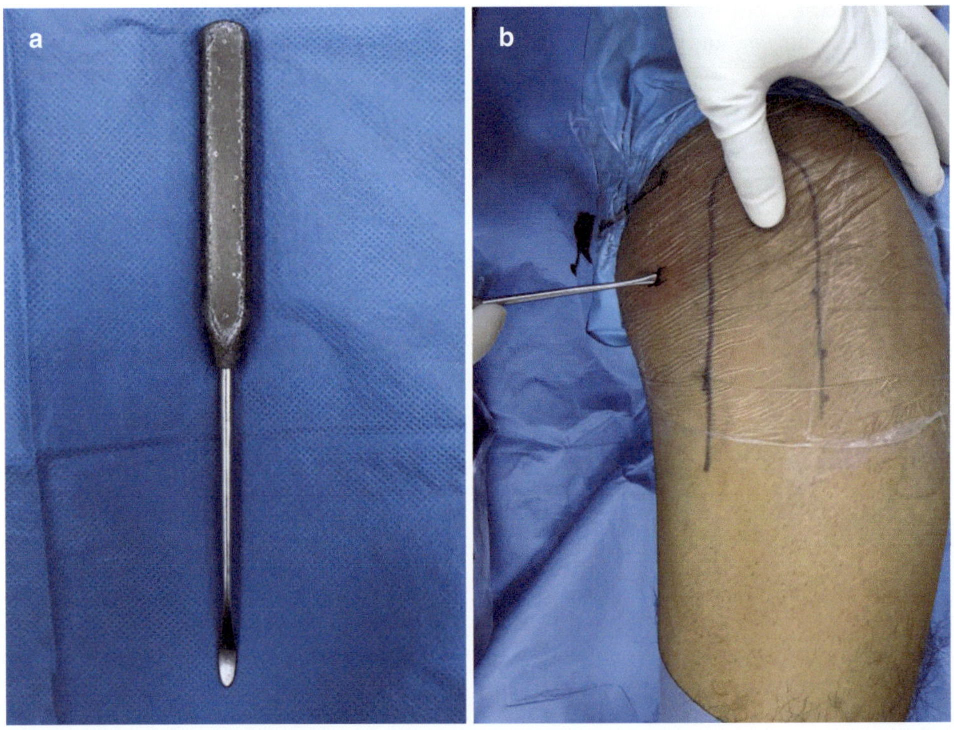

Fig. 4.8 Insert a hand stripper directly over the prominence of the GT to develop a space between the subcutaneous tissue and the ITB

the space superficial to the ITB is further developed with the shaver (Fig. 4.9).

- The shaver is removed and radiofrequency device is inserted through the posterosuperior trochanteric portal (PSTP). ITB is cut from anterior to posterior (Fig. 4.10) to release the contracture tissues until the ITB is cut completely (Fig. 4.11). The space between the severed ends of ITB can also be seen in the postoperative magnetic resonance imaging (MRI) (Fig. 4.12).
- After the contractures are removed, the leg is slowly moved through a full range of motion (ROM) of the hip to confirm no clicking sound.
- In presence of any bleeding point, cautery can be used. Once the surgeon is satisfied, fluid is aspirated and the skin is sutured to close the portals.

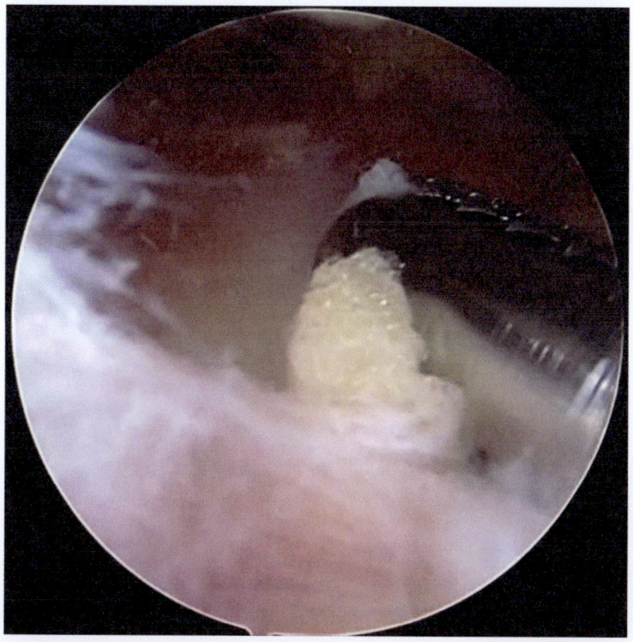

Fig. 4.9 The fat and fibrous tissues are cleaned in the operating space by a shaver

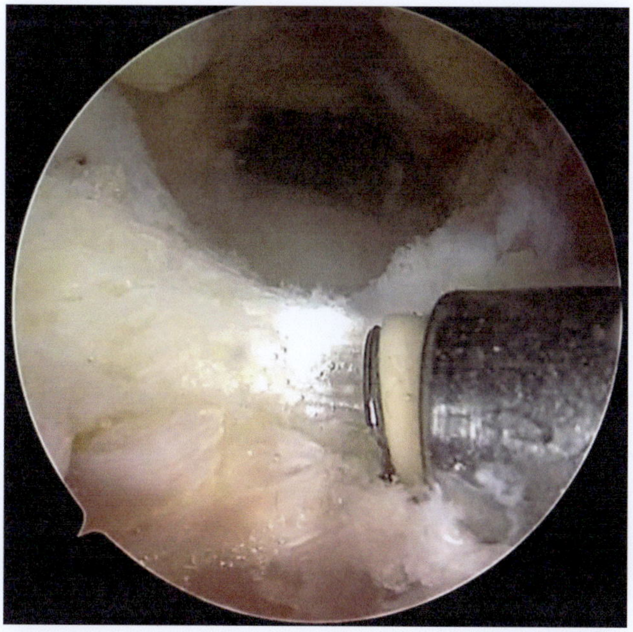

Fig. 4.10 The radiofrequency device is inserted through the posterosuperior trochanteric portal (PSTP). The ITB is initially partially cut from anterior to posterior

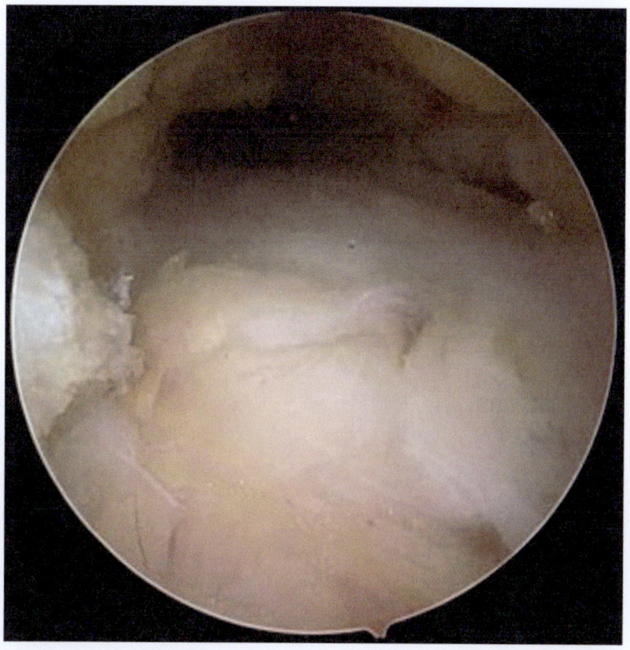

Fig. 4.11 The ITB is cut completely

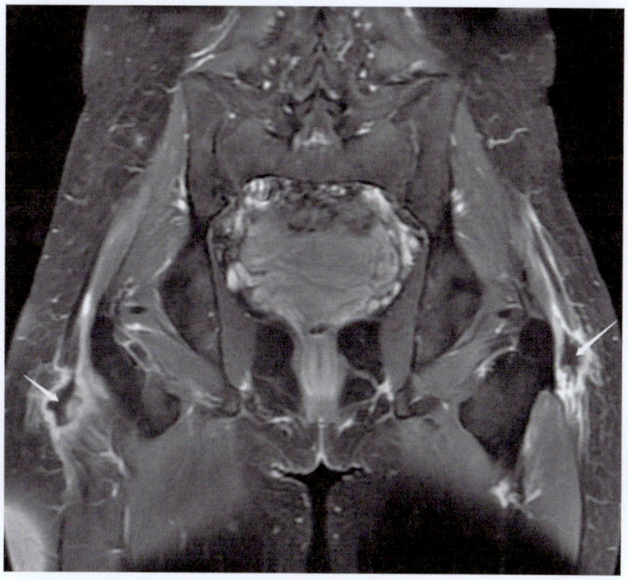

Fig. 4.12 The postoperative magnetic resonance imaging (MRI). The space between the severed ends of ITB (arrow)

4.2.4.5 Complications

- The sciatic nerve lesion during the operation.
- Postoperative hematoma formation.

4.2.4.6 Postoperative Care

- Rehabilitation exercises are begun on the first postoperative day and continued for 3 months.
- Straight line movement, squat with the knees together, sit with legs crossed, and hip abduction exercises.
- These exercises are performed 3–5 times a day with 20–30 repetitions depending on the patient's endurance.

4.2.5 Summary

- Arthroscopic surgery could be an effective procedure for ESH, due to less operating time, small scar, fast postoperative recovery, and complete contracture release.

4.3 Endoscopic Gluteus Maximus Tendon Release for External Snapping Hip

Kan Ouyang and Jian Xu

4.3.1 Introduction

- Gluteal muscle contracture (GMC) is a clinical syndrome due to multiple etiologies in which hip movements may be severely limited. It is characterized by degeneration, necrosis, and fibrosis of the gluteal muscles and fascia [2, 25–29]. It is caused by either congenital or acquired factors, usually associated with repeated intramuscular injection into the gluteal region during childhood. GMC is not uncommon and exists worldwide, involving the United States, France, Italy, Poland, Australia, Spain, China, and India [30]. It is more prevalent in Asian than Caucasian patients. An incidence of 1–2.5% in childhood has been reported. The onset of GMC is usually bilateral, and boys have a higher incidence rate than girls [31]. Patients with GMC typically present with hip abduction and external rotation when crouching. The knees cannot be brought together and are separated in a frog-leg position. Clinical examination is good enough for the diagnosis. MRI may furthermore confirm the diagnosis by manifesting an intramuscular fibrotic cord extending to the thickened distal tendon with atrophy of the gluteus maximus muscle and posteromedial displacement of the iliotibial tract.
- GMC is associated with increased tension of the ITB and GM over the GT. Complete GMC release with open technique has been proven to be an effective way while conservative treatment is not helpful. Open surgery provides clear exposure and easy access to the area but leaves undesirable postoperative scars on the incision. Arthroscopic GMC release is associated with significantly smaller incisions, less postoperative pain, and fewer complications to open technique [27, 31, 32].

4.3.2 Indications

- Patients categorized level II or above should be treated operatively according to Zhao et al. [28] (Table 4.1).
- Patients can be treated by surgery if non-operative treatment does not help.

Table 4.1 Classification of gluteal muscle contracture

Category according to level	
Level I (mild)	The extorsion of lower limb is mild, the abduction contracture is less than 15° with both hip and knee joint in 90° of flexion or adduction range is less than 20° with no flexion. Ober's sign and frog squatting sign are weakly positive. The limp gait is not apparent with lateral inclination of pelvis on anteroposterior radiograph being less than 10°
Level II (moderate)	The extorsion of lower limb is moderate, the abduction contracture ranges from 15° to 60° with both hip and knee joint in 90° of flexion or adduction range is less than 10° with no flexion. Ober's sign and frog squatting sign are positive. The limp gait is apparent with lateral inclination of pelvis on anteroposterior radiograph being less than 20°
Level III (severe)	The extorsion of lower limb is severe, the abduction contracture is more than 60° with both hip and knee joint in 90° of flexion or adduction range is less than 0° with no flexion. Ober's sign and frog squatting sign are strongly positive. The limp gait is remarkably apparent with lateral inclination of pelvis on anteroposterior radiograph being more than 20°

4.3.3 Contra-Indications

- Infection
- Neurological disorders affecting lower limbs
- Hip dysplasia

4.3.4 Author's Preferred Technique

4.3.4.1 Pre-operative Planning

In general, arthroscopic procedures for GMC require safety for sciatic nerve. The outline of sciatic nerve and greater trochanter should be marked in case of nerve injury. The arthroscopy planning starts with the proper material selection, adequate portals and patient positioning, and medical indication.

Required instruments: 4.0 mm, 30° arthroscope, lightweight camera, joint shaver system with full-radius blades, surgical instrument set, such as probes, baskets, graspers, and an arthroscopic radiofrequency system.

4.3.4.2 Patient and Medical Team Positioning

The patient is positioned in a lateral position while under general anesthesia or spinal anesthesia. Always patients have both hips affected, we can operate on one side first following by the other side by turning and repositioning the patient.

4.3.4.3 Portal Design

The greater trochanter, anterior and posterior borders of the contracted gluteal muscle, and the sciatic nerve are outlined. A two- or three-portal technique is used to perform the operation, namely the inferior, anterosuperior (AS), and posterosuperior (PS) portals (Fig. 4.13). With the hip in neutral position, we place the inferior portal, which is used for introduction of the arthroscope, 3 cm directly inferior to the greater trochanter. The AS and PS portals, which are used as the drainage or the working portals for instruments, such as motorized shavers or the radiofrequency device, are placed superior to the greater trochanter. The AS portal is placed anterior to the anterior border of the contracted gluteal muscle, whereas the PS portal is placed posterior to the posterior border of the contracted gluteal muscle. When the surgeon faces the patient's back, the PS portal is used as the working portal and the AS portal is used as outflow portal. When the surgeon faces the patient's abdomen, the AS portal is used as working portal and the PS portal is used as outflow portal. By these ways, the surgeon can complete the operations for both hips just by repositioning of the patient without the need to change the positions of the surgeon and the monitor.

4.3.4.4 Step-by-Step Description of the Technique

During arthroscopic-assisted release, the potential space between the gluteal muscle group and the subcutaneous fat is enlarged using blunt dissection with a periosteal elevator. Continuous inflow of normal saline (containing 1 mg adrenaline per 3000 mL normal saline) into this potential space creates a good working space and the adrenaline will reduce bleeding during the procedure. The three-step technique is used to release the superficial contracture tissues and the deeper tissues. The contracture tissues, which appear silvery and silk-like under the arthroscope, are cut off and vaporized with radiofrequency (Figs. 4.14 and 4.15). The first step involves releasing the thickened fascia and scarring contracture bands of the tensor fasciae latae muscle with radiofrequency. The extent of release is started from the

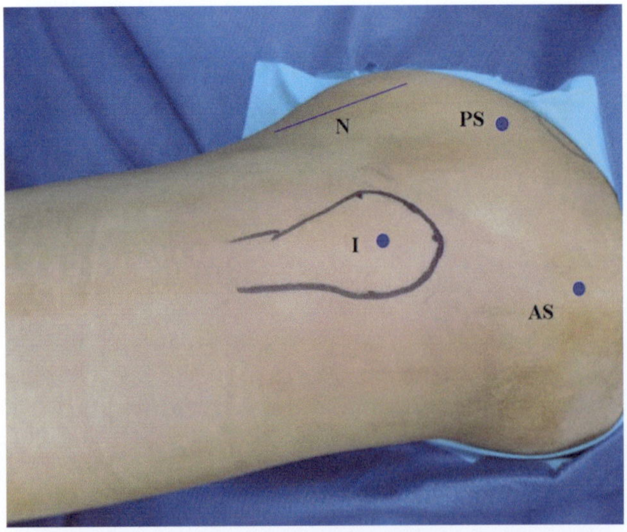

Fig. 4.13 The photograph shows the important anatomic landmarks on the patient during surgery. *AS* anterosuperior portal, *PS* posterosuperior portal, *I* inferior portal, *N* sciatic nerve

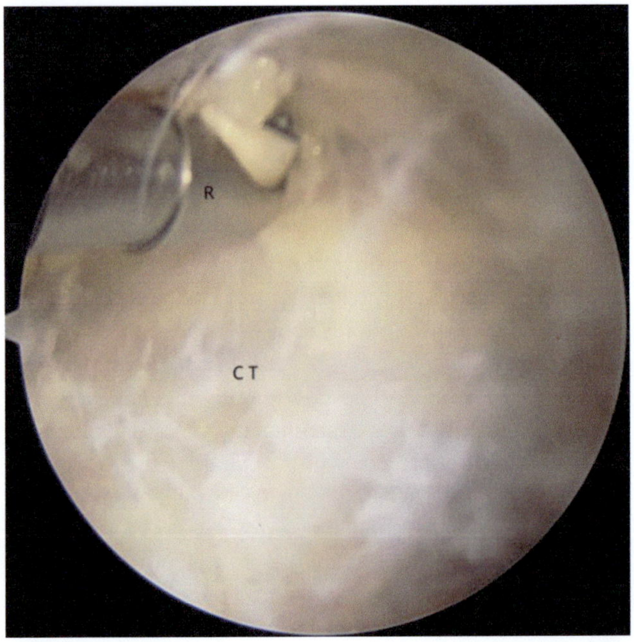

Fig. 4.14 The photograph shows the contracture tissues. *CT* contracture tissues, *R* radiofrequency

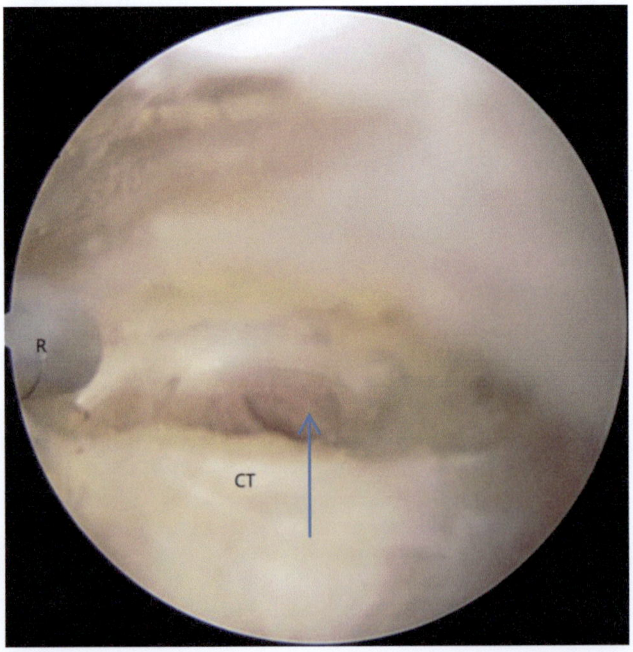

Fig. 4.15 The photograph shows the partial released contracture tissues (at the arrow). *CT* contracture tissues, *R* radiofrequency

ASIS and continues toward the greater trochanter. The second step is started from the anterior edge of gluteus maximus and continued to the linea aspera, distally along the femur. Finally, in the third step, the gluteus medius and gluteus minimus are released. In some severe cases, the external rotator muscles and posterior hip joint capsule are also released. Good hemostasis is maintained throughout surgery to allow clear observation of the surgical site during the entire procedure and to prevent hematoma formation after the operation. This is achieved by coagulation of any bleeding point using radiofrequency energy, increasing the pressure of saline inflow, and adding adrenaline to the saline solution.

4.3.4.5 Complications and Management

- Postoperative hematoma
- Wound complications
- Inadequate release
- Gluteal muscle weakness
- Sciatic nerve damage

4.3.4.6 Postoperative Care

After surgery, the patients are asked to lie in a lateral position to compress one side with their own body weight and a 2-kg ice bag is placed on the other side. The position is switched every 1 or 2 h to ensure good hemostasis. The exudation of fluid from the wound is observed during the first 24 h and thus wound dressings are changed at regular intervals. Functional exercises are started 24 h after surgery, including (1) crouching with both knees close to each other, (2) abducting and adducting the lower limbs while lying in a lateral position, and (3) lying on the back, bringing the knees to the chest, clasping the hands to the front of the shin, and internally rotating the hips while keeping the pelvis as flat as possible. These exercises are performed to prevent scar formation and muscle atrophy.

4.3.4.7 Outcomes

Currently, arthroscopic release is the gold standard for the treatment of GMC. Arthroscopy provides a clear field of view in which the contracture band is well exposed and could be easily released with a hook knife cut and radiofrequency coblation, without extensive muscle dissection [33, 34]. Meanwhile, complete hemostasis is achieved by radiofrequency coblation, reducing the risk of postoperative bleeding and hematoma. Patients are reported to get significantly improved outcome following arthroscopic GMC release [30, 33, 34].

4.3.5 Summary

The arthroscopic GMC release is quite safe and effective; the only caution required is safety for sciatic nerve. Adequate release should be considered involving tensor fasciae latae muscle, gluteus maximus, gluteus medius, and gluteus minimus. Complete hemostasis is needed to avoid complications.

4.4 Endoscopic Management of Recalcitrant Trochanteric Bursitis

Xintao Zhang and Zuru Liang

4.4.1 Introduction

- Trochanteric bursitis (TB) is a common orthopedic condition characterized by chronic lateral hip pain (exacerbated by active abduction, passive adduction, and direct palpation) [35, 36].
- The causes of trochanteric bursitis include microtrauma, traction leading to impaired vascularity, and impingement or spasm/contracture of the overlying iliotibial band [37].
- Most patients with TB are successfully treated with non-operative managements that include activity modification, weight loss, non-steroidal anti-inflammatory medications, physical therapy, and corticosteroid injection [38–41].
- Surgical intervention with open or endoscopic techniques may be necessary in recalcitrant trochanteric bursitis (RTB) that do not respond to non-operative treatment [39, 42].
- Endoscopic minimally invasive procedures have been described for the treatment of RTB: isolated bursectomy, and/or ITB release and resulted in good patient outcomes [37, 38, 43–50].
- But high-level evidence based research is lacking like using control groups or compared to open surgery [39]. (The studies are poor in terms of evidence level hierarchy.) The added value of endoscopic treatment of RTB is needed to be further studied.

4.4.2 Indications

- Patients present with positive findings in Ober test, Patrick-FABER test, and tenderness to palpation over the greater trochanter and have correlating MRI findings of inflammation in the anatomic location of the trochanteric bursa.
- Patients diagnosed with TB have continued bursal pain and limitation of function of the hip joint, and failed at least 6 months of non-operative management, including corticosteroid injection.

4.4.3 Contra-indications

- Patients diagnosed with other hip pathology causing lateral hip pain, including hip joint osteoarthritis, synovitis, labral tears, femoroacetabular impingement, or referred pain from the lumbar spine.
- Infectious bursitis.

4.4.4 Author Preferred Technique

4.4.4.1 Pre-operative Planning

- The Harris Hip Score (HSS) and Visual Analogue Scale (VAS) of every patient are collected.
- In general, endoscopic management for RTB starts with the proper instrument selection, adequate portals and patient positioning, and medical indication.
- Required instruments: 4 mm, 30° arthroscope, light-weight camera, shaver, surgical instrument set, such as probes, baskets, and graspers, and an arthroscopic radiofrequency system. (General/local anesthesia.)

4.4.4.2 Patient and Medical Team Positioning

- The patient is placed in the lateral decubitus position stabilized with beanbags, with the operative leg draped free to allow an assistant to abduct the leg to release the tension on the ITB and soft tissues.
- To standardize endoscopic orientation, the ideal position for the surgeon is at the back of the patient, facing the buttocks aspect. The first assistant is positioned on the oppo-

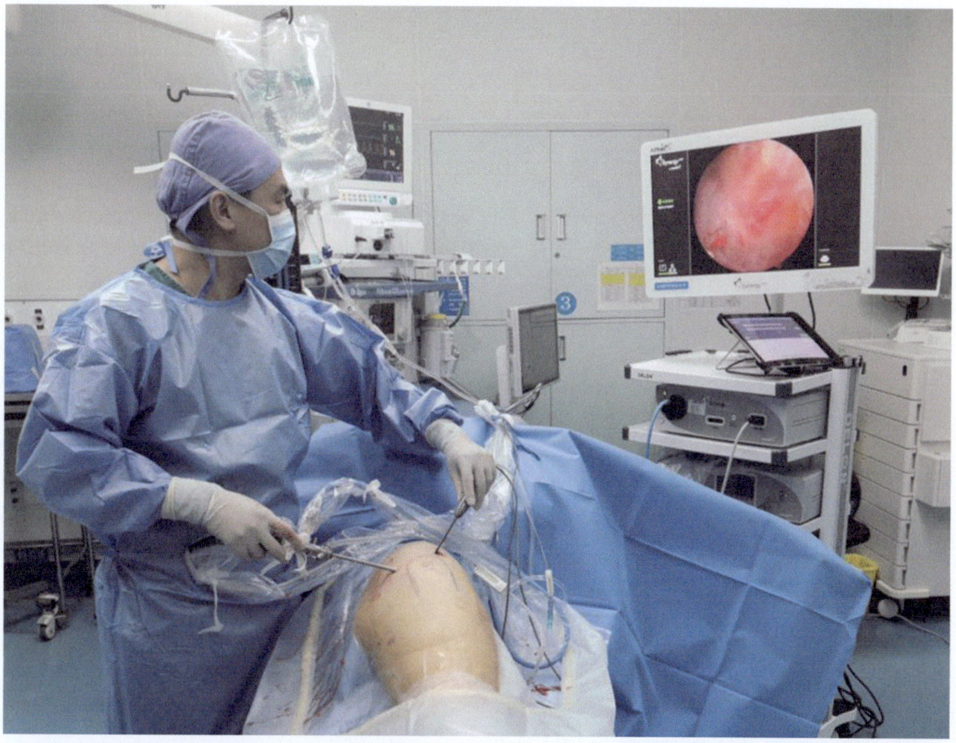

Fig. 4.16 The surgeon is at the back of the patient, facing the buttocks aspect. The first assistant is positioned on the opposite side of the surgeon

site side of the surgeon and is responsible for stabilizing the pelvis if necessary (Fig. 4.16).

- The arthroscopic rack with a video screen and all the other electronic equipment and arthroscopic accessories are positioned at the opposite side of the surgeon.
- Surgery can be performed under general/spinal/local anesthesia.

4.4.4.3 Portal design

- The greater trochanter (GT) is marked on the skin. Two portals are created just right over the top of the GT: The viewing portal is created parallel to the rear edge of the GT, and the working portal is marked parallel to the front edge of the GT (Fig. 4.17). The inter-

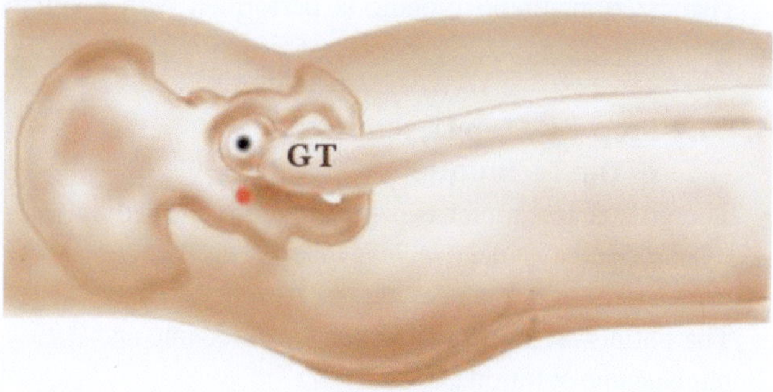

Fig. 4.17 Illustration of a right hip in the supine position demonstrating an outline of skin incision for direct lateral approach (red dotted line). The skin incision is located over the center of the greater trochanter (black dotted line). The interval of two skin incisions is approximately 5–8 cm

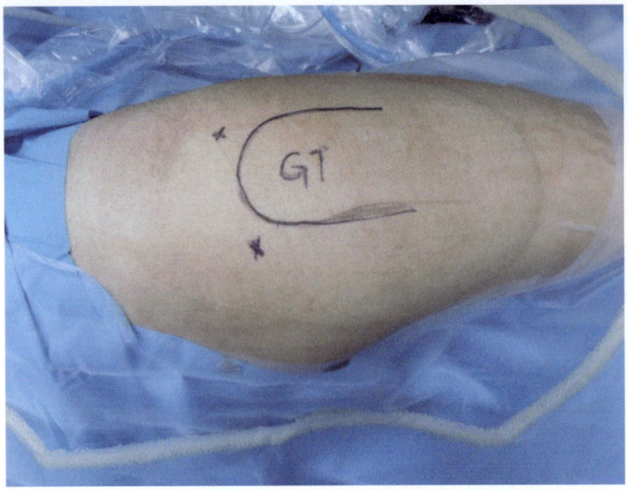

Fig. 4.18 The patient is placed in the lateral decubitus position. The GT is marked on the skin. Two portals are created just right over the top of the GT (cross symbol). The interval of two skin incisions is approximately 5–8 cm

val of two incisions is approximately 5–8 cm (Fig. 4.18).

- By convention, the posterior portal is placed first. The anterior portal is then placed under direct arthroscopic visualization. Prepositioning is performed with a spinal needle.

4.4.4.4 Step-by-Step Description of the Technique

- The greater trochanter is palpated and identified by fluoroscopy, and a spinal needle is inserted until it touches the trochanteric prominence.
- The portals are infiltrated with a 1% lidocaine and 0.25% bupivacaine solution.
- After the needle is withdrawn by 2 or 3 mm, approximately 40 mL of saline solution is injected into the bursa. The spinal needle is left in place for localization purposes.
- A 30°4 mm arthroscope is utilized with fluid irrigation using an epinephrine—saline mixture to facilitate access into this potential space and improve hemostasis.
- The subcutaneous fascia and soft tissues overlying the ITB over the trochanter are debrided by a shaver and/or an arthroscopic radiofrequency probe.
- Once the ITB is well visualized, a 3–4 cm longitudinal ITB incision is performed using the shaver and probe, releasing the ITB and allowing access to the trochanteric bursa. It should be confirmed by hip rotation under endoscopic visualization that there is no longer rubs on the ITB, causing impingement over the greater trochanter.
- Splitting the fibers exposes the bursa. Then an extensive greater trochanteric bursectomy is performed by use of the arthroscopic shaver and radiofrequency probe, exposing the greater trochanter and the gluteus medius. Rotate the leg internally to help fully visualize the bursa space. Coagulation by the radiofrequency probe is used to minimize bleeding and to assist with visualization. Care must be taken with extreme internal rotation to avoid extensively debriding the posterior tissues, placing the sciatic nerve at risk. Rotate the hip internally and externally to verify that the bursectomy is complete and that all adhesions are removed.
- After the bursectomy is completed, excessive fluid is expressed from the portals. And the operative site is injected with 80 mg of methylprednisolone and 20 mL of 0.25% bupivacaine.
- Methylprednisolone acetate (1 mL, 40 mg) and bupivacaine (10 mL) are injected into the area of the resection with an 18-gauge spinal needle. The wounds are dressed, and a compression dressing is applied.

4.4.4.5 Complications and Management

- Minor complications included ecchymosis in the lateral thigh, hematomas, and recurrence.

4.4.4.6 Postoperative Care

- During the postoperative period, local ice therapy is applied for 24 h. And the patient is allowed progressive weight bearing as tolerated with gentle passive and active range of motion for 2 weeks, followed by progression to full activity by 4–6 weeks.

4.4.5 Summary

- Most of the cases of TB will improve with appropriate non-operative measures, but some patients may develop RTB. Studies have shown that endoscopic ITB release and trochanteric bursectomy is a safe and effective treatment that can improve pain and function in patients with RTB.

4.5 Endoscopic Management of Gluteus Medius/Minimus Tendinopathy or Tear

Yan Xu

4.5.1 Introduction

- Greater trochanteric pain syndrome (GTPS) features lateral-sided hip pain and includes a heterogeneous group of conditions, including trochanteric bursitis, external coxa saltans, and gluteus medius and minimus tendinopathy or tear. Present in more than half of GTPS cases, gluteus medius and minimus tendon pathologies are the most common cause of lateral-sided hip pain, ranging from tendinosis to full-thickness tendon tear [51–53].
- Gluteus medius and minimus tearing is mostly chronic and degenerative in nature. It typically affects females between the fourth and sixth decades of life [51–53]. The prevalence of gluteus medius and minimus tendinopathy or tear increases with age and can reach as high as 80% after the age of 70 [54].
- Gluteal tendon tears were incidental findings during surgical procedures and were first described by Bunker et al. and Kagan et al. in late 1990s [55, 56]. Since then, various open and endoscopic procedures have been proposed for the direct repair of gluteus medius and minimus tendon tear, with endoscopic repair increasingly recognized as a safe and efficacious management approach [57–66]. For massive irreparable tears, both open and endoscopic procedures using tendon transfer techniques have also been described [67, 68].
- The gluteus medius and gluteus minimus muscles act mainly to abduct and medially rotate the thigh. Hence, they are often collectively referred to as the "hip abductors" or "rotator-cuff of the hip." A thorough understanding of the anatomic attachment of these muscles is critical for optimal surgical outcomes (Figs. 4.19 and

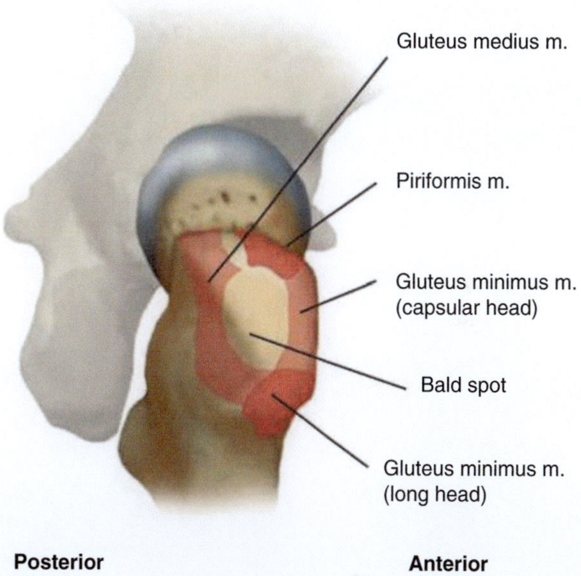

Fig. 4.19 Illustration of a superolateral view of the right proximal femur in a cadaveric specimen demonstrating the attachment sites of the gluteus medius tendon, the two heads of the gluteus minimus muscle, and the piriformis muscle as well as the bald spot of the greater trochanter. (Reproduced from Federer et al. [69, 70])

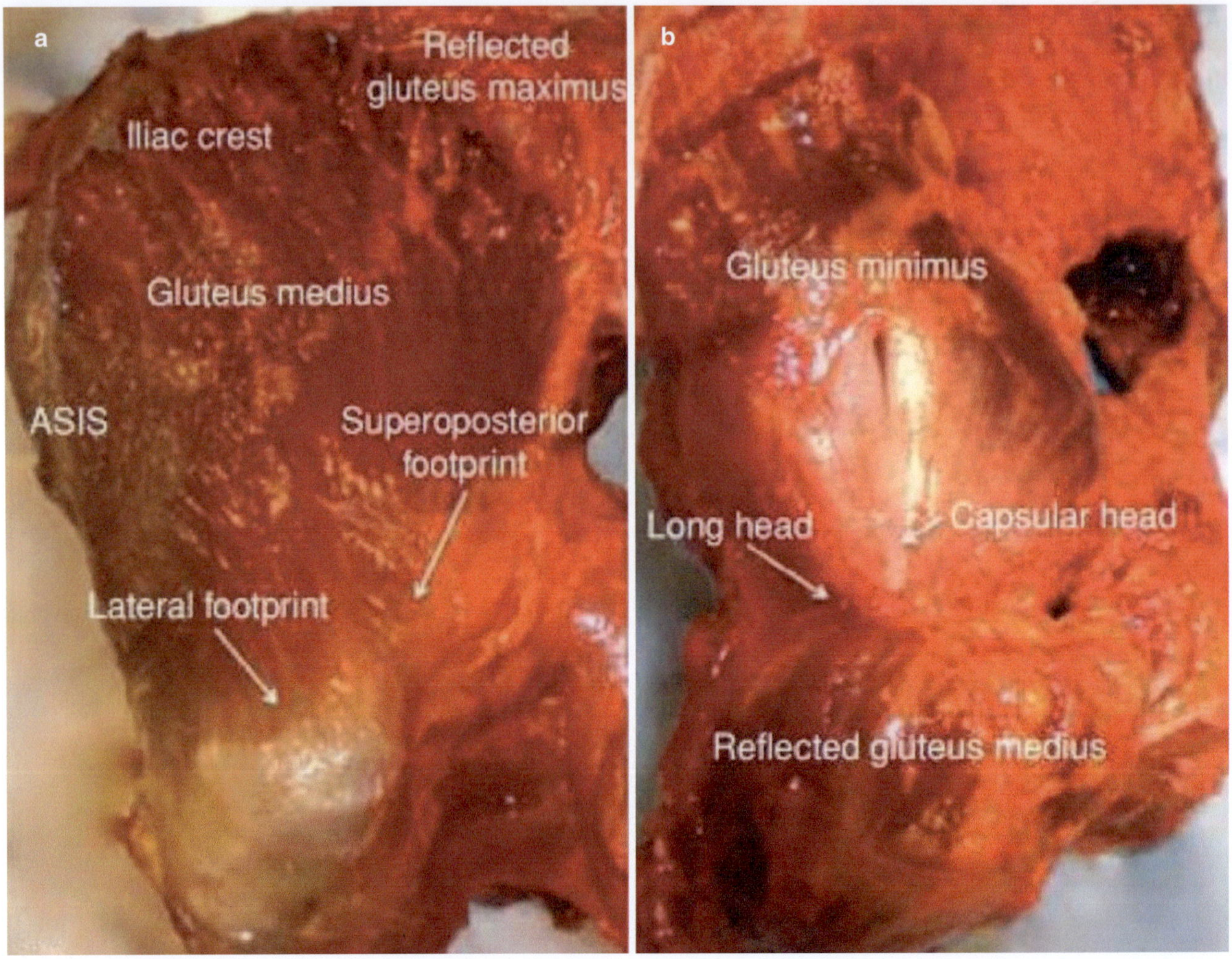

Fig. 4.20 (**a**) On this left hip, the gluteus medius originates along the iliac crest and inserts at the lateral and superoposterior footprint on the greater trochanter. The ASIS is the origin of the TFL, whose fascia distally becomes the ITB, traversing down to its distal insertion at the lateral aspect of the tibial tubercle. (**b**) The gluteus medius is reflected over the greater trochanter. The capsular head of the gluteus minimus attaches to the anterior greater trochanter whereas the long head inserts into the anterior and inferior greater trochanter. *ASIS* anterior superior iliac spine, *TFL* tensor fascia latae, *ITB* iliotibial band. (Reproduced from Federer et al. [69, 70])

4.20). The gluteus medius originates from the posteroinferior edge of the iliac crest and inserts on the lateral and superoposterior facets of the greater trochanter. It consists of anterior, middle, and posterior parts. The anterior part and a section of the middle part attach to the lateral facet, while the posterior part and the remainder of the middle part insert on the superoposterior facet. The gluteus minimus originates along the middle gluteal line between the anterior inferior iliac spine and the posterior inferior iliac spine, attaching distally to the anterior facet and the joint capsule [71].

4.5.2 Indications

- Symptomatic tears unresponsive to conservative management

4.5.3 Contra-indications

- Large, retracted full-thickness tears
- Advanced fatty degeneration of gluteus medius and minimus muscle

In cases of significant tendon retraction or severe muscle atrophy with fatty infiltration, reconstruction using tendon transfer techniques, typically done in an open fashion, is considered more appropriate [66–68, 72].

4.5.4 Author Preferred Techniques

4.5.4.1 Pre-operative Planning

- A comprehensive assessment of pertinent imaging studies is performed to indicate the size of tear, with MRI being the primary evaluation method. Ultrasound may serve as a suitable alternative in patients for whom MRI is contraindicated or unrevealing.

- Required instruments: 70° arthroscope, 8.25 × 9-mm twist-in cannulas, double- or triple-loaded suture anchors, suture passers, suture retrievers, knotless fixation devices, epinephrine (1 mg/3 L saline), and fluid inflow pump.
- The location of the greater trochanter is marked for reference.

4.5.4.2 Patient Positioning

- The patient is positioned supine on an arthroscopic traction table with the operative leg slighted abducted, which helps expand peritrochanteric space by reducing iliotibial band tension.
- The C-arm enters contralaterally and is centered over the greater trochanter.

4.5.4.3 Portal design

- Four portals are used in this procedure, including the standard anterolateral (AL) and midanterior (MA) portals, along with a posterolateral (PL) portal and a distal anterolateral accessory (DALA) portal (Fig. 4.21). The PL portal and the DALA portal are located approximately 3 cm proximal and 3 cm distal, respectively, to the greater trochanter along the long axis through the center of the trochanter.

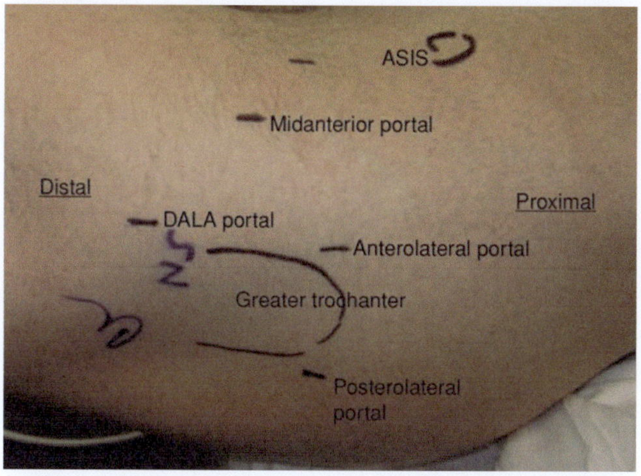

Fig. 4.21 The portal placement on a left hip shown relative to the palpable ASIS and greater trochanter. *DALA* distal anterolateral accessory portal, *ASIS* anterior superior iliac spine. (Reproduced from Poultsides et al. [73])

4.5.4.4 Step-by-Step Description of the Techniques

- Arthroscopy of the hip joint is first performed to check for and address any concomitant intra-articular pathology. Once intra-articular procedures are completed, all instruments are removed and traction is released.
- The peritrochanteric compartment is first accessed through the placement of DALA portal under fluoroscopy. A cannula is introduced and a 70° arthroscope is then inserted into the peritrochanteric space. Vastus lateralis, which signifies the inferomedial border of the peritrochanteric compartment, should be visualized if the arthroscope is properly positioned.
- The fluid pump pressure is set at 40 mmHg. Epinephrine can be used in the inflow to control bleeding.
- The AL portal is created, through which a shaver is introduced. Trochanteric bursectomy is then conducted to better visualize the gluteal tendon insertion sites.
- The gluteal tendons are checked with a probe for any superficial tearing or undersurface delamination. Once the lesion is identified, appropriate surgical procedures are selected, respectively, for low-grade partial tears (25%), and full-thickness tears [63].

Micropuncture and Knotless Suture Staple Technique for Low-Grade Partial Tears

- Low-grade partial tears can be addressed using a knotless technique, which negates the need for suture passing and knot tying.
- The PL portal is established. A cannula is introduced through this portal and a microfracture awl is inserted through the cannula. Multiple holes are made with the awl on the lateral facet of the greater trochanter, in order to promote tendon healing by increasing exudation of marrow contents. The depth of puncture into the bone should be 3–5 mm.
- A metal punch is twisted through the tendon and driven into the lateral facet of trochanter, creating a pilot hole for anchor placement. An anchor is then advanced

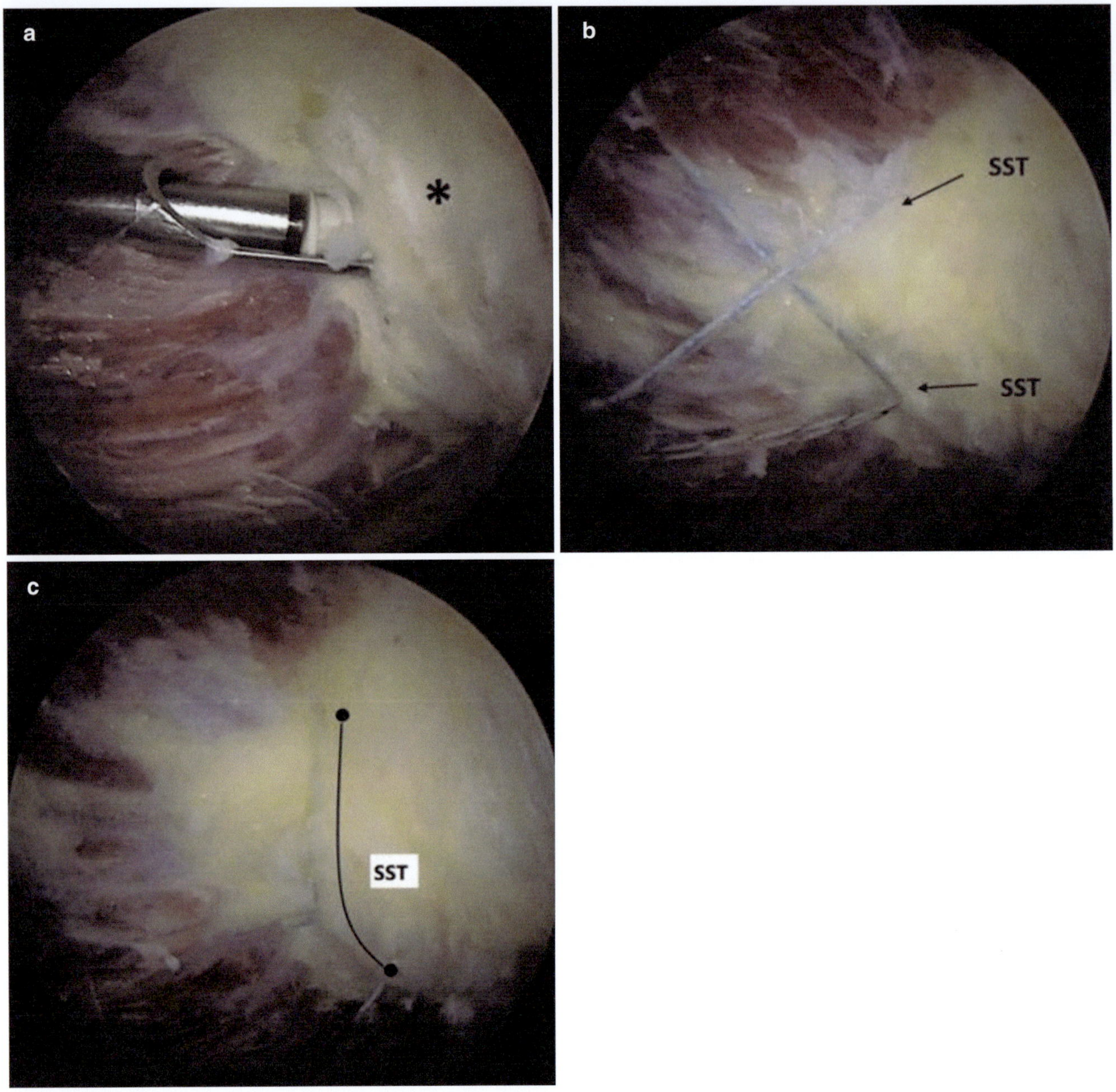

Fig. 4.22 Right hip positioned supine with 30° of abduction; all arthroscopic views are from the DALA portal. (**a**) Placement of 3.0-mm PEEK Knotless SutueTak (Arthrex) anchor within gluteal tendon footprint at area of confirmed undersurface partial tear. *Gluteus medius tendon. (**b**) Crisscross configuration of 2 knotless repair anchors placed within the superoposterior facet. (**c**) Completed gluteus medius repair using suture staple technique. *DALA* distal anterolateral accessory portal, *SST* suture staple repair stitch. (Reproduced from Lall et al. [74–76])

through the tendon and placed into the pilot hole (Fig. 4.22a). A total of two pairs of anchors are needed. The posteroproximal, anteroproximal, posterodistal, and anterodistal anchors are sequentially placed in this manner.

- It is important to note that, as a general rule, the operative leg should be maximally internally rotated while placing the posterior anchors and kept neutral while placing the anterior anchors.
- Each pair of anchors is then linked together, producing a suture staple construct (Fig. 4.22b, c) [64].

Transtendinous Repair Technique for High-Grade Partial Tears

- In cases of high-grade partial tears, which are predominantly undersurface tears in nature, a transtendinous technique is adopted.
- A beaver blade is introduced through the AL portal and a longitudinal incision is made within the tendon (Fig. 4.23a). The arthroscope is advanced through the incision to visualize the undersurface tear (Fig. 4.23b). Devitalized tissues on the deep side of the tendon are debrided with a shaver inserted through the AL portal. The lateral facet of the trochanter is further freshened with a burr to a bleeding bed for optimal healing.
- The PL portal is established, through which double- or triple-loaded anchors are inserted through the tendon split and placed perpendicular to the bone surface (Fig. 4.23c). The number and distribution of anchors are dependent on the size and pattern of tear.
- One limb of suture is passed through each of the anterior and posterior leaflets of the tendon (Fig. 4.23d). The AL portal can be used for retrieving and docking the sutures once the sutures are passed. After this process is repeated for every anchor, the sutures are tied, achieving a side-to-side repair (Fig. 4.23e) [65].

4.5.4.5 Double-Row Fixation Technique for Complete Tears

- Double-row fixation is usually reserved for full-thickness tears. This technique involves the placement of four or six suture anchors.
- Once a full-thickness tear is identified, the severity of retraction and fatty degeneration is assessed to determine

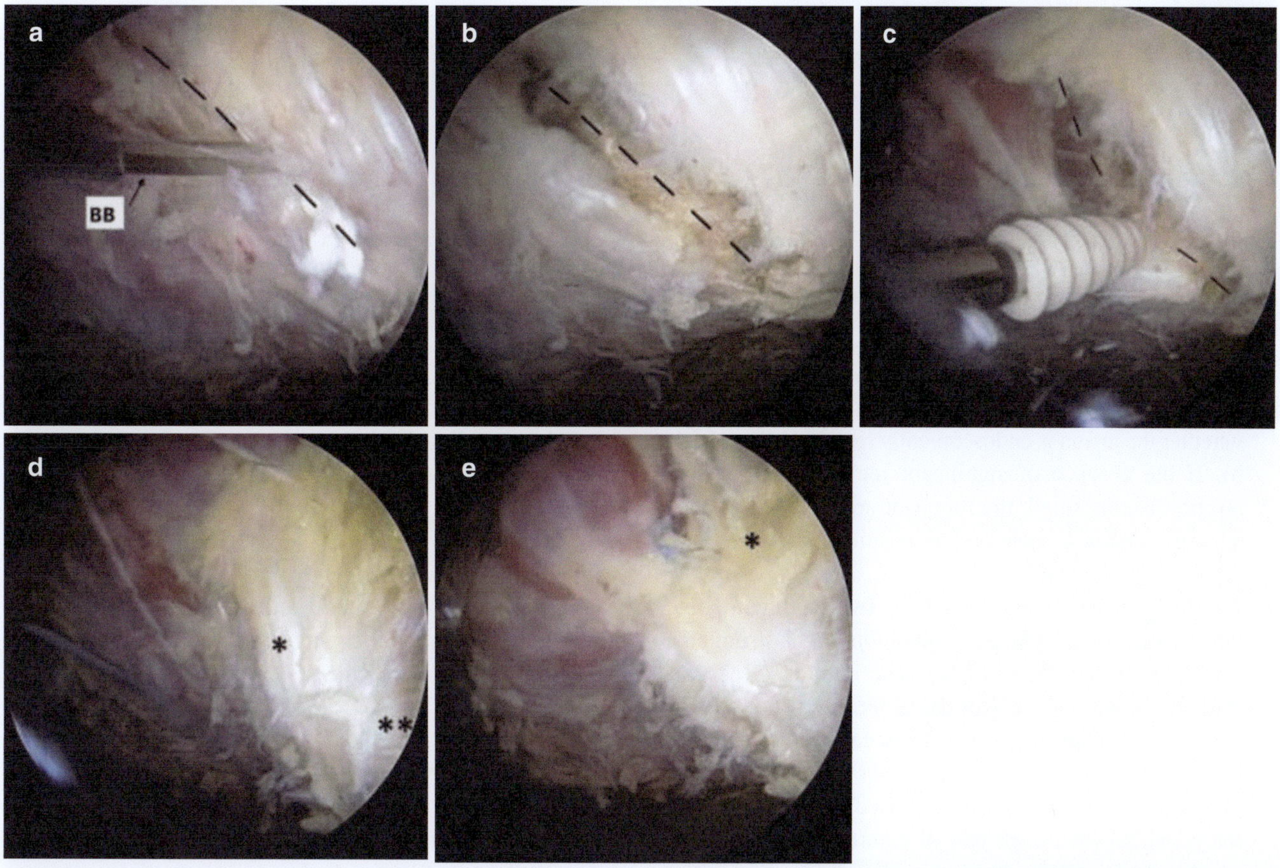

Fig. 4.23 Right hip positioned supine with 30° of abduction; all arthroscopic views are from the DALA portal. (**a**) Arthroscopic beaver blade splits into high-grade partial-thickness tearing of the abductor tendon. (**b**) Arthroscopic view of transtendinous access to greater trochanteric footprint. (**c**) After decortication of bony footprint, arthroscopic view of double-loaded corkscrew anchor (Arthrex) being placed at the superoposterior greater trochanteric facet. (**d**) Arthroscopic view of sutures tails being passed in a side-to-side configuration along transtendinous split, proximal to distal direction. (**e**) Arthroscopic view showing completed repair of gluteus medius tendon using the transtendinous technique. *BB* arthroscopic beaver blade, *DALA* distal anterolateral accessory portal. Dotted line, transtendinous window. *Gluteus medius tendon. **Vastus lateralis tendon. (Reproduced from Lall et al. [74–76])

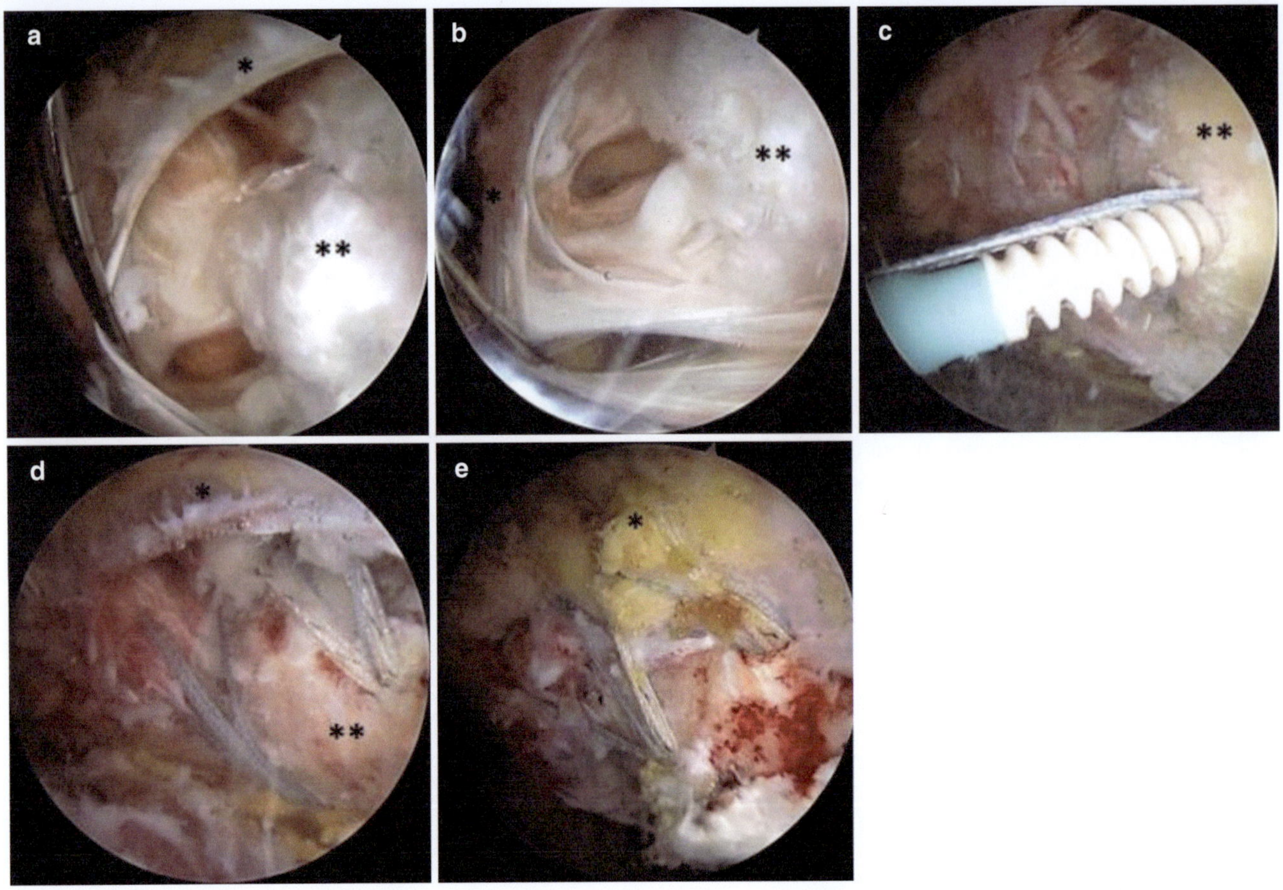

Fig. 4.24 Right hip positioned supine with 30° of abduction; all arthroscopic views are from the DALA portal. (**a**, **b**) Full-thickness, retracted gluteus medius tear is identified and probed, exposing insertional facet of the greater trochanter. (**c**) After diseased tendon debridement and footprint decortication, shown here is placement of double-loaded corkscrew suture anchor (Arthrex) within superoposterior greater trochanteric facet. (**d**) Passage of suture tails in horizontal mattress fashion from anterior to posterior direction. (**e**) Arthroscopic view showing completed repair using a double-row suture-bridge configuration. *DALA* distal anterolateral accessory portal. *Gluteus medius tendon. **Greater trochanter. (Reproduced from Lall et al. [74–76])

whether the lesion is endoscopically reparable (Fig. 4.24a, b). If the absence of significant retraction and muscle atrophy is confirmed, the footprint area is then prepared and the tendon is debrided in a similar fashion to the repair of partial tears.

- The PL portal is then established. Two or three double-loaded anchors are placed through this portal, from anterior to posterior (Fig. 4.24c). The sutures are passed through the tendon in a mattress fashion and knots are tied (Fig. 4.24d). One suture limb from each knot is retained to be passed into anchors in the distal row.
- One additional knotless anchor is used for every anchor in the proximal row. Each pair of suture limbs is incorporated into a knotless anchor, creating a suture-bridge configuration (Fig. 4.24e) [60, 72].

4.5.4.6 Complications and Management

- Wound complications.
- Retears.

Endoscopic repair results in significantly lower rates in wound complications, retear, and deep vein thrombosis, possibly due to less soft-tissue dissection and earlier postoperative mobilization with the endoscopic approach [77, 78].

4.5.4.7 Postoperative Care

- The rehabilitation protocol for hip abductor tears depends on the degree of tear and the security of repair.
- Generally, patients with low-grade partial tears are instructed to wear a hip brace and use crutches for

2 weeks. Physical therapy is initiated the day after surgery.
- Patients with high-grade partial tears and complete tears are instructed to wear a hip brace and use crutches for 6 and 8 weeks, respectively. Rehabilitation may begin at 6 weeks postoperatively.
- Precaution against contact activities and forced stretching should be taken for at least 4 months postoperatively.

4.5.4.8 Outcome

- Endoscopic repair of hip abductors has been shown to be a viable technique, according to short- and mid-term outcomes. Significant improvement in pain relief and strength restoration has been reported with excellent patient satisfaction [77–82].
- Similar outcomes were reported between open and endoscopic approaches, although future randomized studies are required to draw a more definitive conclusion [83].
- No disparities in clinical outcomes after gluteus medius repair were found between men and women [84]. Muscular fatty degeneration is associated with inferior clinical outcomes [85].

4.5.5 Summary

- With the advancement in endoscopic technology and operative experience, the endoscopic repair of gluteus medius and minimus tendon tears has been increasingly proven as a reliable management approach in selected patients.
- Randomized or prospective studies on surgical outcomes are needed to validate our current attitude toward this procedure.

References

1. Chang KS, Cheng YH, Wu CH, et al. Dynamic ultrasound imaging for the iliotibial band/snapping hip syndrome. Am J Phys Med Rehabil. 2015;94(6):e55–6.
2. Yuan BT, Qu F, Wang SX, et al. Histology and molecular pathology of iliotibial tract contracture in patients with gluteal muscle contracture. Biosci Rep. 2019;39(9):BSR20181351.
3. de Valderrama JAF, de Miguel RE. Fibrosis of the gluteus maximus: a cause of limited flexion and adduction of the hip in children. Clin Orthop Relat Res. 1981;156:67–78.
4. Hang YS. Contracture of the hip secondary to fibrosis of the gluteus maximus muscle. J Bone Joint Surg Am. 1979;61(1):52–5.
5. Chahla J, Nwachukwu BU, Beck EC, et al. Influence of acetabular labral tear length on outcomes after hip arthroscopy for femoroacetabular impingement syndrome with capsular plication. Am J Sports Med. 2019;47(5):1145–50.
6. Vap AR, Mitchell JJ, Briggs KK, et al. Outcomes of arthroscopic management of trochanteric bursitis in patients with femoroacetabular impingement: a comparison of two matched patient groups. Arthroscopy. 2018;34(5):1455–60.
7. Liu YJ, Wang ZG, Wang JL, et al. Clinical classification of gluteal muscle contracture under arthroscopy. China J Orthop Traumatol. 2013;26(6):468–70.
8. Rai S, Meng C, Wang X, et al. Gluteal muscle contracture: diagnosis and management options. SICOT J. 2017;3:1.
9. 刘玉杰, 王志刚, 李众利, 等.关节镜监视下射频汽化治疗注射性臀肌挛缩症的初步报告.中华骨科杂志.2003;23(3):150–2.
10. Liu YJ, Wang Y, Xue J, et al. Arthroscopic gluteal muscle contracture release with radiofrequency energy. Clin Orthop Relat Res. 2009;467(3):799–804.
11. Yoon JY, Kwak HS, Yoon KS, et al. Arthroscopic treatment for external snapping hip. Hip Pelvis. 2014;26(3):173–7.
12. Shrestha A, Wu P, Ge H, et al. Clinical outcomes of arthroscopic surgery for external snapping hip. J Orthop Surg Res. 2017;12(1):81.
13. Rai S, Jin S, Meng C, et al. Arthroscopic release using F and C method versus conventional open release method in the treatment of gluteal muscle contracture: a comparative study. BMC BMC Musculoskelet Disord. 2017;18(1):113.
14. Zini R, Munegato D, De Benedetto M. Endoscopic iliotibial band release in snapping hip. Hip Int. 2013;23(2):225–32.
15. Yen YM, Lewis CL, Kim YJ. Understanding and treating the snapping hip. Sports Med Arthrosc Rev. 2015;23:194–9.
16. Provencher MT, Hofmeister E, Muldoon MP. The surgical treatment of external coxa saltans (the snapping hip) by Z-plasty of the iliotibial band. Am J Sports Med. 2004;32:470–6.
17. Kim CH, Lee SK, Kim JH, Yoon PW. External snapping hip: classification based on magnetic resonance imaging features and clinical correlation. Hip Int. 2020;23:1120–5.
18. White RA, Hughes MS, Burd T, Hamann J, Allen WC. A new operative approach in the correction of external coxa saltans: the snapping hip. Am J Sports Med. 2004;32:1504–8.
19. Polesello GC, Queiroz MC, Domb BG, Ono NK, Honda EK. Surgical technique: endoscopic gluteus maximus tendon release for external snapping hip syndrome. Clin Orthop Relat Res. 2013;471:2471–6.
20. Zhu D, Zhiwei C, Ying L, et al. Comparison of arthroscopic versus open surgery on external snapping hip caused by gluteal muscle contracture. Hip Int. 2018;28:173–7.
21. Zoltan DJ, Clancy WG Jr, Keene JS. A new operative approach to snapping hip and refractory trochanteric bursitis in athletes. Am J Sports Med. 1986;14:201–4.
22. Brignall CG, Stainsby GD. The snapping hip. Treatment by Z-plasty. J Bone Joint Surg Br. 1991;73:253–4.
23. Kunac N, Trsek D, Medancić N, Starcević D, Haspl M. Endoscopic treatment of the external snapping hip syndrome: surgical technique and report of two cases. Acta Clin Croat. 2012;51:661–6.
24. Ilizaliturri VM, Martinez-Escalante FA, Chaidez PA, et al. Endoscopic iliotibial band release for external snapping hip syndrome. Arthroscopy. 2006;22:505–10.
25. Chiang CL, Tsai MY, Chang WN, Chen CK. Aberrant femoral torsion presenting with frog-leg squatting mimicking gluteal muscle contracture. Clin Orthop Relat Res. 2012;470(4):1165–70.
26. You T, Yang B, Zhang XT, et al. A possible prediction of dystocia at the time of cesarean delivery: gluteal muscle contracture, a single center experience from China. Medicine (Baltimore). 2020;99(7):e19138.
27. Zhang T, Xu S, Li H, He X, Zhang F. Comparison of the clinical effects of arthroscopic surgery vs. open surgery for grade II gluteal muscle contracture in adults. Exp Ther Med. 2018;16(1):364–9.
28. Zhao CG, He XJ, Lu B, Li HP, Wang D, Zhu ZZ. Classification of gluteal muscle contracture in children and outcome of different treatments. BMC Musculoskelet Disord. 2009;10:34.
29. Zhou R, Ren S, Li C, Zhang X, Zhang W. miR-29a is a potential protective factor for fibrogenesis in gluteal muscle contracture. Physiol Res. 2020;69(3):467–79.
30. Huang JB, Ge H, Zhang YL, et al. The role of arthroscopic release of gluteal muscle contracture in improving patellofemoral instability. J Orthop Surg Res. 2019;14(1):159.
31. Liu YJ, Wang Y, Xue J, Lui PP, Chan KM. Arthroscopic gluteal muscle contracture release with radiofrequency energy. Clin Orthop Relat Res. 2009;467(3):799–804.
32. Zhang X, Jiang X, He F, et al. Arthroscopic revision release of gluteal muscle contracture after failed primary open surgery. Int Orthop. 2017;41(8):1521–6.
33. Dai Z, Chen Z, Liao Y, Tang Z, Cui J. Comparison of arthroscopic versus open surgery on external snapping hip caused by gluteal muscle contracture. Hip Int. 2018;28(2):173–7.
34. Fu D, Yang S, Xiao B, Wang H, Meng C. Comparison of endoscopic surgery and open surgery for gluteal muscle contracture. J Pediatr Orthop. 2011;31(5):e38–43.
35. Speers CJ, Bhogal GS. Greater trochanteric pain syndrome: a review of diagnosis and management in general practice. Br J Gen Pract. 2017;67(663):479–80.
36. Williams BS, Cohen SP. Greater trochanteric pain syndrome: a review of anatomy, diagnosis and treatment. Anesth Analg. 2009;108(5):1662–70.
37. Fox JL. The role of arthroscopic bursectomy in the treatment of trochanteric bursitis. Arthroscopy. 2002;18(7):E34.
38. Drummond J, Fary C, Tran P. The outcome of endoscopy for recalcitrant greater trochanteric pain syndrome. Arch Orthop Trauma Surg. 2016;136(11):1547–54.
39. Reid D. The management of greater trochanteric pain syndrome: a systematic literature review. J Orthop. 2016;13(1):15–28.
40. Koulischer S, Callewier A, Zorman D. Management of greater trochanteric pain syndrome: a systematic review. Acta Orthop Belg. 2017;83(2):205–14.
41. Barratt PA, Brookes N, Newson A. Conservative treatments for greater trochanteric pain syndrome: a systematic review. Br J Sports Med. 2017;51(2):97–104.
42. Pretell J, et al. Distal fascia lata lengthening: an alternative surgical technique for recalcitrant trochanteric bursitis. Int Orthop. 2009;33(5):1223–7.
43. Vap AR, et al. Outcomes of arthroscopic management of trochanteric bursitis in patients with femoroacetabular impingement: a comparison of two matched patient groups. Arthroscopy. 2018;34(5):1455–60.

44. Mitchell JJ, et al. Endoscopic trochanteric bursectomy and iliotibial band release for persistent trochanteric bursitis. Arthrosc Tech. 2016;5(5):e1185–9.
45. Govaert LH, et al. Endoscopic bursectomy and iliotibial tract release as a treatment for refractory greater trochanteric pain syndrome: a new endoscopic approach with early results. Arthrosc Tech. 2012;1(2):e161–4.
46. Wiese M, et al. Early results of endoscopic trochanter bursectomy. Int Orthop. 2004;28(4):218–21.
47. Zeman P, et al. Clinical results of endoscopic treatment of greater trochanteric pain syndrome. Acta Chir Orthop Traumatol Cechoslov. 2017;84(3):168–74.
48. Bradley DM, Dillingham MF. Bursoscopy of the trochanteric bursa. Arthroscopy. 1998;14(8):884–7.
49. Farr D, et al. Arthroscopic bursectomy with concomitant iliotibial band release for the treatment of recalcitrant trochanteric bursitis. Arthroscopy. 2007;23(8):905.e1–5.
50. Baker CL Jr, et al. Arthroscopic bursectomy for recalcitrant trochanteric bursitis. Arthroscopy. 2007;23(8):827–32.
51. Kenanidis E, Kyriakopoulos G, Kaila R, Christofilopoulos P. Lesions of the abductors in the hip. EFORT Open Rev. 2020;5(8):464–76.
52. LaPorte C, Vasaris M, Gossett L, Boykin R, Menge T. Gluteus medius tears of the hip: a comprehensive approach. Phys Sportsmed. 2019;47(1):15–20.
53. Mosier BA, Quinlan NJ, Martin SD. Peritrochanteric Endoscopy. Clin Sports Med. 2016;35(3):449–67.
54. Chi AS, Long SS, Zoga AC, Read PJ, Deely DM, Parker L, Morrison WB. Prevalence and pattern of gluteus medius and minimus tendon pathology and muscle atrophy in older individuals using MRI. Skelet Radiol. 2015;44(12):1727–33.
55. Bunker TD, Esler CN, Leach WJ. Rotator-cuff tear of the hip. J Bone Joint Surg Br. 1997;79(4):618–20.
56. Kagan A 2nd. Rotator-cuff tear of the hip. J Bone Joint Surg Br. 1998;80(1):182–3.
57. Voos JE, Rudzki JR, Shindle MK, Martin H, Kelly BT. Arthroscopic anatomy and surgical techniques for peritrochanteric space disorders in the hip. Arthroscopy. 2007;23(11):1246.e1–5.
58. Thaunat M, Noël E, Nové-Josserand L, Murphy CG, Sbiyaa M, Sonnery-Cottet B. Endoscopic management of gluteus medius tendon tears. Sports Med Arthrosc Rev. 2016;24(1):11–8.
59. Parker EA, Meyer AM, Laskovski JR, Westermann RW. Endoscopic gluteus Medius repair with an ITB-sparing versus ITB-splitting approach: a systematic review and meta-analysis. Orthop J Sports Med. 2020;8(5):2325967120922196.
60. Domb BG, Carreira DS. Endoscopic repair of full-thickness gluteus medius tears. Arthrosc Tech. 2013;2(2):e77–81.
61. Thaunat M, Chatellard R, Noël E, Sonnery-Cottet B, Nové-Josserand L. Endoscopic repair of partial-thickness undersurface tears of the gluteus medius tendon. Orthop Traumatol Surg Res. 2013;99(7):853–7.
62. Byrd JW. Gluteus medius repair with double-row fixation. Arthrosc Tech. 2013;2(3):e247–50.
63. Lall AC, Schwarzman GR, Battaglia MR, Chen SL, Maldonado DR, Domb BG. Greater trochanteric pain syndrome: an intraoperative endoscopic classification system with pearls to surgical techniques and rehabilitation protocols. Arthrosc Tech. 2019;8(8):e889–903.
64. Hartigan DE, Mansor Y, Perets I, Walsh JP, Mohr MR, Domb BG. Knotless "suture staple" technique for endoscopic partial thickness abductor tendon repair. Arthrosc Tech. 2018;7(10):e975–80.
65. Domb BG, Nasser RM, Botser IB. Partial-thickness tears of the gluteus medius: rationale and technique for trans-tendinous endoscopic repair. Arthroscopy. 2010;26(12):1697–705.
66. Davies JF, Davies DM. Surgical technique for the repair of tears to the gluteus Medius and Minimus tendons of the hip. JBJS Essent Surg Tech. 2014;4(2):e11.
67. Whiteside LA. Surgical technique: gluteus maximus and tensor fascia lata transfer for primary deficiency of the abductors of the hip. Clin Orthop Relat Res. 2014;472(2):645–53.
68. Thaunat M, Roberts T, Bah A, Vieira TD, Haidar I, Bauwens PH. Endoscopic transfer of gluteus maximus and tensor fascia Lata for primary hip abductor deficiency. Arthrosc Tech. 2020;9(9):e1235–9.
69. Federer AE, Mather RC, Bush-Joseph CA, Nho SJ. Hip arthroscopy anatomy and access peritrochanteric compartment. In: Clohisy JC, Beaule PE, Della Valle CJ, et al., editors. The adult hip: hip preservation surgery. Philadelphia: Wolters Kluwer Health; 2015. p. 298–308. Figure 27.1; p. 299.
70. Federer AE, Mather RC, Bush-Joseph CA, Nho SJ. Hip arthroscopy anatomy and access peritrochanteric compartment. In: Clohisy JC, Beaule PE, Della Valle CJ, et al., editors. The adult hip: hip preservation surgery. Philadelphia: Wolters Kluwer Health; 2015. p. 298–308. Figure 27.4; p. 305.
71. Gottschalk F, Kourosh S, Leveau B. The functional anatomy of tensor fasciae latae and gluteus medius and minimus. J Anat. 1989;166:179–89.
72. Byrd JWT. Arthroscopic management of abductor tears. In: Byrd JWT, Bedi A, Stubbs AJ, editors. The hip: AANA advanced arthroscopic surgical techniques. Thorofare: SLACK Incorporated; 2016. p. 221–30.
73. Poultsides LA, Kelly BT. Hip arthroscopy—disorders of the trochanteric space—bursitis and abductor tears. In: Clohisy JC, Beaule PE, Della Valle CJ, et al., editors. The adult hip: hip preservation surgery. Philadelphia: Wolters Kluwer Health; 2015. p. 326–41. Figure 30.3; p. 327.
74. Lall AC, Schwarzman GR, Battaglia MR, Chen SL, Maldonado DR, Domb BG. Greater trochanteric pain syndrome: an intraoperative endoscopic classification system with pearls to surgical techniques and rehabilitation protocols. Arthrosc Tech. 2019;8(8):e889–903. Figure 5; p. e894
75. Lall AC, Schwarzman GR, Battaglia MR, Chen SL, Maldonado DR, Domb BG. Greater trochanteric pain syndrome: an intraoperative endoscopic classification system with pearls to surgical techniques and rehabilitation protocols. Arthrosc Tech. 2019;8(8):e889–903. Figure 6; p. e895
76. Lall AC, Schwarzman GR, Battaglia MR, Chen SL, Maldonado DR, Domb BG. Greater trochanteric pain syndrome: an intraoperative endoscopic classification system with pearls to surgical techniques and rehabilitation protocols. Arthrosc Tech. 2019;8(8):e889–903. Figure 7; p. e896
77. Alpaugh K, Chilelli BJ, Xu S, Martin SD. Outcomes after primary open or endoscopic abductor tendon repair in the hip: a systematic review of the literature. Arthroscopy. 2015;31(3):530–40.
78. Chandrasekaran S, Lodhia P, Gui C, Vemula SP, Martin TJ, Domb BG. Outcomes of open versus endoscopic repair of abductor muscle tears of the hip: a systematic review. Arthroscopy. 2015;31(10):2057–67.e2.
79. Voos JE, Shindle MK, Pruett A, Asnis PD, Kelly BT. Endoscopic repair of gluteus medius tendon tears of the hip. Am J Sports Med. 2009;37(4):743–7.
80. Domb BG, Botser I, Giordano BD. Outcomes of endoscopic gluteus medius repair with minimum 2-year follow-up. Am J Sports Med. 2013;41(5):988–97.
81. Chandrasekaran S, Gui C, Hutchinson MR, Lodhia P, Suarez-Ahedo C, Domb BG. Outcomes of endoscopic gluteus medius repair: study of thirty-four patients with minimum two-year follow-up. J Bone Joint Surg Am. 2015;97(16):1340–7.
82. Perets I, Mansor Y, Yuen LC, Chen AW, Chaharbakhshi EO, Domb BG. Endoscopic gluteus medius repair with concomitant arthroscopy for labral tears: a case series with minimum 5-year outcomes. Arthroscopy. 2017;33(12):2159–67.

83. Meghpara MB, Yelton MJ, Annin S, Shapira J, Rosinsky PJ, Maldonado DR, Lall AC, Domb BG. Mid-term outcomes of endoscopic gluteus medius repair with concomitant arthroscopic labral treatment: a propensity-matched controlled study. Arthroscopy. 2020;36(11):2856–65.
84. Meghpara MB, Bheem R, Haden M, Rosinsky PJ, Shapira J, Maldonado DR, Lall AC, Domb BG. Differences in clinical presentations and surgical outcomes of gluteus medius tears between men and women. Am J Sports Med. 2020;26:363546520966335.
85. Thaunat M, Clowez G, Desseaux A, Murphy CG, Sbiyaa M, Noël E, Sonnery-Cottet B. Influence of muscle fatty degeneration on functional outcomes after endoscopic gluteus medius repair. Arthroscopy. 2018;34(6):1816–24.

Endoscopy of the Deep Gluteal Space

5

Tun Hing Lui, Luis Perez Carro,
Moises Fernandez Hernando, Luis Cerezal Pesquera,
Natalia Fernandez Escajadillo,
Jose Antonio Fernandez-Divar, Ana Alfonso Fernandez,
Victor M. Ilizaliturri Jr, Ruben Arriaga,
Carlos Suarez-Ahedo, Tiao Su, Guangxing Chen,
and Yan Xu

Abstract

Deep gluteal syndrome (DGS) is defined as the presence of pain in the subgluteal space caused from non-discogenic and extra-pelvic entrapment of the sciatic nerve in which piriformis syndrome is the most common cause. The whole sciatic nerve trajectory in the deep gluteal space can be addressed by an endoscopic surgical technique, allowing the treatment of the diverse causes of sciatic nerve entrapment. Ischiofemoral impingement is a rare cause of posterior hip pain featured by the contact between the lesser trochanter and the ischium. If conservative treatment fails to relieve symptoms, endoscopic lesser trochanter osteoplasty can be considered. Hamstring injuries affect both athletes and middle-aged individuals and may cause significant impairment. The spectrum of hamstring injuries ranges from muscle strains to avulsion injuries. Non-operative management has been proposed for muscle strains and low-grade partial tears of the hamstring origin, whereas surgery is recommended in the setting of more refractory cases of proximal avulsions, with open surgical repair with suture anchors being the gold standard. With the advent of hip arthroscopy and refinement of endoscopic techniques, endoscopic hamstring repair has come to be considered as an effective and safe alternative to open repair. In this chapter, the endoscopic techniques are outlined.

Keywords

Hip endoscopy · Sciatic nerve entrapment · Deep gluteal syndrome · Piriformis syndrome · Deep gluteal space Sciatic nerve · Neurolysis · Ischiofemoral impingement Lesser trochanter osteoplasty · Hamstring · Biceps femoris · Semimembranosus · Semitendinosus Ischial bursectomy

The corresponding author of section 5.1 is Luis Perez Carro, Email: lpcarro@gmail.com
The corresponding author of section 5.2 is Carlos Suarez-Ahedo, Email: drsuarezahedo@gmail.com
The corresponding author of section 5.3 is Guangxing Chen, Email: cgx7676@hotmail.com
The corresponding author of section 5.4 is Yan Xu, Email: yanxu@139.com

T. H. Lui (✉)
Department of Orthopaedics and Traumatology, North District Hospital, Hong Kong, China

The Second Affiliated Hospital, Shenzhen University, Shenzhen, China

L. P. Carro · N. F. Escajadillo · J. A. Fernandez-Divar
A. A. Fernandez
Orthopedic Surgery Department Clinica Mompia, Santander, Cantabria, Spain

M. F. Hernando · L. C. Pesquera
Department of Radiology, Diagnóstico Médico Cantabria (DMC), Santander, Cantabria, Spain

V. M. Ilizaliturri Jr · R. Arriaga
National Rehabilitation Institute of Mexico, Mexico City, Mexico

C. Suarez-Ahedo
National Rehabilitation Institute of Mexico, Mexico City, Mexico

Hospital Medica Sur, Mexico City, Mexico

T. Su · G. Chen
Center for Joint Surgery, Southwest Hospital, Army Medical University, Chongqing, China

Y. Xu
Institute of Sports Medicine, Peking University Third Hospital, Beijing, China

© The Author(s), under exclusive license to Springer Nature Singapore Pte Ltd. 2021
T. H. Lui (ed.), *Endoscopy of the Hip and Knee*, https://doi.org/10.1007/978-981-16-3488-8_5

5.1 Endoscopic Management of Deep Gluteus Syndrome

5.1.1 Introduction

- The subgluteal space refers to the potential space between the middle and deep gluteal aponeurosis layers containing cellular and fatty tissue [1, 2].
- Deep gluteal syndrome (DGS) is defined as the presence of pain in the subgluteal space resulted from non-spinal and extra-pelvic causes of sciatic nerve entrapment.
- DGS is most commonly presented as buttock or hip pain with tenderness in the retro-trochanteric and gluteal regions. The patients with DGS can also present with unilateral or sometimes bilateral sciatic-like pain which is exacerbated with hip rotation with the hip flexed and knee extended. Less commonly, the patients may experience sitting intolerance of more than 20–30 min, limping, sensation loss or disturbance in the affected lower limb, lumbago, and night pain which is better at daytime.
- Surgical treatment is indicated for DCS recalcitrant to non-operative treatment. Whether open or endoscopic approach to be utilized depends on the clinical and radiological diagnosis.
- The whole course of the sciatic nerve in the deep gluteal space can be accessed endoscopically, allowing endoscopic treatment of various causes of sciatic nerve entrapment.
- Endoscopic sciatic nerve decompression is effective to improve function and reduce hip pain in cases of sciatic nerve entrapment in the deep gluteal space.

5.1.2 Indications

- Entrapment of the sciatic nerve along its course in the deep gluteal space, from the greater sciatic notch to the quadratus femoris.
- A comprehensive history and physical examination can pinpoint the anatomical site of sciatic nerve entrapment which can be confirmed radiologically.
- The sciatic nerve neuropathy as a result of the following reported etiologies can be triggered by prolonged sitting or stretching, direct contusion to the gluteal region, overuse or pelvic/spinal instability.

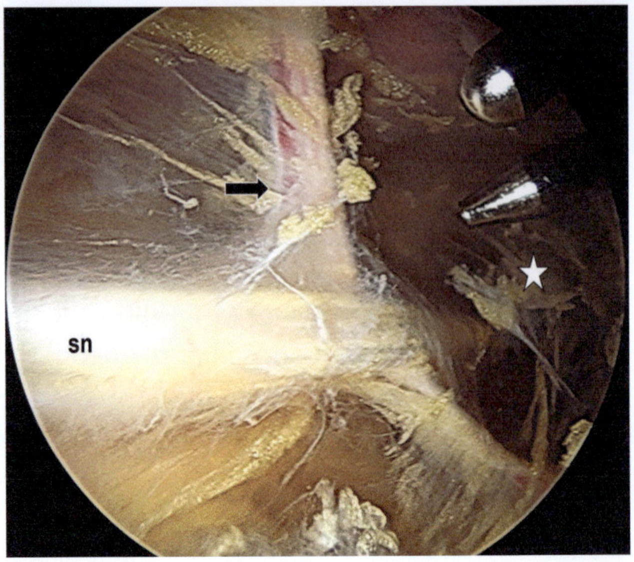

Fig. 5.1 Right hip. Endoscopy shows a vascular band (Black arrow) piercing the sciatic nerve causing tethering. *SN* Sciatic nerve. White star: Distal

5.1.2.1 Fibrous and Fibrovascular Bands

- Constricting fibrous bands are common causes of sciatic nerve entrapment in DGS which can limit or block sciatic nerve motion during hip and knee movements. Macroscopically, the bands can be primarily divided into pure fibrous, pure vascular, and fibrovascular bands [3] (Fig. 5.1).
- The bands can also be classified according to its anatomical location along the sciatic nerve. Proximal bands locate near the greater sciatic notch. The distal bands locate in the ischial tunnel between the quadratus femoris and origins of the hamstrings. The middle bands locate at the level of the piriformis and obturator internus-gemelli complex. The bands can be either medial or lateral to the sciatic nerve in all these locations.
- The bands can be classified according to the pathomechanism:
  - **Compressive or bridge-type bands (type 1)**, which limit the movement compressing the nerve from anterior to posterior (type 1A) or from posterior to anterior (type 1B).
  - **Adhesive bands or horse-strap bands (type 2)**. These bands can tether the sciatic nerve laterally from the greater trochanter (type 2A) or medially from the sacrotuberous ligament (type 2B).

- **Bands anchored to the sciatic nerve with undefined distribution (type 3)**. These bands have inconsistent distribution and tether the nerve multidirectionally.

5.1.2.2 Piriformis Syndrome

- In the past, DCS and piriformis syndrome were considered to be the same disease entity. In fact, piriformis syndrome is just one of the diverse orthopedic and non-orthopedic etiologies of sciatic nerve entrapment causing gluteal pain.
- Potential patholgies in the piriformis syndrome:
  - **Piriformis muscle hypertrophy**: Asymmetrically hypertrophied piriformis muscle can displaced the sciatic nerve anteriorly resulting in DGS.
  - **Dynamic sciatic nerve entrapment** by the piriformis muscle.
  - **Anomalous trajectory** of the sciatic nerve (anatomical variations).

5.1.2.3 Gemelli-Obturator Internus Syndrome

- As the sciatic nerve runs deep to the piriformis muscle and then superficial to the superior gemelli/obturator internus, action of these two muscle groups may result in scissoring effect to the sciatic nerve resulting in dynamic nerve entrapment.

5.1.2.4 Quadratus Femoris and Ischiofemoral Pathology

- Ischiofemoral impingement syndrome (IFI) is an under-recognized extra-articular impingement of the hip which is defined as the presence of hip pain associated with diminished space between the proximal femur and the ischial tuberosity. Diminished ischiofemoral space compared to healthy controls (the ischiofemoral space measures 23 ± 8 mm and femoral space 12 ± 4 mm) and altered signals of the quadratus femoris muscle due to muscle edema, rupture or atrophy are the characteristic MRI findings [4]. It should be noted that the ischiofemoral space is a gait-related dynamic area with various contributing and predisposing factors [5].

5.1.2.5 Hamstring Conditions

- **Ischial tunnel syndrome**: The sciatic nerve can be entrapped close to the ischial tuberosity during hip motion as a result of various pathologies of the hamstring origin in the ischial tuberosity. The pathologies can appear isolated or in combination and include acute, chronic or recurrent, partial or complete hamstring strain; detachment of tendon origin; acute or chronic avulsion fracture of the tendon origin or its nonunion; apophysitis; unfused apophysis; calcified tendinosis or tendinopathy of the proximal hamstrings tendons and contusion [6].

5.1.3 Contra-Indications for Endoscopy

- Infections.
- Patients have concomitant condition that requires major orthopedic or open procedures, e.g. osteotomies.

5.1.4 Author Preferred Technique

Endoscopic decompression of the sciatic nerve in the subgluteal space is technical demanding and should be reserved for experienced hip arthroscopists familiar with the gross and endoscopic anatomy of this region [2, 7].

5.1.4.1 Pre-operative Planning

- For patients with buttock pain without obvious diagnosis, spinal or intra-pelvic pathologies should be excluded by appropriate imaging studies. The active piriformis and seated piriformis stretch tests are more sensitive and specific than other tests to diagnose sciatic nerve entrapments especially when they are performed in combination [8].
- In deep gluteal syndrome, study of sciatic nerve stiffness associated with limb movements by ultrasound strain elastography can provide crucial information about the degree of nerve entrapment with specificity of 93.5%, sensitivity of 88.9%, and accuracy of 90.6% [9].
- Non-operative treatment of deep gluteal syndrome includes rest, anti-inflammatory drugs, muscle relaxants, physiotherapy, and ultrasound guided injections and should be targeted to the suspected entrapment site. Operative treatment should only be indicated for patients not responded to non-operative treatment. Whether open or endoscopic approach to be utilized depends on the clinical and radiological diagnosis. The response to ultra-

Table 5.1 Diagnosis and treatment algorithm for deep gluteal syndrome

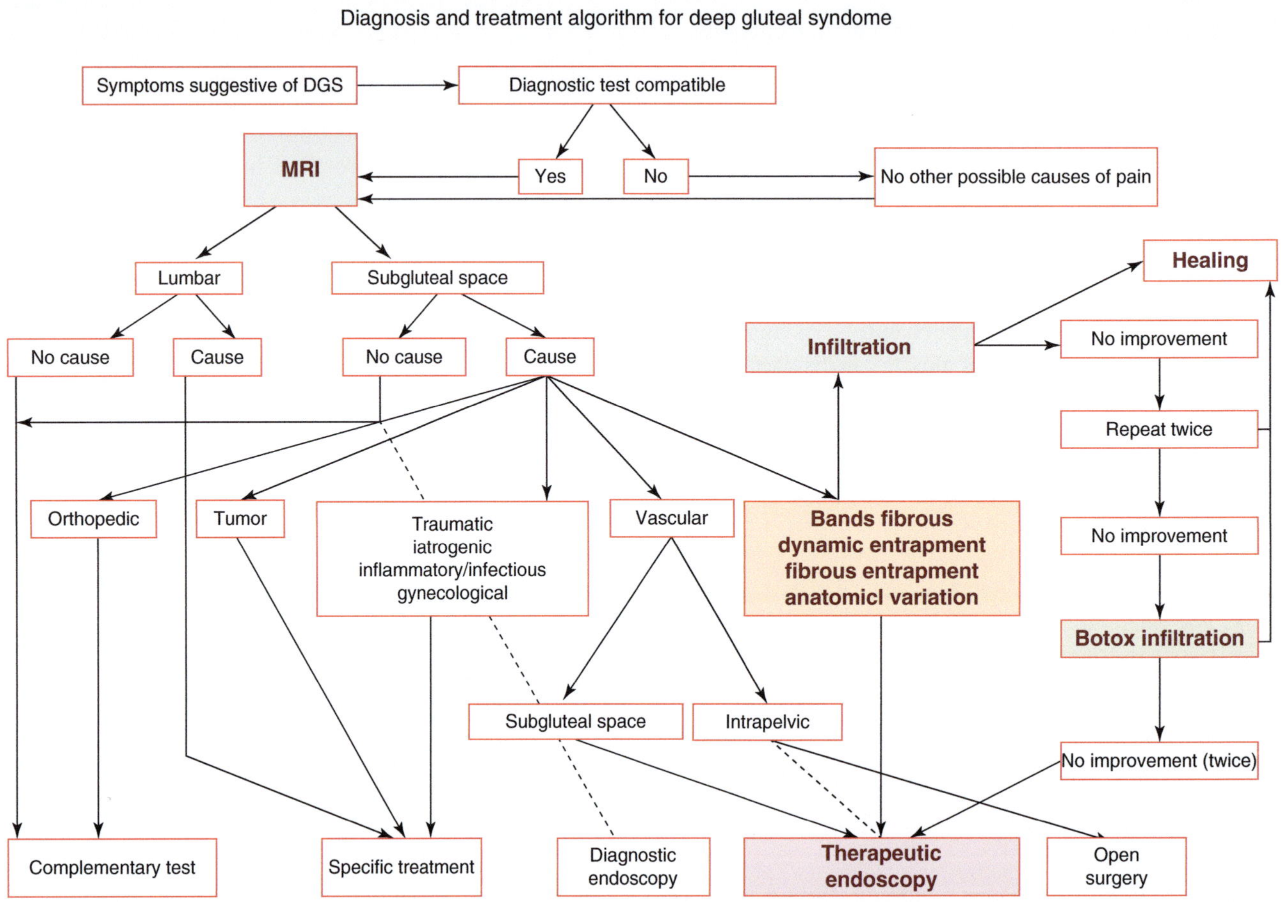

sound guided injections can give hint to the operative outcome (Table 5.1).

Instruments/Equipment/Implants Required

- 70° arthroscope. Sometimes, extra-long scope is needed for large sized patients.
- Arthroscopic shaver or dissection scissors.
- Radiofrequency probe. It is important to keep the irrigation fluid flow during utilization of the radiofrequency probe. The temperature profile during activation of a monopolar radiofrequency device was confirmed to be safe at a distance of 3–10 mm from the sciatic nerve with activation times of 3, 5, and 10 s [10]. The standard radiofrequency mode for vessel cauterization is a 3 s interval of activation with continuous irrigation.
- Fluoroscopy. Frequent confirmation of proper position of the endoscopic view by intra-operative fluoroscopy is important.

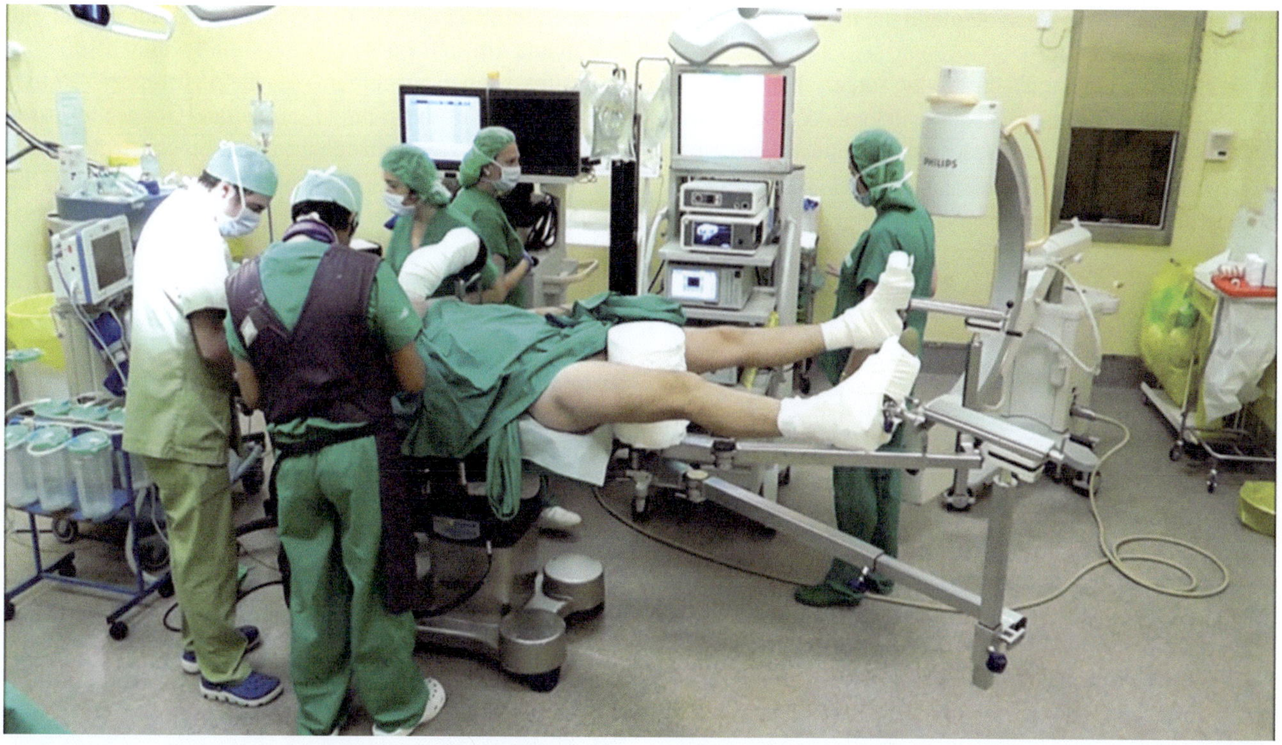

Fig. 5.2 Patient positioning: The patient is positioned supine in a traction table with standard preparation for hip arthroscopy. Traction is not applied and there is 20° of contralateral tilt. The leg (Right in this case) is position in 15–20° abduction and 20–40° internal rotation in order to open the space between the iliotibial band and the greater trochanter

5.1.4.2 Patient Positioning

- The patient is positioned supine in a traction table with standard preparation for hip arthroscopy. No traction is applied and there is 20° of contralateral tilt (Fig. 5.2).
- The operated hip is positioned in 15–20° abduction and 20–40° internal rotation so that the space between the greater trochanter and the iliotibial band (ITB) is opened up.
- If indicated, the procedure may be performed concomitant to a central and/or peripheral compartments hip arthroscopy. However, if possible, it is better to perform the hip arthroscopy in the other operation settings so that post-operative sciatic nerve stretch injury by traction during hip arthroscopy can be avoided.

5.1.4.3 Portals Design

- The subgluteal space is the posterior extension of the peritrochanteric space between the greater trochanter and the iliotibial band. Therefore, access to this space is gained through those portals traveling through the peritrochanteric space. Two groups of portals can be used to approach the peritrochanteric space: (1) standard anterolateral, anterior, and posterolateral hip arthroscopy portals redirected to the peritrochanteric space and (2) the proximal anterolateral accessory portal, distal anterolateral accessory portal, peritrochanteric space portal, and auxiliary posterolateral portal specifically designed for access of the peritrochanteric space [11] Auxiliary distal portals at the level of the lesser trochanter are crucial for endo-

scopic treatment of Ischiofemoral impingement (IFI) [12] (Figs. 5.3 and 5.4).
- We interchange portals during the surgery but for instrumentation we use proximal anterolateral accessory portal, distal anterolateral accessory portal, and auxiliary posterolateral portal. The viewing portal is usually the peritrochanteric portal.

5.1.4.4 Step-by-Step Description of the Technique

Approach to Peritrochanteric Space

- The peritrochanteric space portal is made first. A 5.0-mm metallic cannula is placed between the ITB and the lateral aspect of the greater trochanter, and the cannula tip can be swept proximally and distally to ensure proper placement of the instrument. Proper positioning of the cannula immediately over the vastus ridge of the greater trochanter can be confirmed fluoroscopically (Fig. 5.5). Endoscopic examination of the space starts from the gluteus maximus insertion at the linea aspera (Fig. 5.6). It may need to remove the fibrous tissue bands in this in order to visualize the coalescence.

Distal Dissection

- Sciatic nerve decompression should be started at distal site and proximal nerve decompression should only be performed after complete distal decompression. Inspection of the sciatic nerve starts distal to the quadra-

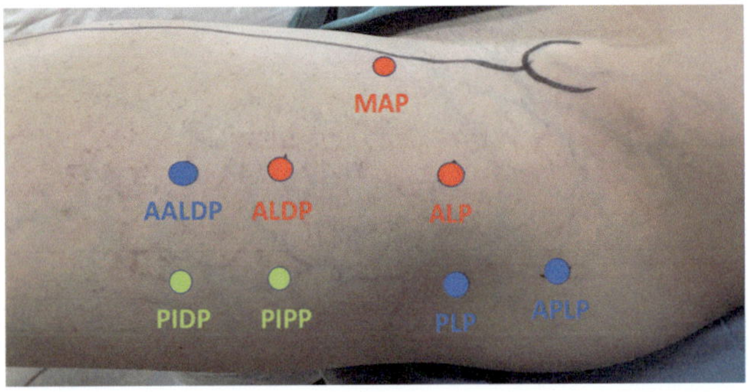

Fig. 5.3 Left gluteal region showing portal placement for subgluteal endoscopy. Midanterior portal (MAP). Accessory anterolateral distal portal (AALDP). Anterolateral distal portal (ALDP). Anterolateral portal (ALP). Posterolateral portal (PLP). Auxiliary posterolateral portal (APLP). Auxiliary distal portals at the level of the lesser trochanter (Ischiofemoral impingement (IFI) portals) are crucial for ischiofemoral impingement decompression. Posterior ischiofemoral distal portal (PIDP). Posterior ischiofemoral proximal portal (PIPP)

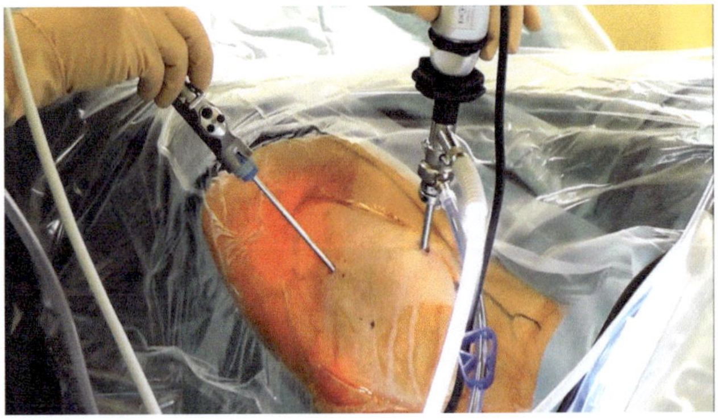

Fig. 5.5 Left Hip. Approach to peritrochanteric space. The midanterior portal is the viewing portal and the anterolateral distal portal is the working portal

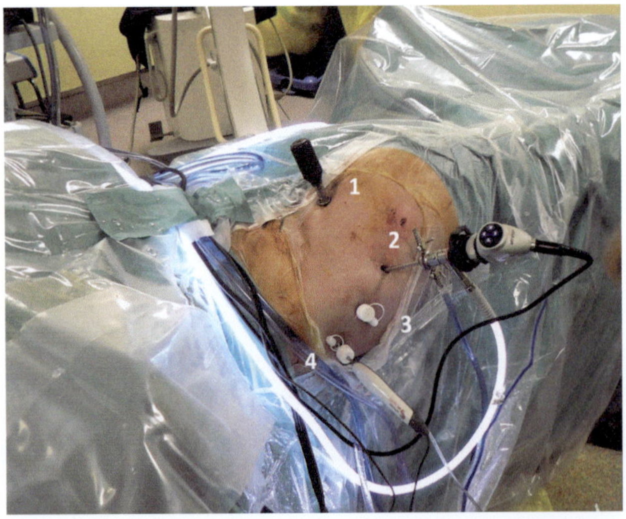

Fig. 5.4 Right gluteal region showing portal placement for subgluteal endoscopy. (1) Midanterior portal, (2) anterolateral distal portal, (3) posterolateral portal, (4) auxiliary posterolateral portal

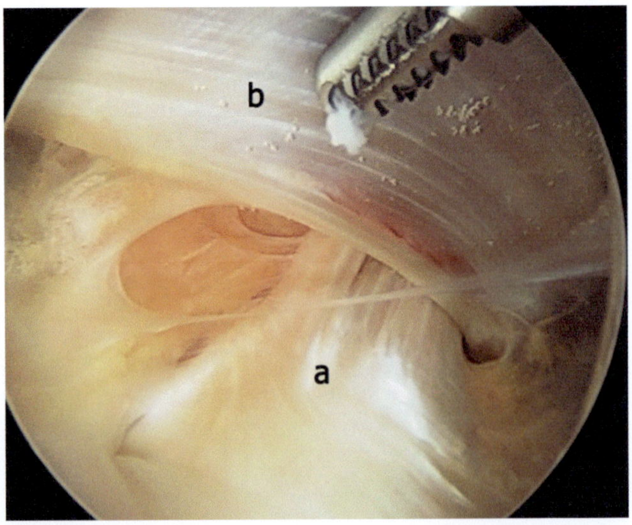

Fig. 5.6 Endoscopic view right hip. The peritrochanteric portal is the viewing portal. Endoscopic assessment begins at the gluteus maximus insertion at the linea aspera. (**a**) Gluteus maximus insertion, (**b**) Vastus lateralis

tus femoris, just above the gluteal sling (Fig. 5.7). The ischial tunnel hamstring origin and sacrotuberous ligament is inspected and any fibrous adhesions should be released from the sciatic nerve. The lateral, medial, and retrosciatic aspects of the sciatic nerve should be examined to ensure complete distal release and the posterior cutaneous nerve should be identified. A blunt dissector, e.g. a switching rod, can be used for adhesiolysis of the sciatic nerve and determine tension of the nerve (Fig. 5.8).

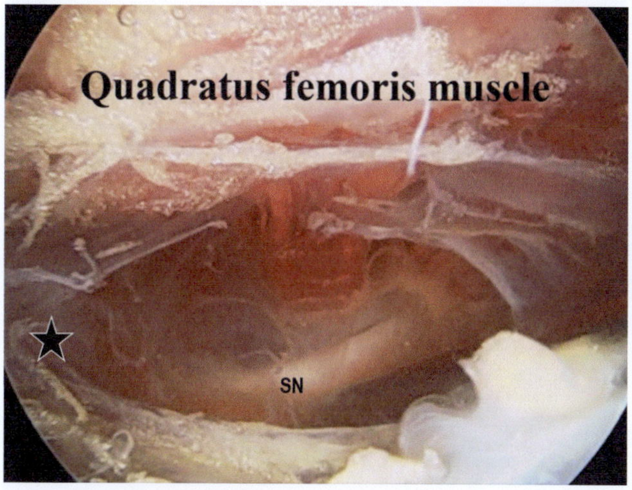

Fig. 5.7 Right hip. Inspection of the sciatic nerve starts distal to the quadratus femoris, just above the gluteal sling. The portion of the sciatic nerve posterior to the quadratus femoris is visualized and the color of the nerve, the epineural blood flow, and the epineural fat is noted. *SN* Sciatic nerve. Black star: Distal

- The portion of the sciatic nerve posterior to the quadratus femoris is examined for its color, epineural blood flow, and epineural fat. Noticeable epineural blood flow and epineural fat can be observed in normal sciatic nerve, whereas an abnormal sciatic nerve will appear white and lack of epineural blood flow. The epineural fat in many cases is diminished or completely obliterated. Whenever possible, the epineural fat should be preserved during nerve dissection [13].

Lesser Trochanter Approach for IFI Syndrome

- The operative goal in IFI syndrome is to re-establish a normal ischiofemoral space (IFS) and a complete resection of the lesser trochanter may not be needed. The posterolateral trans-quadratus approach seems to be the most appropriate approach to achieve this goal [6, 12]. Assessment of the sciatic nerve and hamstring repair if indicated can also be performed via this approach.

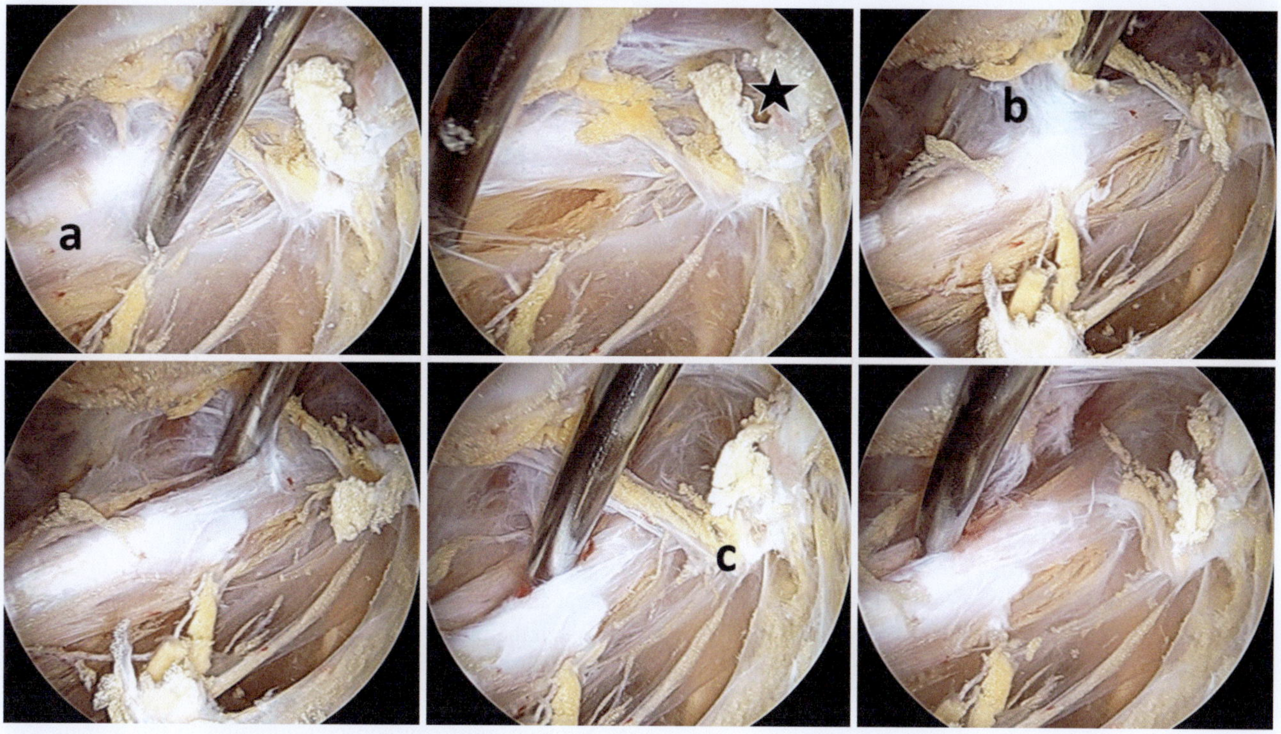

Fig. 5.8 Left hip. Sciatic nerve release. A blunt dissector, such as a switching stick, can be employed for release of scar bands expose the sciatic nerve and determine the tension. (**a**) Sciatic nerve, (**b**) Adhesive band or horse-strap bands (type 2), (**c**) Compressive or bridge-type bands (type 1). Black star: Proximal

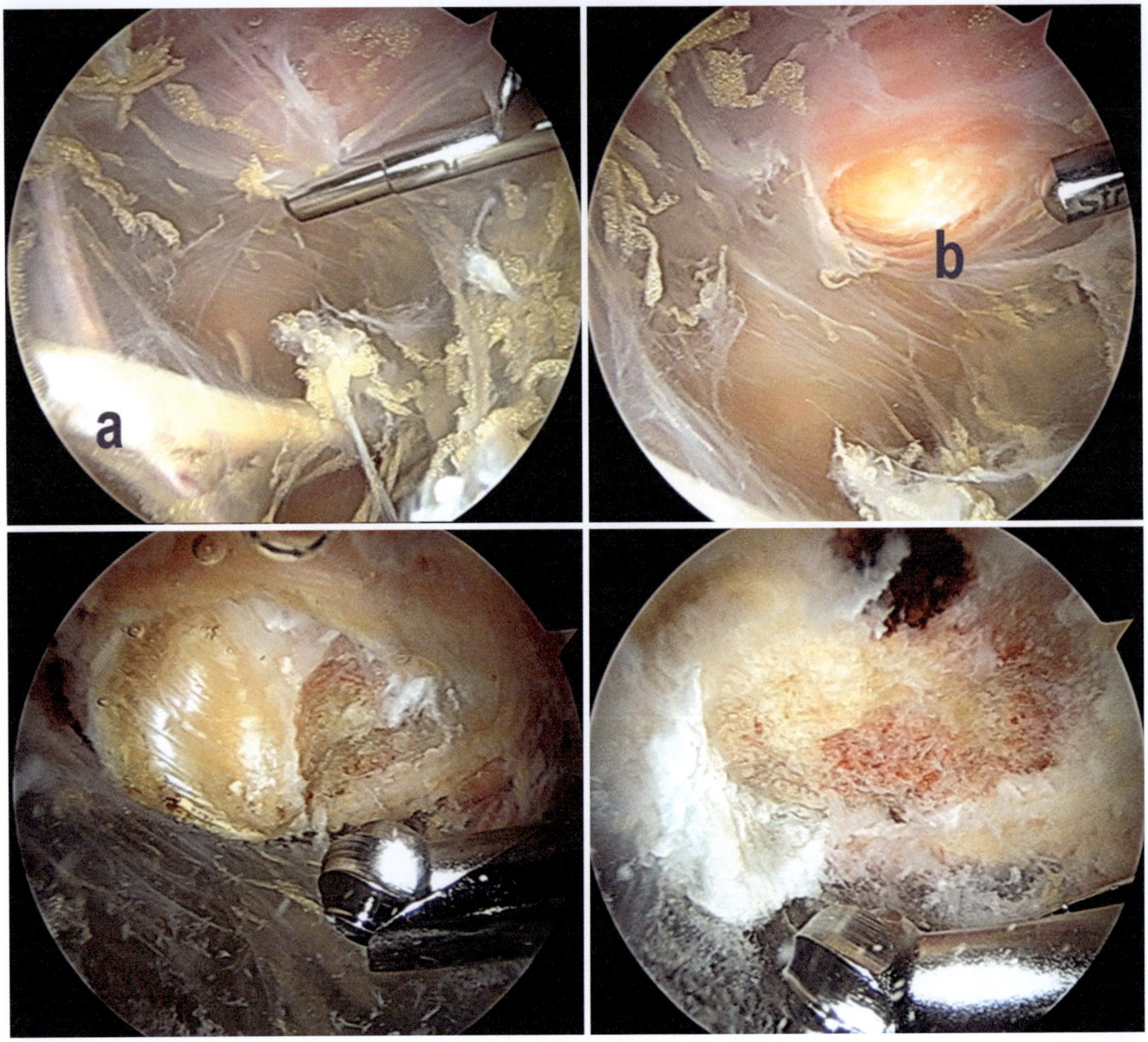

Fig. 5.9 Right hip. Endoscopic view showing ischiofemoral impingement decompression. Access to resection of the lesser trochanter through the posterolateral trans-quadratus approach. (**a**) Sciatic nerve, (**b**) Lesser trochanter

- The lesser trochanter can be approached through a small window in the quadratus femoris muscle (Fig. 5.9). This window is located between the medial circumflex femoral artery (proximal) and first perforating femoral artery (distal). The proximal and distal edges of the muscle should be preserved in order to avoid injury to these arteries. Ischioplasty when needed can also be performed via this approach. The aim of the osteoplasty of the posterior one-third of the lesser trochanter is to obtain an IFS of 17 mm or more, preserving non-impinging bone and the iliopsoas insertion.

Proximal Dissection

- Dissection can be proceeded proximally after the distal dissection. The arthroscope is rotated proximally and the vastus lateralis fibers are identified and can be traced toward its insertion on the vastus tubercle. The scope is rotated anteriorly and superiorly, and the gluteus minimus tendon is seen anteriorly. When the scope is advanced anteriorly over the gluteus minimus, the gluteus medius tendon and its attachment to the greater trochanter can be seen.
- Finally, the piriformis muscle can be seen, and any abnormal anatomical variants of the muscle are identified.
- When the piriformis tendon is located, the tendons of the gemellus and obturator internus muscles can be possibly identified.
- Surgeon must pay constant attention to the branches of the inferior gluteal artery which are in vicinity of the piriformis muscle. Looking back proximally, in the region of the obturator internus a superficial arterial branch of the

inferior gluteal artery crosses the sciatic nerve laterally between the piriformis and superior gemellus muscles and must be cauterized and released with a radiofrequency probe prior to inspection of the piriformis. Sometimes, a large vessel or a confluence of vessels is present and ligation of the vessels is required.

- In many cases, a thick tendon can be present in the deep surface of the piriformis muscle belly and overlies the sciatic nerve. The lower border of the piriformis muscle can be shaved with an arthroscopic shaver in order to expose the piriformis tendon.
- The tendon is then carefully grasped with an arthroscopic scissors and the scissors is pulled laterally along the tendon towards its insertion at the greater trochanter. This maneuver can ensure that only the tendon is released.
- Alternatively, the tendon can be released by a radiofrequency probe with a 3 s interval of activation and continuous irrigation (Fig. 5.10).
- The possible variations of anatomical relationship between the piriformis muscle and the sciatic nerve should be identified (Beton and Anson classification types B-F).
- The possible anatomical variations of obturator internus should also be checked and released if it is found to compress on the sciatic nerve. Finally, the nerve is probed up to the sciatic notch.
- The sciatic nerve is then assessed dynamically with internal/external rotation motion in flexed and fully extended positions of the operated hip. The kinematic excursion of the nerve is assessed and the presence of any dynamic nerve impingement is noted.

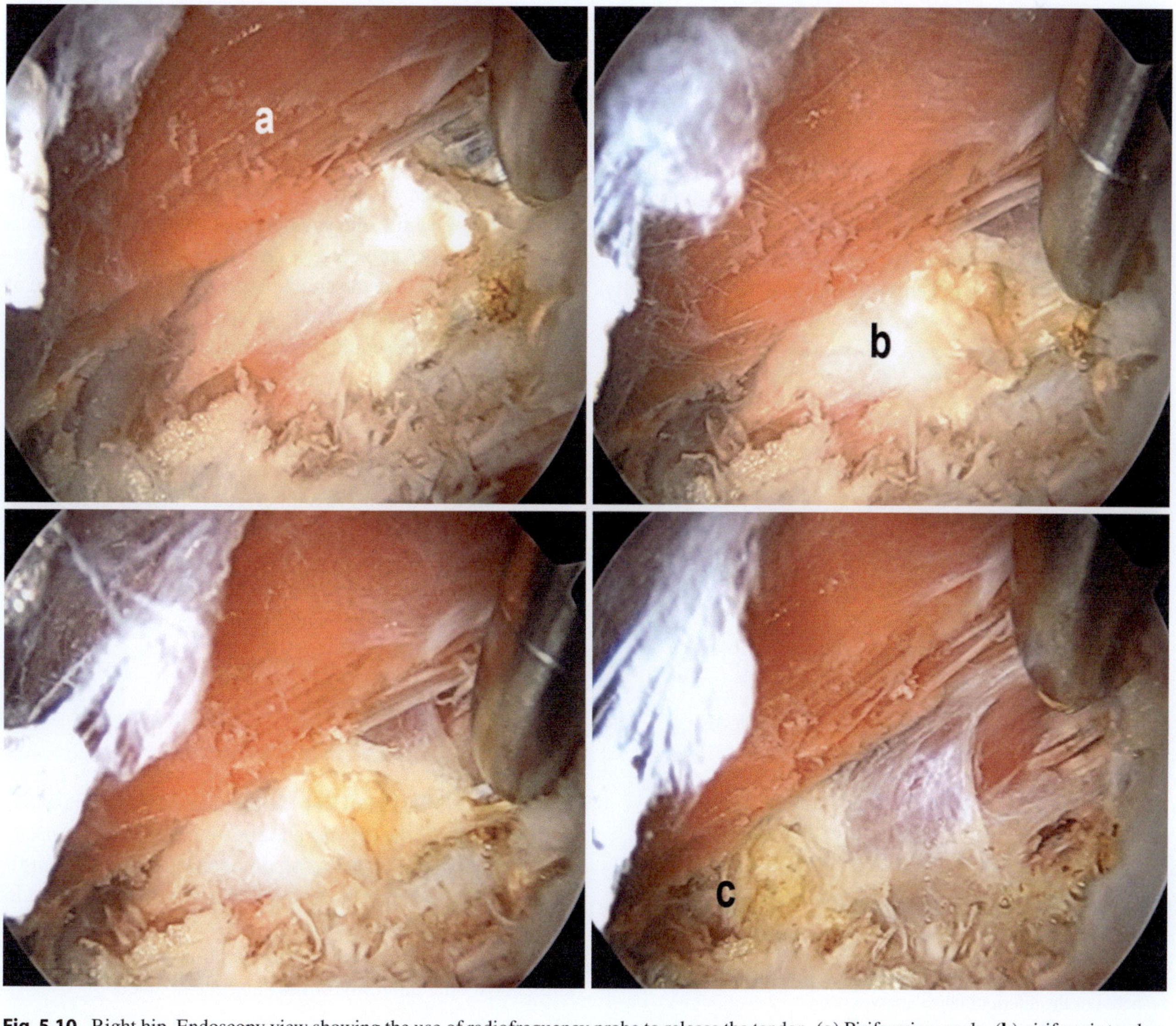

Fig. 5.10 Right hip. Endoscopy view showing the use of radiofrequency probe to release the tendon. (**a**) Piriformis muscle, (**b**) piriformis tendon, (**c**) stump of the piriformis tendon after tenotomy

5.1.4.5 Complications and Management

- Complications include hematoma collection as a result of early post-operative NSAIDs utilization and excessive post-operative activity. This risk can be minimized by usage of tranexamic acid with the same protocol as in hip and knee arthroplasty and keeping the drain for post-operative 18 h (Fig. 5.11).
- The most significant complication is damage to the sciatic nerve. Scar formation around the nerve can be controlled with antiadhesions gels in order to prevent painful scar neuropathy.
- Another significant complication is abdominal (retroperitoneal) fluid extravasation. This risk can be minimized by keeping the fluid inflow pressure to a minimum while allows the endoscopic work. If no clinical contra-indication, hypotensive anaesthesia can be adopted to allow good endoscopic visualization under low pressure fluid inflow. Other safety measures include constant monitoring of the patient by the anaesthetists to look for any signs of abdominal (retroperitoneal) fluid distension or any drop in body temperature.

5.1.4.6 Post-operative Care

- The aim of post-operative rehabilitation is to improve mobility and maintain hip range of motion. Any type of stretching of the sciatic nerve that may lead to neuralgia or neuropraxia should be avoided. The rehabilitation course for patient to return to previous activity usually takes about 24 weeks to be completed. The degree of safe excursion of the sciatic nerve is determined by the hip and knee positions. With the hip in flexion, abduction and external rotation, the sciatic nerve tends to slide along the posterior border of the greater trochanter [14]. Passive hip circumduction exercise with the hip in 45 degrees flexion and maximal external rotation can be started on post-operative Day 1. This hip position engages the greater trochanter against the ischium and mobilizes the sciatic nerve laterally. The knee should be flexed during the curcumduction exercise to relax the sciatic nerve tensión. Nervce gliding and piriformis stretching exercises can be done as pain tolerated. Standard physiotherapy protocol can be started as early as post-operative 6 weeks.

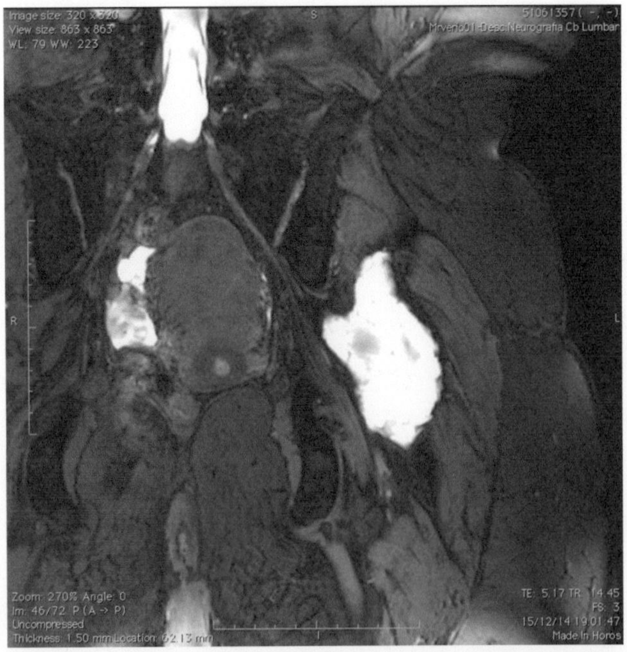

Fig. 5.11 Hematoma in the left deep gluteal space due to bleeding of branches of the inferior gluteal artery

5.1.4.7 Outcome

- Overall, 33 studies evaluating the operative (Open and endoscopic) management of deep gluteal syndrome were identified in the literature [15–17].
- Although most of the identified studies were case reports and series, the reported operative outcome consistently showed improvement in pain and a low incidence of complications, particularly for endoscopic surgery.
- The incidence of complications from these procedures was low. Overall, the incidence of major complications including deep infection is less than 1% in open procedures and 0% in endoscopic procedures. The incidence of minor complications is 8% in open procedures and less than 1% in endoscopic procedures.
- We have reviewed and evaluated our results and endoscopic findings of 52 patients (52 hips) (38 female −14 male) (28 right −24 left) with deep gluteal syndrome treated by endoscopic sciatic nerve release in the subgluteal space between November 2011 and April 2015. 39 patients reported good to excellent results. The averaged mHHS improved from 52 to 79 after surgery. 13 patients reported to have symptoms improved but not to the degree of good outcome and need to continue narcotic use after surgery [6].

5.1.5 Summary

There is an explosion of knowledge related to the diagnosis and treatment of the disease entities in the subgluteal space.

Endoscopic sciatic nerve decompression is a useful surgical approach to improve function and diminish hip pain in subgluteal sciatic nerve entrapments but requires significant hip arthroscopy experience with familiarity with the gross and endoscopic anatomy of the subgluteal space.

5.2 Endoscopic Management of Piriformis Syndrome

Victor M. Ilizaliturri Jr, Ruben Arriaga and Carlos Suarez-Ahedo

5.2.1 Introduction

Piriformis syndrome (PS) can be defined as the compression or the irritation of the sciatic nerve by the adjacent piriformis muscle in the gluteal area [18]. This compression of the sciatic nerve leads a cause of Non-discogenic Sciatica [19]. Previously it has been shown that it accounts from 0.3% to 6.0% of all reported cases of sciatica and low back pain [19]. However, Piriformis Syndrome (PS) is a cause of Deep Gluteal Syndrome (DGS), because the entrapment of the sciatic nerve has been commonly attributed to compression from fibrovascular structures, the muscle/tendon complex of the piriformis, obturator internus/gemelli and/or proximal hamstrings.

Freiberg et al. [20] proposed the compression of the nerve trunk by the piriformis muscle, later in 1974 Robinson [21] coined the term piriformis syndrome.

More recently, Martin et al. [22] have described a detailed clinical history and diagnostic tests for this condition.

Literature on PS, sciatica and other conditions associated with low back pain or posterior buttock pain, is vast and it is apparent that there are still issues of uncertainty and controversy related to the proper diagnosis and treatment of this condition [23–27].

Decompression of the sciatic nerve at the level of the piriformis muscle has been described as treatment for symptomatic sciatic nerve entrapment. This has been done traditionally through an open posterior approach with varying results [22]. More recently endoscopic decompression and neurolysis of the sciatic nerve has been described positioning the patient in supine position using anterior lateral and posterior lateral portals with standard and 70° arthroscopes [27–30]. Jackson in 2016 [31] described an Endoscopic Sciatic Nerve Decompression in the Prone Position. The lateral decubitus position has been described by Ilizaliturri et al. [32] and Knudsen et al. [33].

5.2.2 Endoscopic Decompression

Endoscopic Decompression is an effective approach that allows the treatment of deep gluteal syndrome [34]. Many advantages have been described for this technique compared with the open surgical technique, however, requires a high level of arthroscopic proficiency.

5.2.3 Indication

Surgery is indicated when pain is not relieved by conservative measures, including physical activity change, physical therapy, local steroid injections on the piriformis muscle, for at least 3 months [35].

5.2.4 Contra-Indication

Moreover, not all patients with are good surgical candidates; therefore, it is important to understand, on the basis of the cause and investigations, which patients benefit most from surgical management. The most common contra-indications are the presence of lumbar spine pathology that originates of the sciatic pain (disc hernia), sciatic nerve entrapment before the exit through the sciatic notch, intraabdominal pathology that compresses the sciatic nerve.

5.2.5 Surgical Technique

Positioning of the patient depends on surgeon's preference. Hip traction is not usually needed, but if hip arthroscopy is required, it is recommended to perform before sciatic neurolysis [33]. Nerve conduction and EMG are usually monitored intraoperatively and can demonstrate changes and improvement after sciatic nerve decompression [36]. The operative side is prepared

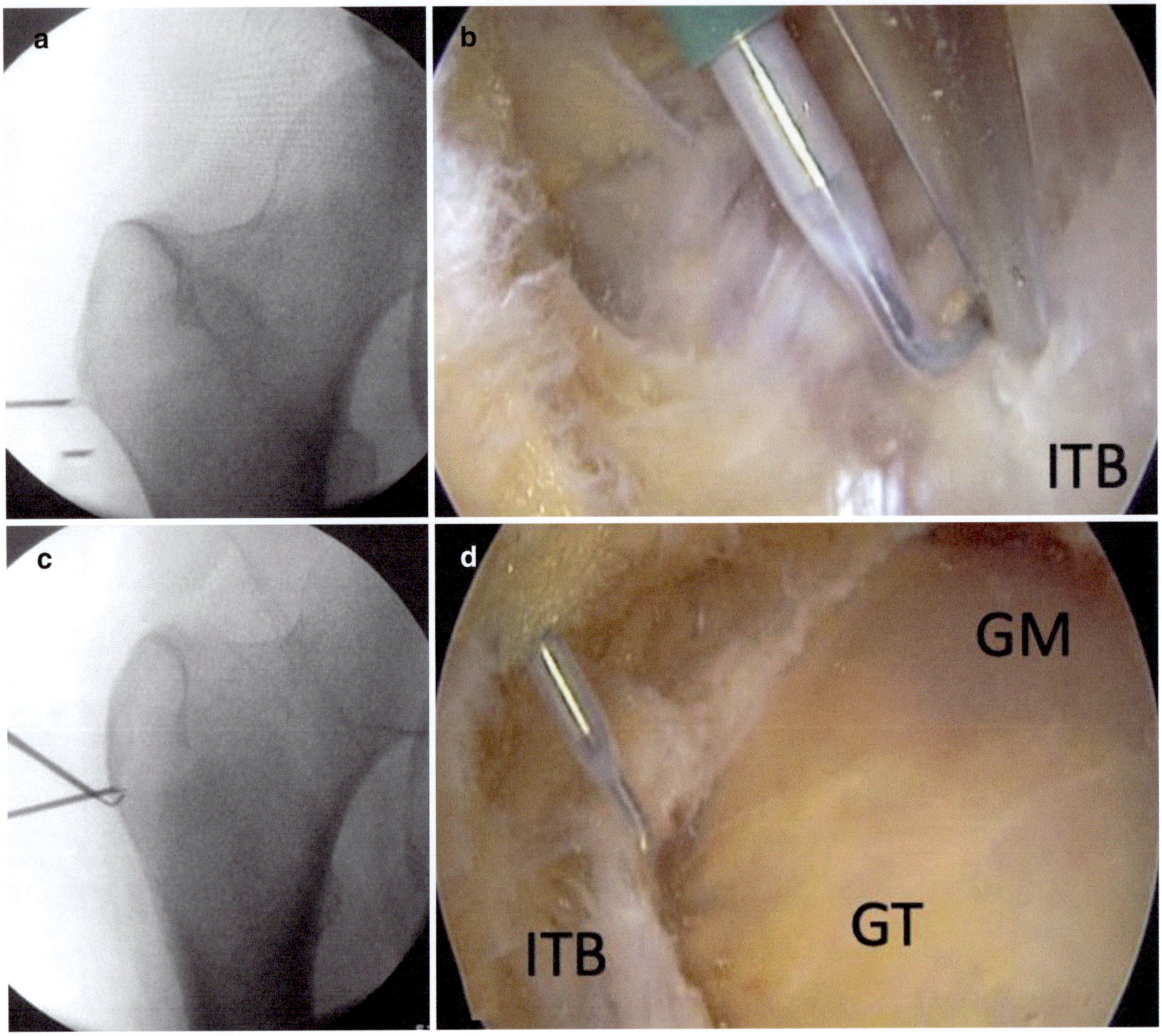

Fig. 5.12 (**a**) Fluoroscopic view of the spinal needle positioned over the Great Trochanter (GT) Right Hip. (**b**) Endoscopic view of the entry point of the needle over the Iliotibial band (ITB), a radiofrequency hook probe is in position to release the ITB. (**c**) Fluoroscopic view of the radiofrequency hook probe beside the needle before release the ITB. (**d**) Endoscopic view of an oval window was performed on the ITB. The GT and gluteus medius (GM) are observed through the defect

and draped to allow for free mobility of the lower extremity. The greater trochanter is marked on the skin and a spinal needle is positioned at the lateral aspect of the greater trochanter using fluoroscopy (Fig. 5.12). A "10-step technique" described by Martin [36] allows for a complete and safe sciatic nerve decompression. Two portals are usually needed (anterolateral and posterolateral portals for supine position, posterosuperior and posteroinferior portals for lateral decubitus position) and a third portal (auxiliary portal) can be used.

A standard length 4.0 mm 30-degrees arthroscope is introduced at the peritrochanteric space. A shaver is introduced to perform the bursectomy and inflow with saline is started with the pump varying from 30 mmHg to 60 mmHg [32, 33, 36]. Hemostasis using a radiofrequency wand is performed during this step. Once the Quadratus femoris is clearly identified (internal rotation of the hip during this step facilitate adequate identification). Fluoroscopy can be used to confirm the position at the piriformis tendon insertion and it can be released (Fig. 5.13). Blunt dissection following the obturator internus muscle is performed until the sciatic nerve is identified. Flexion and extension of the hip is carried out to confirm mobility of the sciatic nerve. Endoscopic neurolysis is performed if indicated. The fibrovascular bands and adhesions compressing or restricting mobility of the sciatic nerve are identified, gently dissected and resected using the radiofrequency ablation device, shaver or arthroscopic scissors. Dynamic evaluation of sciatic nerve kinematics with direct visualization is performed at this step to verify the complete sciatic neurolysis (fluoroscopy can be used) (Fig. 5.14). Finally, hemostasis is verified, arthroscopic fluid can be removed by placing a spinal needle at a safe distance from the nerve [33] and the portal incisions are closed and draped.

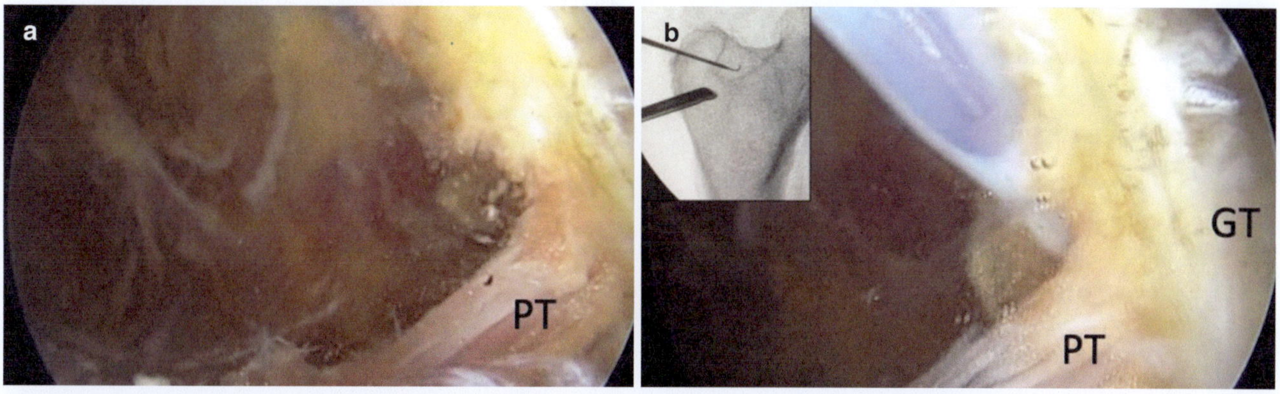

Fig. 5.13 Endoscopic view of the release of the Piriformis tendon (PT). (**a**) Insertion of the PT on the GT. (**b**) A radiofrequency hook probe is utilized to release the PT from the back of the GT. The fluoroscopic image shows the position of the radiofrequency hook probe and the arthroscope in relation with the GT

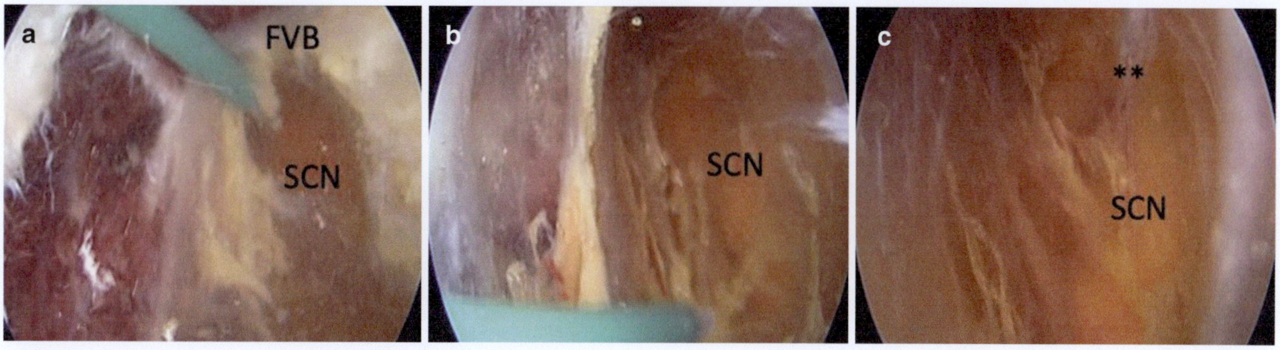

Fig. 5.14 (**a**, **b**) Endoscopic view of the Sciatic Nerve (SCN) entrapped in a Fibrovascular Band (FVB). (**b**) As a radiofrequency hook probe is used to release the FVB. (**c**) After decompression of the sciatic nerve the FVB are no longer observed and vasa-nervorum is observed (double asterisk) on the SCN after the decompression

5.2.6 Summary

With recent advances in hip arthroscopy and better understanding of PS, reports in the literature are varied, most are case reports and small series with variable results. The largest cohorts were published by Fishman et al. [27], Indrekvam & Sudmann [37], Benson & Schutzer [38], and Filler [39]. The results from these 4 studies, respectively, showed an improvement achieving more than 50% symptom relief. Endoscopic decompression of sciatic nerve allows improved visualization and less soft tissue and muscle damage. However, previous training in cadavers before practicing the endoscopic technique in patients is mandatory to minimize damage to the important arteriovenous and neural structures.

Pearls and Pitfalls of the endoscopic release of the piriformis tendon and sciatic nerve exploration
Lateral release of the piriformis tendon (at its insertion on the greater trochanter) indicated in the case of a single sciatic nerve that passes deeply to the muscle belly of the piriformis.
When the sciatic nerve pierces through the muscle belly of the piriformis it must be released at the site of compression; the same is true for a bifurcated nerve that passes around or pierces the muscle belly of the piriformis.
Adequate hemostasis is mandatory at every step of the procedure to obtain an adequate view of every structure.
The pump pressure is initially set at 30 mmHg but can be safely increased to 80 mmHg.
Nerve monitoring may be needed at least for the initial learning curve for this procedure.
Fluoroscopy guidance is advisable.
Inexperience with proximal GT anatomy can negatively affect the outcome

5.3 Endoscopic Management of Ischiofemoral Impingement

Tiao Su and Guangxing Chen

5.3.1 Introduction

Ischiofemoral impingement (IFI) is characterized by the narrowing space between the lesser trochanter (LT) and the lateral border of the ischium leading to the entrapment of soft tissue structure like quadratus femoris, hamstring and sciatic nerve, etc. Although it was first described 40 years ago, IFI commonly remained misdiagnosed in clinical experience because it is a rare cause of hip pain [40, 41].

The management of patients diagnosed with IFI ranges between conservative treatment and surgical procedures [41, 42]. Patients who failed conservative treatments such as physiotherapy or activity modification often requires surgical management. Excision of the LT using an open approach is a classic operative procedure for IFI to restore normal ischiofemoral space (IFS) and quadratus femoris space (QFS) [42]. However, with the development of endoscopic techniques and devices, some authors recently recommended the entire procedure being operated endoscopically [12, 43, 44].

To sum up, the accuracy of diagnose of patients with suspected IFI depends on a comprehensive history, clinical evaluation, and radiologic assessment. The management options consist of conservative treatment and surgical procedures.

5.3.2 Indications

Patients with posterior hip pain who meet all of the following criteria:

- IFS ≤ 17 mm and QFS ≤ 8 mm.
- Soft tissue involvement: quadratus femoris edema, hamstring tendonitis, ischial bursitis, and sciatic nerve irritation
- Physical examination: irritated posterolateral hip pain with adduction and extension.
- Eliminate other intra-articular and intra-pelvic etiologies for posterior hip symptom.
- Failed conservative treatments for 3 months.

5.3.3 Contra-Indications

- Severe osteoporosis
- Local infection

5.3.4 Author Preferred Technique *(Anterior Approach)*

5.3.4.1 Pre-operative Planning

- Required instruments: 70-degree high-definition arthroscope, lightweight camera, shaver system, pump system, probe, arthroscopic burr, high-flow endoscopic sheath, and an arthroscopic radiofrequency system.

5.3.4.2 Patient Positioning

- The patient is placed supine on a hip distraction table. The involved hip is positioned in 50° of flexion, 20° adduction, and maximal external rotation. The contralateral hip is abducted and externally rotated (Fig. 5.15).

5.3.4.3 Portal Design

- Two portals are used: proximal anterolateral and distal (Fig. 5.16). Proximal anterolateral portal is placed 2 cm

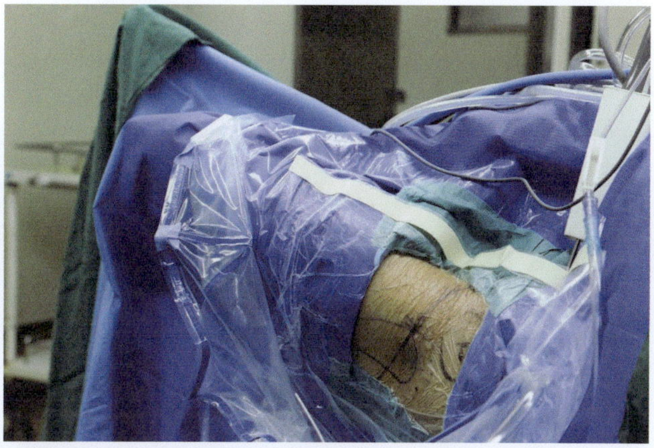

Fig. 5.15 Patient positioning for IFI: hip flexion, adduction, and maximal external rotation

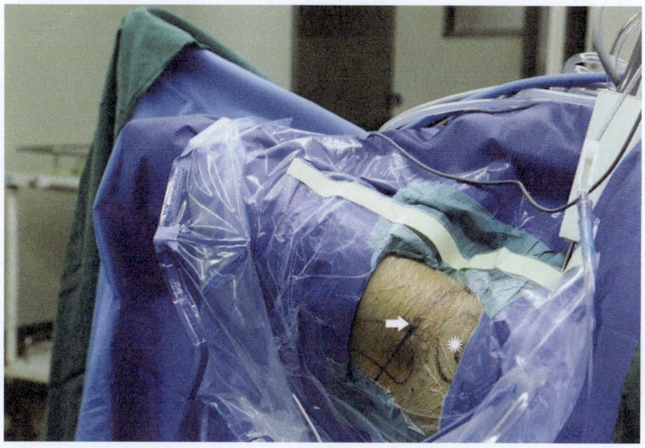

Fig. 5.16 Arthroscopic portals for the access to lesser trochanter: proximal anterolateral (star) and distal (arrow) portal

anterior and 2 cm superior to the tip of the greater trochanter. Distal portal is the main operation portal which is placed 3–5 cm distally to the proximal anterolateral portal.

5.3.4.4 Step-by-Step Description of the Technique

- A 70° arthroscope is inserted into the proximal anterolateral portal, while the distal accessory portal is primarily responsible for operative procedure like probing or recontouring with a burr.
- Partially detach the distal iliopsoas tendon insertion. 60% of the iliopsoas insertion is tendinous and 40% of the insertion is muscular. The tendinous part is released to expose the LT while the muscular insertion is left intact (Fig. 5.17).
- Resect the entire lesser trochanter with arthroscopic burr to restore a functionally normal ischiofemoral space (Fig. 5.18).

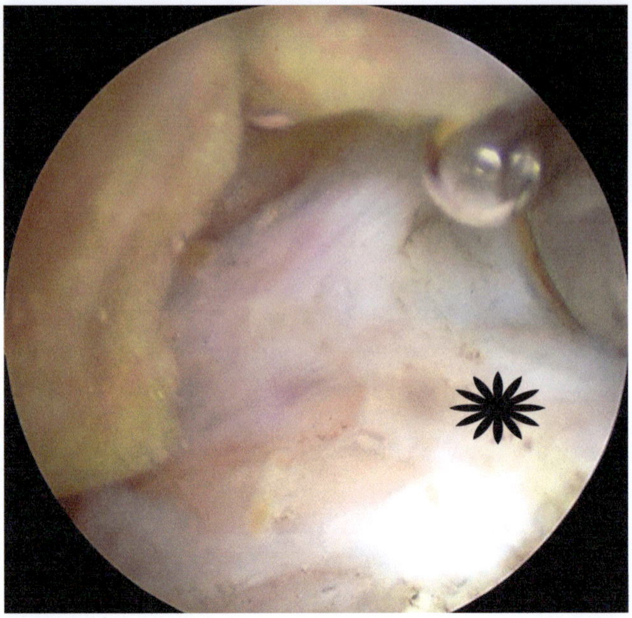

Fig. 5.17 Arthroscopic image of the iliopsoas tendon (star), which is partially resected for the access to lesser trochanter

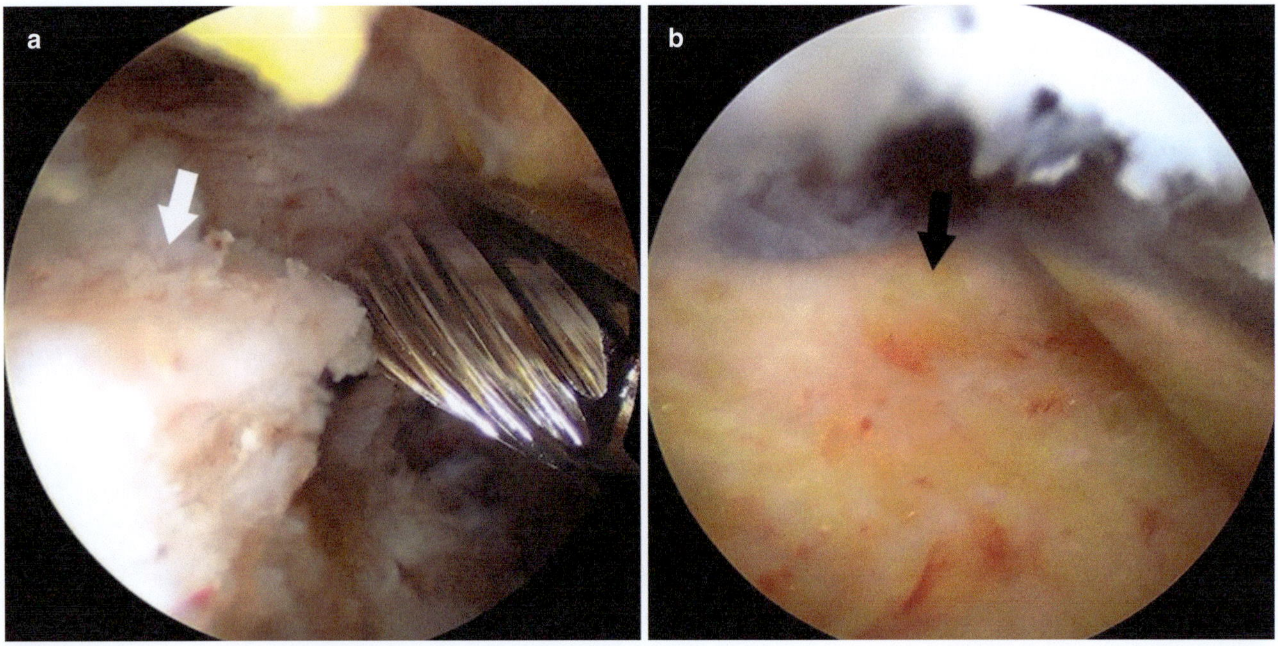

Fig. 5.18 Arthroscopic images of the lesser trochanter (**a**) before and (**b**) after osteoplasty. The lesser trochanter (white arrow) should be leveled to the surrounding medial femoral cortex (black arrow)

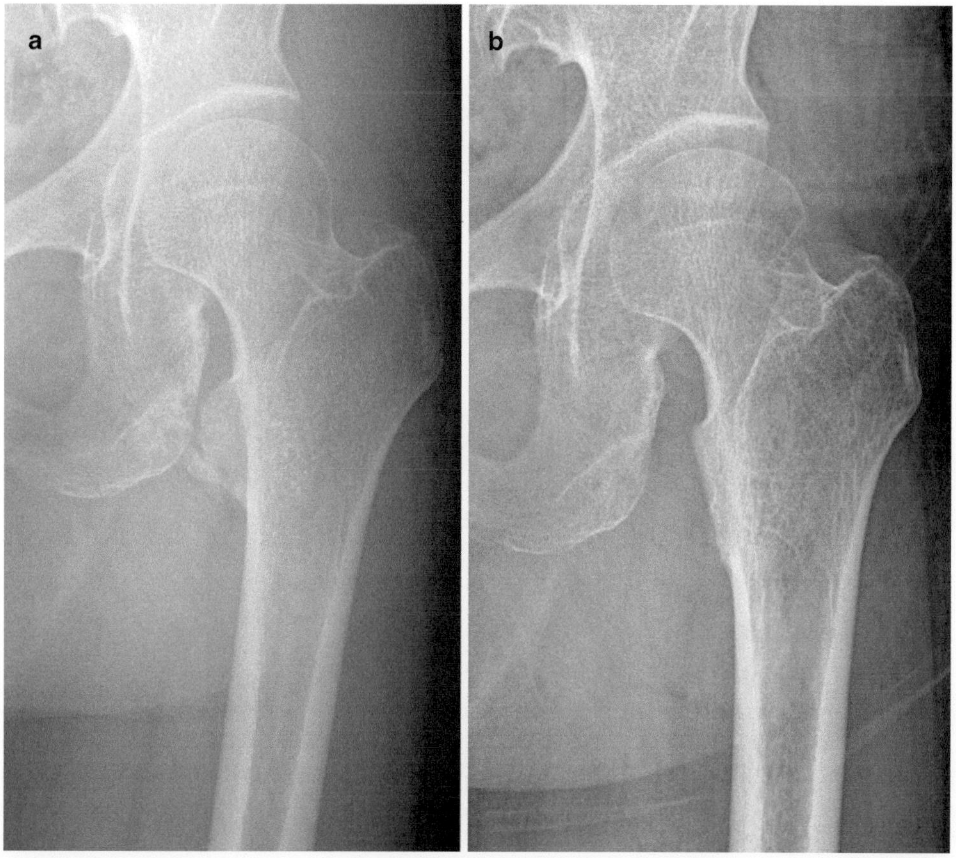

Fig. 5.19 Pre-operative (**a**) and post-operative (**b**) X-ray image showing adequate decompression of the lesser trochanter

- Use fluoroscopy to ensure adequate decompression of the lesser trochanter which should be leveled to the surrounding medial femoral cortex (Fig. 5.19).
- Dynamic examination of hip adduction-extension and internal-external rotation under fluoroscopy are performed to guarantee adequate lesser trochanter decompression.

5.3.4.5 Complications

- Hip flexor weakness which is able to restore due to the remaining intact iliopsoas tendon insertion.
- Femoral fracture if lesser trochanter is over resected.
- Neurovascular injury, which is rare.

5.3.4.6 Post-operative Care

- 20-lb flat-foot weightbearing using crutches for 2 weeks and then transited from partial to full weight bearing for the following 4 weeks.
- No straight leg raise training for 6 weeks to protect the remaining iliopsoas tendon insertion.
- No limitation of hip extension and abductor strengthening. Hip flexor strengthening is usually allowed 6 weeks post-operatively.

5.3.4.7 Outcome

- Endoscopic lesser trochanter decompression is able to relief patients' symptoms with rare complication for experienced hip arthroscopists.
- There are two approaches for endoscopic lesser trochanterplasty: anterior and posterior. Both approaches show successful outcome in various reports [12, 43–45].
- As previously described, the advantages of anterior approach are concluded as follow: (1) Resection of quadratus femoris is avoided. (2) It lowers the risk of injury of the medial femora circumflex artery and the sciatic nerve.
- Conversely, the advocates of posterior approach believe that it provides more direct exposure of the lesser trochanter, especially the posterior part. However, with sufficient

hip external rotation and abduction, the anterior approach is able to achieve the similar access.

- Consider that iliopsoas tendon is partially detached, the main concern of post-operative complication focuses on the reduction of hip flexion strength [46, 47]. Nonetheless, a recent study found no residual hip flexor weakness in 1-year follow-up post-operatively [46].
- To sum up, the anterior approach is safe and efficient due to decreased risk of neurovascular injury and the reproducible means for lesser trochanter osteoplasty and iliopsoas release for IFI.

5.3.5 Summary

With the imaging criteria being well-established, ischiofemoral impingement is diagnosed more frequently than ever. Surgical correction is recommended when conservative treatments fail, because it is safe and efficient with favorable outcome.

- Besides detailed pre-operative planning and adequate anatomy knowledge, sufficient surgical experience of the surgeon is required in order to achieve a good surgical outcome.

5.4 Endoscopic Hamstring Repair and Ischial Bursectomy

Yan Xu

5.4.1 Introduction

- Hamstring injuries are common among recreational and elite athletes, constituting up to 29% of all injuries in an array of sports. The overwhelming majority of hamstring injuries are muscle belly injuries, with only 3–11% of all hamstring injuries being proximal avulsions [48–50].
- The mechanism of injury for proximal avulsions is through an eccentric contraction of the hamstring with ipsilateral hip hyperflexion and knee extension, which typically occurs during sports that involve ballistic movements such as waterskiing [48, 49, 51].
- The hamstring muscle complex consists of the biceps femoris, semitendinosus, and semimembranosus, with the biceps femoris being the most frequently injured. The biceps femoris and semitendinosus arise from the inferomedial aspect of the ischial tuberosity as a conjoint tendon, and the semimembranosus originates anterolaterally on the lateral aspect of the ischium (Figs. 5.20 and 5.21) [52, 53].
- Hamstring injuries traditionally have been classified as mild (Grade I), moderate (Grade II), or severe (Grade III). Grade I injuries are characterized by overstretching with minimal loss of structural integrity of the musculotendinous unit. Grade II injuries are defined as partial or incomplete tears while Grade III injuries are complete ruptures [49, 54].
- Most hamstring strains respond well to nonsurgical treatment and do not require surgical intervention [49–51]. Proximal hamstring avulsions, however, have been shown to benefit from surgical management as compared with conservative treatment. Acute repairs are generally considered superior to chronic repairs [51, 55–59].
- Endoscopic proximal hamstring repair technique was first developed by Dierckman and Guanche in 2012, after which several modified techniques were subsequently described. Although studies comparing the outcomes of endoscopic hamstring repair with those of traditional open procedures are currently lacking, this technique has been shown to be an effective approach in pain relief and functional restoration [60–69].

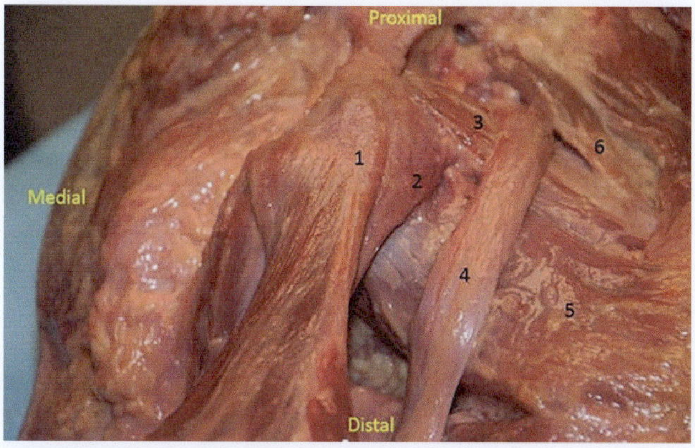

Fig. 5.20 Normal anatomy of proximal hamstring insertion sites, posterior view. *1* conjoined tendon, *2* semimembranosus tendon, *3* inferior gemellus, *4* sciatic nerve, *5* quadratus femoris, *6* piriformis (Reproduced from Philippon et al. [52])

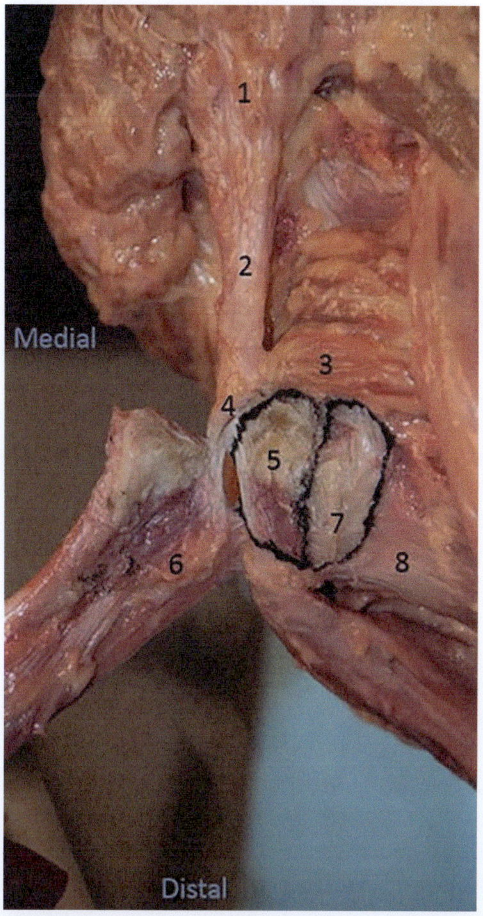

Fig. 5.21 Normal anatomy of proximal hamstring insertion sites, posterolateral view. *1* Sacrum, *2* sacrotuberous ligament, *3* inferior gemellus, *4* medial bony prominence, *5* conjoined footprint, *6* conjoined tendon (reflected), *7* semimembranosus footprint, *8* quadratus femoris (Reproduced from Philippon et al. [52])

5.4.2 Indications

- Three-tendon avulsion with or without retraction.
- Two-tendon avulsion with >2 cm of retraction.
- Persistent pain or weakness in partial tear despite extensive nonsurgical management [51, 60–69].

5.4.3 Contra-Indications

- Incision site infection
- Overt hemostatic abnormality

5.4.4 Author Preferred Technique

5.4.4.1 Pre-operative Planning

- A thorough evaluation of pertinent imaging studies, including plain X-rays and MRI, is required to rule out apophyseal avulsions and to assess for the degree of tear and presence of retraction.
- Required instruments: 30-degree arthroscope, extended-length arthroscopic cannulas, double- or triple-loaded suture anchors, wire passers, penetrators, needle-passing devices, and fluid inflow pump.
- Outline the ischium and mark portal sites in advance.

5.4.4.2 Patient Positioning

- The patient is positioned prone after the induction of anesthesia, with the operating table rotated 180° to place the head of the table at patient's caudal end. The non-operative foot is fixed to the operating table with a safety strap while the operative foot hangs freely over the table's distal edge for the time being.
- It is worth noting that the table is kept flat, as opposed to slight flexion for open techniques, in order to maintain the subgluteal space, which may be compromised by excessive flexion of the hip joint.
- Then, the operating table is tilted to the contralateral side for around 15° with the C-arm centered over the ischium, thus creating an en face image of the ischium by aligning the inferior pubic ramus with the ischium in the same perpendicular plane. The operative foot is then abducted 45° and placed on a well-padded sterile Mayo stand. This maneuver increases the distance between the sciatic nerve and the ischium and expands the volume of ischiofemoral space, thereby permitting a safer endoscopic working environment (Fig. 5.22). The operative hip and thigh are subsequently prepared and draped.
- The surgeon and assistant are positioned between the ipsilateral leg and operating table. The arthroscopic instruments are placed contralaterally.

5.4.4.3 Portal Design

- Four portals are used in this technique. The midcentral portal, which is located 2 cm distal to the inferior border of ischial tuberosity along the vertical axis through the center of the tuberosity, is made first. The medial portal is positioned 4 cm medial and 2 cm superior to the midcentral portal and is established second. The lateral portal is established next, which lies 4 cm lateral and 2 cm superior to the midcentral portal. Finally, the suture management portal is made 3 cm proximal to the midpoint of inferior border of the tuberosity along the vertical axis. This portal is primarily for suture management purposes, as its name indicates. Hence, it may be estab-

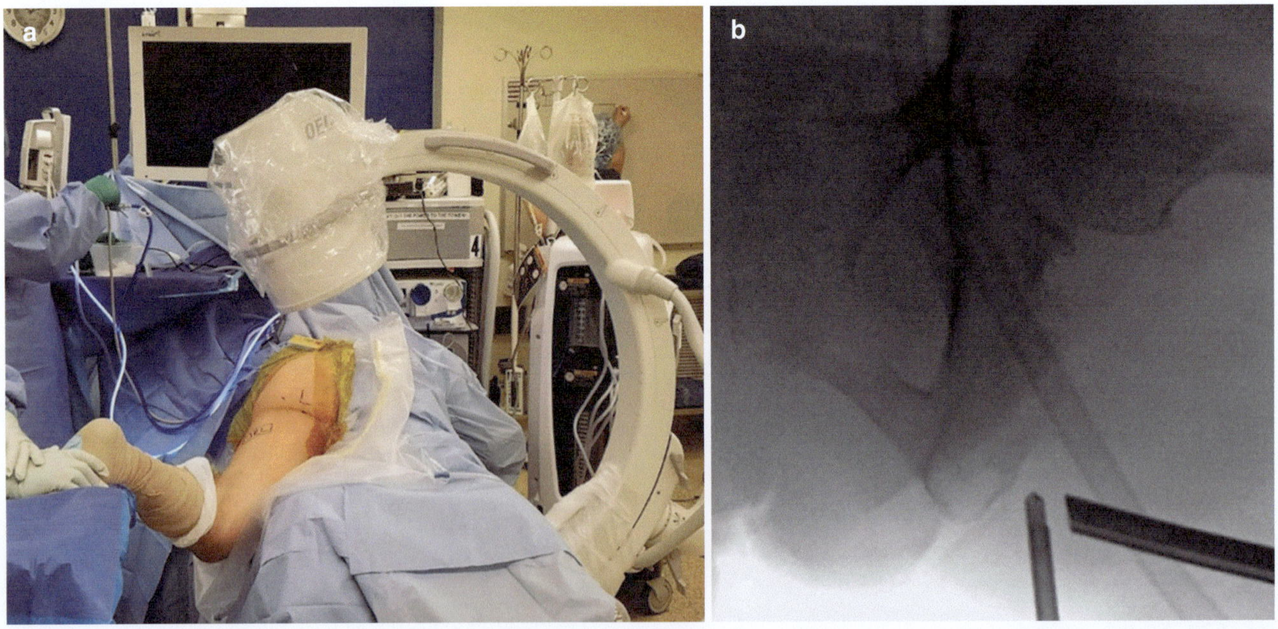

Fig. 5.22 (**a**) Positioning of the operative extremity. (**b**) An en face image of the ischium (Reproduced from Laskovski et al. [62])

lished last, after tendon incision and ischial debridement (Fig. 5.23).

- This sequential order of portal placement is further supported by findings from a cadaveric study, reporting that the midcentral portal enables a clear visualization of the sciatic nerve and both the midcentral and medial portals are within safe distances from adjacent nerves [70].

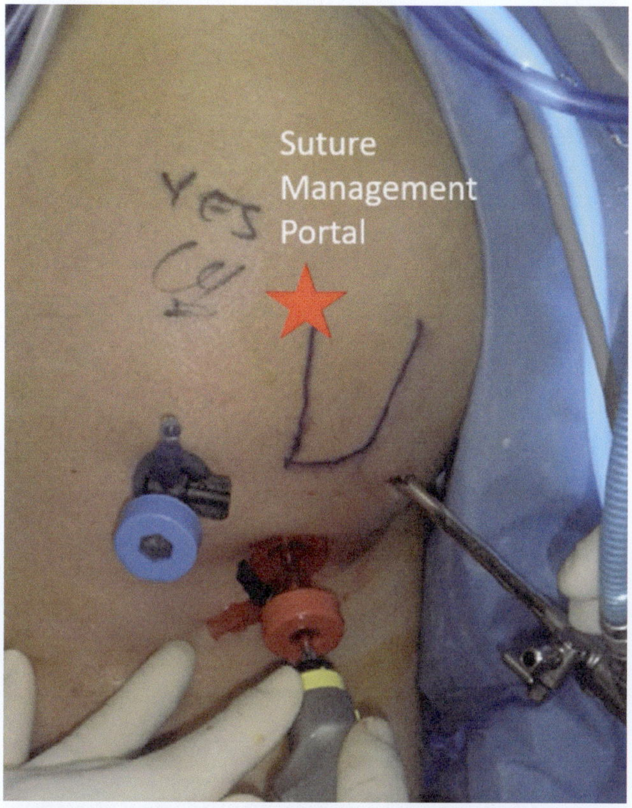

Fig. 5.23 Portal placement for endoscopic hamstring repair. Superior, medial, lateral, and inferior are at the top, right, left, and bottom of the figure, respectively (Reproduced from Laskovski et al. [62])

5.4.4.4 Step-by-Step Description of the Technique

- The midcentral portal is established first. An 18-gauge needle is used to assist in localization of the ischial tuberosity. Fluoroscopy is utilized to ensure that the needle tip obtains a centered position on the ischium. Once confirmed, a cannula is then introduced, through which a 30-degree arthroscope is inserted.
- The fluid inflow pump is used with the fluid pressure set at 25 mmHg.
- The medial portal is made under direct endoscopic visualization with a spinal needle, which is replaced by a switching stick once access to hamstring origin is obtained. A cannula is subsequently placed, penetrating the gluteus maximus fascia.
- After the borders of ischial tuberosity are identified, the subgluteal space is then developed. The medial aspect of the ischium is delineated with electrocautery and shaver whereas the lateral portion is exposed using blunt dissection with a switching stick, since the sciatic nerve lies laterally and anteriorly to the tuberosity.
- The lateral portal is established next under direct visualization. The technique for the placement of this portal is similar to the technique described for the medial portal.
- The sciatic nerve is dissected as dissection moves on anteriorly and laterally. Overlying soft tissue bands are carefully released, thus mobilizing and protecting the sciatic nerve during tendon exposure and repair.
- The hamstring origin on the ischial tuberosity is inspected and probed to evaluate the extent of tear.
- Incomplete tears appear normal upon inspection but exhibit excessive mobility when probed. In these cases, the avulsed tendon is split off longitudinally with an endoscopic knife and then removed (Fig. 5.24).

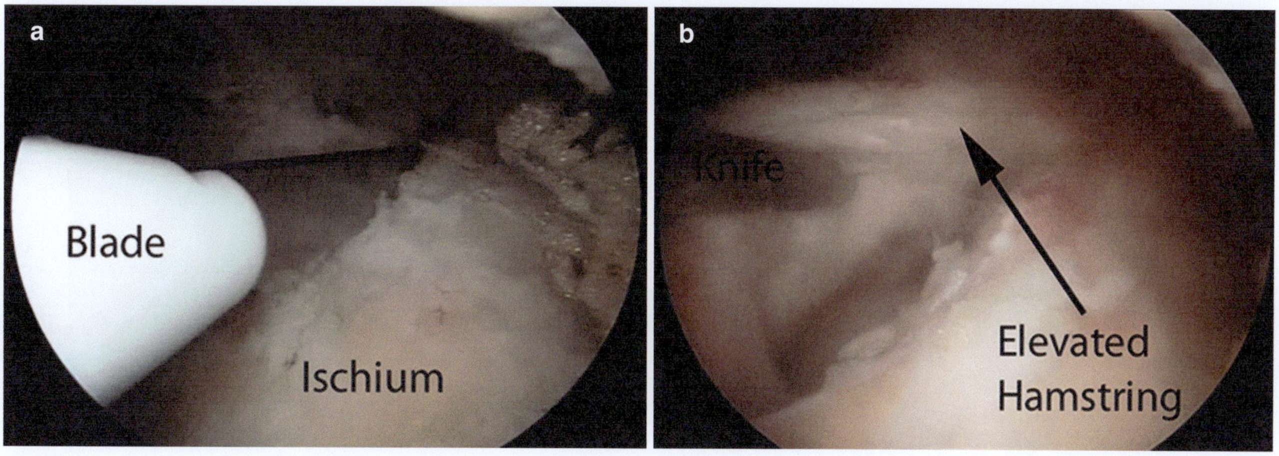

Fig. 5.24 (**a**) Knife incision at the proximal end of the ischium. (**b**) Detached lateral hamstring complex (Reproduced from Guanche [64])

- The hamstring footprint is debrided and denuded to bleeding bone with a shaver, in order to create an ideal healing environment (Fig. 5.25).
- The suture management portal is made under endoscopic visualization. Double- or triple-loaded suture anchors may be used. One suture anchor per centimeter of detachment is usually indicated.
- Mattress sutures are passed through each avulsed tendon, after which a transport cannula is introduced and knots are tied (Fig. 5.26). Finally, the arthroscope is removed and the wound is closed.

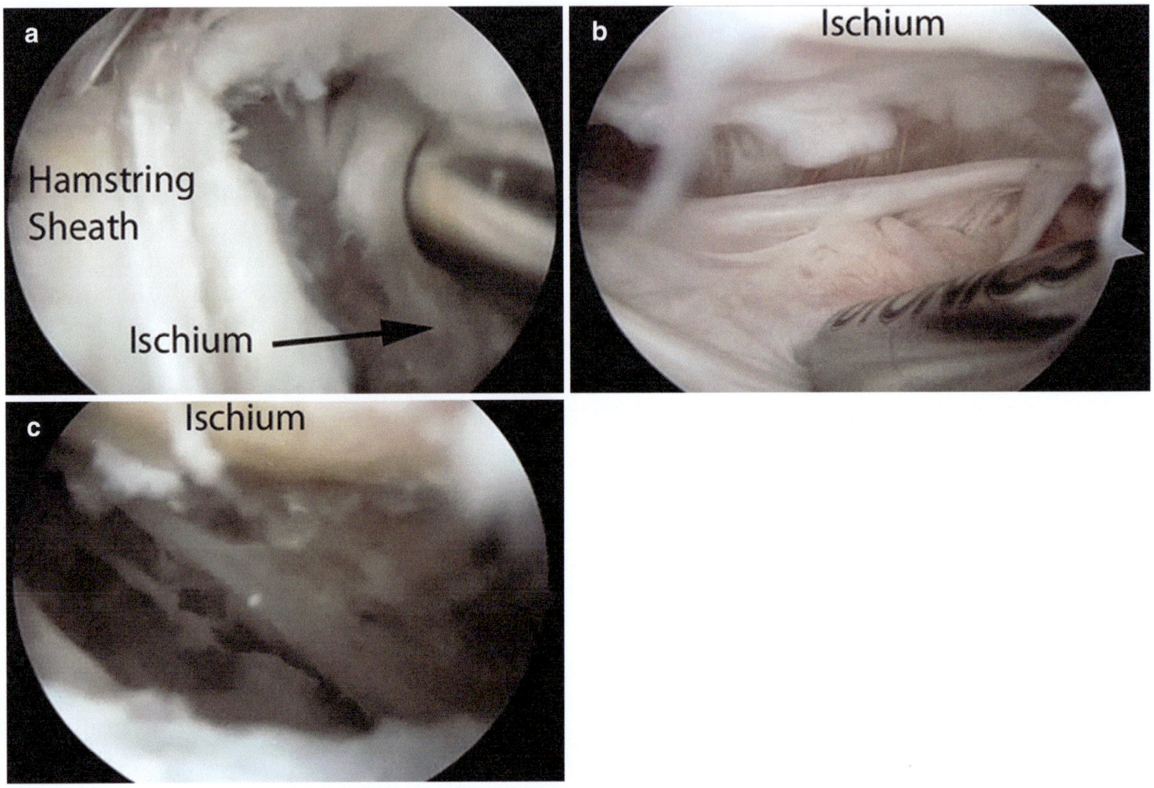

Fig. 5.25 (**a**) Debridement of the lateral aspect of ischium. (**b**) Ischial bursa prior to debridement. (**c**) Ischial bursa after debridement (Reproduced from Guanche [64])

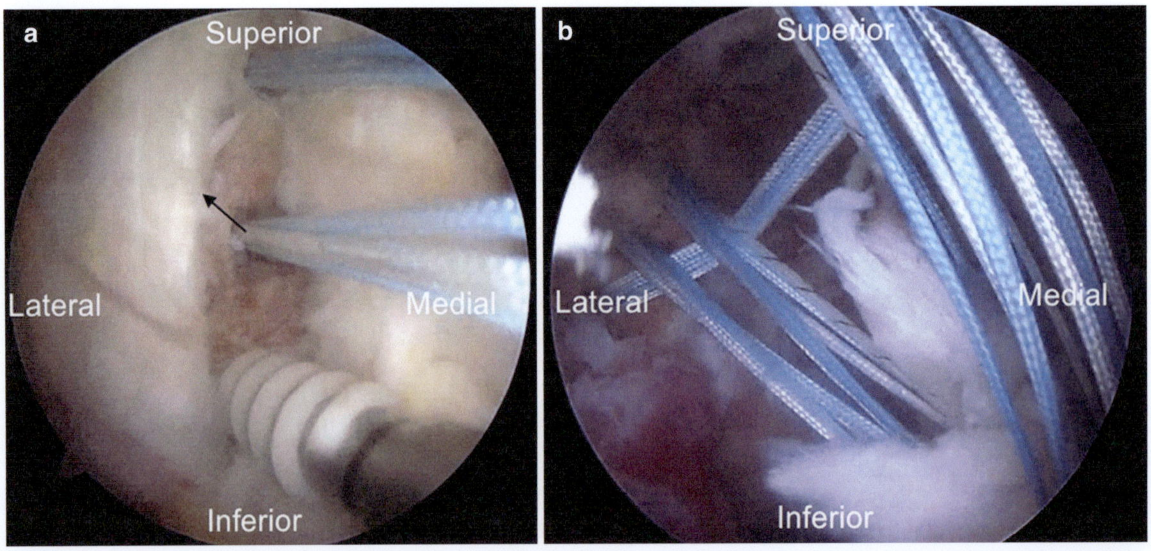

Fig. 5.26 (**a**) Anchors are being placed longitudinally for a side-to-side repair of an incomplete tear. (**b**) Sutures limbs are brought through the suture management portal, which helps maintain an orderly surgical field. The left leg is the operative extremity with the scope in the midcentral portal and the medial portal as the working portal (Reproduced from Laskovski et al. [62])

5.4.4.5 Complications and Management

- Iatrogenic nerve injury
- Wound infection
- Re-rupture and reoperation
- Fluid extravasation into the pelvis [55, 60, 61]

Open repair results in a complication rate of 23.17% [55]. Neurological and septic complications are theoretically lessened with the adoption of endoscopic approach, as nervous structures are better protected and incision sites are no longer in proximity to the perianal zone in this fashion [61–63].

5.4.4.6 Post-operative Care

- A hinged knee brace is applied to keep the ipsilateral knee flexed at 90° for the first 4 weeks, after which gradual extension of the knee is allowed to achieve maximum knee extension and full weight bearing by 6–8 weeks. Crutches are also used to avoid weight bearing for the first few weeks.
- Physical therapy is started when full weight bearing is achieved, primarily focusing on stretching and range of motion during the initial stage. Hamstring strengthening may be initiated at 10–12 week, with subsequent return to full play at around 4 months post-operatively [62].

5.4.4.7 Outcome

- Since endoscopic hamstring repair is a relatively novel surgical approach, few studies regarding clinical outcomes after this procedure are available.
- One study on the short-term outcomes after endoscopic hamstring repair reported significant improvement in pain, range of motion, strength, and return to sports regardless of injury type and surgery timing [60]. Another study reported an overall satisfaction of 94% and found no statistical difference in functional outcomes between open and endoscopic techniques, although no definitive conclusion could be made due to the limited number of patients [58].

5.4.5 Summary

- Though most proximal hamstring repairs are by far still performed using the traditional open approach, the efficacy and safety of endoscopic proximal hamstring repair techniques are increasingly demonstrated and supported in the past few years.
- Despite the many benefits of endoscopic approach as treatment for hamstring injuries, this technique remains relatively obscure to newcomers in this particular field, due to its steeping learning curve and high technical demands.
- Further studies directly comparing the clinical outcomes between endoscopic and open procedures are critical to the evolvement of treatment algorithm for hamstring injuries.

References

1. Martin HD, Shears SA, Johnson JC, Smathers AM, Palmer IJ. The endoscopic treatment of sciatic nerve entrapment/deep gluteal syndrome. Arthroscopy. 2011;27(2):172–81.
2. Perez-Carro L, Hernando MF, Cerezal L, Saenz Navarro I, et al. Gross and endoscopic posterior hip anatomy. In: Martin H, Gómez-Hoyos J, editors. Posterior hip disorders. Cham: Springer; 2019. p. 1–27.
3. Hernando MF, Cerezal L, Perez-Carro L, Abascal F, Canga A. Deep gluteal syndrome: anatomy, imaging, and management of sciatic nerve entrapments in the subgluteal space. Skelet Radiol. 2015;44(7):919–34.
4. Torriani M, Souto SC, Thomas BJ, Ouellette H, Bredella MA. Ischiofemoral impingement syndrome: an entity with hip pain and abnormalities of the quadratus femoris muscle. AJR Am J Roentgenol. 2009;193(1):186–90.
5. Hernando MF, Cerezal L, Perez-Carro L, et al. Evaluation and management of ischiofemoral impingement: a pathophysiologic, radiologic, and therapeutic approach to a complex diagnosis. Skelet Radiol. 2016;45(6):771–87.
6. Perez-Carro L, Hernando MF, Cerezal L, et al. Deep gluteal space problems: piriformis syndrome, ischiofemoral impingement and sciatic nerve release. Muscle Ligaments Tendons J. 2016;6:384–96.
7. Perez-Carro L, Golano P, Fernandez EN, Ruperez VM, Victor Diego V, Cerezal L. Normal articular anatomy. In: Kim J, editor. Hip magnetic resonance imaging. Springer; 2014. p. 57–72.
8. Martin HD, Kivlan BR, Palmer IJ, Martin RL. Diagnostic accuracy of clinical tests for sciatic nerve entrapment in the gluteal region. Knee Surg Sports Traumatol Arthrosc. 2014;22(4):882–8.
9. Stajic S, Vojvodic A, Perez-Carro L, et al. A challenge for ultrasound elastography. Int J Curr Adv Res. 2018:11773–6.
10. Martin HD, Palmer IJ, Hatem M. Monopolar radiofrequency use in deep gluteal space endoscopy: sciatic nerve safety and fluid temperature. Arthroscopy. 2014;30:60–4.
11. Robertson WJ, Kelly BT. The safe zone for hip arthroscopy: a cadaveric assessment of central, peripheral, and lateral compartment portal placement. Arthroscopy. 2008;24:1019–26.
12. Hatem MA, Palmer IJ, Martin HD. Diagnosis and 2-year outcomes of endoscopic treatment for ischiofemoral impingement. Arthroscopy. 2015;31(2):239–46.
13. Martin HD, Hatem MA, Champlin K, Palmer IJ. The endoscopic treatment of sciatic nerve entrapment/deep gluteal syndrome. Tech Orthop. 2012;27:172–83.
14. Martin HD, Reddy M, Gómez-Hoyos J. Deep gluteal syndrome. J Hip Preserv Surg. 2015;2:99–107.
15. Kay J, de Sa D, Morrison L, Fejtek E, Simunovic N, Martin HD, Ayeni OR. Management of deep gluteal syndrome causing sciatic nerve entrapment: a systematic review. Arthroscopy. 2017;33(12):2263–78.
16. Perez-Carro L, de Diego V, Fernández Escajadillo N, Rupérez Vallejo M, Sumillera M, Sainz I. Tratamiento endoscópico del atrapamiento del nervio ciático en el espacio subglúteo, Síndrome del glúteo profundo/piramidal. Cuad Artrosc. 2012;2:24–33.
17. Aguilera-Bohorquez B, Cardozo O, Brugiatti M, Cantor E, Valdivia N. Manejo endoscópico del atrapamiento del nervio ciático en el síndrome de glúteo profundo: resultados clínicos. Rev Esp Cir Ortop Traumatol. 2018;62:322–7.
18. Kay J, de Sa D, Morrison L, et al. Surgical management of deep gluteal syndrome causing sciatic nerve entrapment: a systematic review. Arthroscopy. 2017;33(12):2263–2278.e1. https://doi.org/10.1016/j.arthro.2017.06.041.
19. Cass SP. Piriformis syndrome: a cause of nondiscogenic sciatica. Curr Sports Med Rep. 2015;14(1):41–4.
20. Freiberg AH, Vinke TH. Sciatica and the sacroiliac joint. J Bone Joint Surg. 1934;16:126–36.
21. Robinson DR. Piriformis syndrome in relation to sciatic pain. Am J Surg. 1947;73:355–8.
22. Martin HD, Kivlan BR, Palmer IJ. Nerve entrapment lesions of the hip and thigh. In: JC DL, Drez Jr D, Miller MD, editors. DeLee and Drez's orthopaedic sports medicine. 4th ed. Saunders Elsevier: Philadelphia, PA; 2015.
23. Hopayian K, Song F, Riera R, et al. The clinical features of the piriformis syndrome: a systematic review. Eur Spine J. 2010;19:2095–109.
24. Lewis AM, Layzer R, Engstrom JW, et al. Magnetic resonance neurography in extraspinal sciatica. Arch Neurol. 2006;63:1469–72.
25. Filler AG, Haynes J, Jordan SE, et al. Sciatica of non-disc origin and piriformis syndrome: diagnosis by magnetic resonance neurography and interventional magnetic resonance imaging with outcome study of resulting treatment. J Neurosurg Spine. 2005;2:99–115.
26. Thomas Byrd JW. Piriformis syndrome. Oper Tech Sports Med. 2005;2:71–9.
27. Fishman LM, Dombi GW, Michaelsen C, et al. Piriformis syndrome: diagnosis, treatment, and outcome—a 10-year study. Arch Phys Med Rehabil. 2002;83:295–301.
28. Filler AG. Piriformis and related entrapment syndromes: diagnosis and management. Neurosurg Clin N Am. 2008;19:609–22.
29. Martin HD, Atem M, Palmer IJ. Endoscopic sciatic nerve decompression: operative technique. Oper Tech Sports Med. 2012;20:325–33.
30. Martin HD, Shears SA, Smathers AM, et al. The endoscopic treatment of sciatic nerve entrapment/deep gluteal syndrome. Arthroscopy. 2011;27:172–81.
31. Jackson TJ. Endoscopic sciatic nerve decompression in the prone position-an ischial-based approach. Arthrosc Tech. 2016;5(3):e637–42.
32. Ilizaliturri VM Jr, Arriaga R, Villalobos FE, Suarez-Ahedo C. Endoscopic release of the piriformis tendon and sciatic nerve exploration. J Hip Preserv Surg. 2018;5(3):301–6.
33. Knudsen JS, Mei-Dan O, Brick MJ. Piriformis syndrome and endoscopic sciatic neurolysis. Sports Med Arthrosc Rev. 2016;24(1):e1–7.
34. Aguilera-Bohorquez B, Cardozo O, Brugiatti M, Cantor E, Valdivia N. Endoscopic treatment of sciatic nerve entrapment in deep gluteal syndrome: Clinical results. Manejo endoscópico del atrapamiento del nervio ciático en el síndrome de glúteo profundo: resultados clínicos. Rev Esp Cir Ortop Traumatol. 2018;62(5):322–7.
35. Ham DH, Chung WC, Jung DU. Effectiveness of endoscopic sciatic nerve decompression for the treatment of deep gluteal syndrome. Hip Pelvis. 2018;30(1):29–36.
36. Martin HD, Hatem MA, Palmer IJ. Surgical technique: endoscopic sciatic nerve release, Chapter 75. In: Nho SJ, et al., editors. Hip arthroscopy and hip joint preservation surgery. New York: Springer Science+Business Media; 2015.
37. Indrekvam K, Sudmann E. Piriformis muscle syndrome in 19 patients treated by tenotomy—a 1- to 16-year follow-up study. Int Orthop. 2002;26:101–3.
38. Benson ER, Schutzer SF. Posttraumatic piriformis syndrome: diagnosis and results of operative treatment. J Bone Joint Surg Am. 1999;81:941–9.
39. Filler AG, Haynes J, Jordan SE, et al. Sciatica of nondisc origin and piriformis syndrome: diagnosis by magnetic resonance neurography and interventional magnetic resonance imaging with outcome study of resulting treatment. J Neurosurg Spine. 2005;2(2):99–115.
40. Johnson KA. Impingement of the lesser trochanter on the ischial ramus after total hip arthroplasty. Report of three cases. J Bone Joint Surg Am. 1977;59(2):268–9.

41. Nakano N, Yip G, Khanduja V. Current concepts in the diagnosis and management of extra-articular hip impingement syndromes. Int Orthop. 2017;41(7):1321–8.
42. Ali A, Whitwell D, Ostlere S. Case report: imaging and surgical treatment of a snapping hip due to ischiofemoral impingement. Skelet Radiol. 2011;40(5):653–6.
43. Jo S, O'Donnell JM. Endoscopic lesser trochanter resection for treatment of ischiofemoral impingement. J Hip Preserv Surg. 2015;2(2):184–9.
44. Wilson MD, Keene JS. Treatment of ischiofemoral impingement: results of diagnostic injections and arthroscopic resection of the lesser trochanter. J Hip Preserv Surg. 2016;3(2):146–53.
45. Safran M, Ryu J. Ischiofemoral impingement of the hip: a novel approach to treatment. Knee Surg Sports Traumatol Arthrosc. 2014;22(4):781–5.
46. Brandenburg JB, Kapron AL, Wylie JD, Wilkinson BG, Maak TG, Gonzalez CD, Aoki SK. The functional and structural outcomes of arthroscopic iliopsoas release. Am J Sports Med. 2016;44(5):1286–91.
47. Howse E, Mannava S, Tamam C, Martin H, Bredella M, Stubbs A. Ischiofemoral space decompression through posterolateral approach: cutting block technique. Arthrosc Tech. 2014;3(6):661–5.
48. van der Made AD, Reurink G, Gouttebarge V, Tol JL, Kerkhoffs GM. Outcome after surgical repair of proximal hamstring avulsions: a systematic review. Am J Sports Med. 2015;43(11):2841–51.
49. Ahmad CS, Redler LH, Ciccotti MG, Maffulli N, Longo UG, Bradley J. Evaluation and management of hamstring injuries. Am J Sports Med. 2013;41(12):2933–47.
50. Guanche CA. Endoscopy of proximal hamstring injuries. In: Byrd JWT, Bedi A, Stubbs AJ, editors. The hip: AANA advanced arthroscopic surgical techniques. SLACK Incorporated; 2016. p. 251–61.
51. Cohen S, Bradley J. Acute proximal hamstring rupture. J Am Acad Orthop Surg. 2007;15(6):350–5.
52. Philippon MJ, Ferro FP, Campbell KJ, Michalski MP, Goldsmith MT, Devitt BM, Wijdicks CA, LaPrade RF. A qualitative and quantitative analysis of the attachment sites of the proximal hamstrings. Knee Surg Sports Traumatol Arthrosc. 2015;23(9):2554–61.
53. Beltran L, Ghazikhanian V, Padron M, Beltran J. The proximal hamstring muscle-tendon-bone unit: a review of the normal anatomy, biomechanics, and pathophysiology. Eur J Radiol. 2012;81(12):3772–9.
54. Clanton TO, Coupe KJ. Hamstring strains in athletes: diagnosis and treatment. J Am Acad Orthop Surg. 1998;6(4):237–48.
55. Bodendorfer BM, Curley AJ, Kotler JA, Ryan JM, Jejurikar NS, Kumar A, Postma WF. Outcomes after operative and nonoperative treatment of proximal hamstring avulsions: a systematic review and meta-analysis. Am J Sports Med. 2018;46(11):2798–808.
56. Rust DA, Giveans MR, Stone RM, Samuelson KM, Larson CM. Functional outcomes and return to sports after acute repair, chronic repair, and allograft reconstruction for proximal hamstring ruptures. Am J Sports Med. 2014;42(6):1377–83.
57. Cohen SB, Rangavajjula A, Vyas D, Bradley JP. Functional results and outcomes after repair of proximal hamstring avulsions. Am J Sports Med. 2012;40(9):2092–8.
58. Bowman EN, Marshall NE, Gerhardt MB, Banffy MB. Predictors of clinical outcomes after proximal hamstring repair. Orthop J Sports Med. 2019;7(2):2325967118823712.
59. Arner JW, Freiman H, Mauro CS, Bradley JP. Functional results and outcomes after repair of partial proximal hamstring avulsions at midterm follow-up. Am J Sports Med. 2019;47(14):3436–43.
60. Kurowicki J, Novack TA, Simone ES, Mease SJ, Festa A, McInerney VK, Scillia AJ. Short-term outcomes following endoscopic proximal hamstring repair. Arthroscopy. 2020;36(5):1301–7.
61. Dierckman BD, Guanche CA. Endoscopic proximal hamstring repair and ischial bursectomy. Arthrosc Tech. 2012;1(2):e201–7.
62. Laskovski JR, Kahn AJ, Urchek RJ, Guanche CA. Endoscopic proximal hamstring repair and ischial bursectomy using modified portal placement and patient positioning. Arthrosc Tech. 2018;7(11):e1071–8.
63. Fletcher AN, Lau BC, Mather RC 3rd. Endoscopic proximal hamstring tendon repair for nonretracted tears: an anatomic approach and repair technique. Arthrosc Tech. 2020;9(4):e483–91.
64. Guanche CA. Hamstring injuries. J Hip Preserv Surg. 2015;2(2):116–22.
65. Domb BG, Linder D, Sharp KG, Sadik A, Gerhardt MB. Endoscopic repair of proximal hamstring avulsion. Arthrosc Tech. 2013;2(1):e35–9.
66. Mehta N, Alter T, Beck EC, Cancienne JM, Bressler LR, Liu JN, Nho SJ. Endoscopic repair of proximal hamstring tear with double-row suture bridge construct. Arthrosc Tech. 2019;8(7):e675–8.
67. Jackson TJ, Trenga A, Lindner D, El-Bitar Y, Domb BG. Endoscopic transtendinous repair for partial-thickness proximal hamstring tendon tears. Arthrosc Tech. 2014;3(1):e127–30.
68. Gómez-Hoyos J, Reddy M, Martin HD. Dry endoscopic-assisted mini-open approach with neuromonitoring for chronic hamstring avulsions and ischial tunnel syndrome. Arthrosc Tech. 2015;4(3):e193–9.
69. Atzmon R, Amar E, Maor D, Rath E. A combined endoscopic and open surgical approach for chronic retracted proximal hamstring avulsion. J Hip Preserv Surg. 2019;6(3):284–8.
70. Bataillie F, Bataillie S, van Beek N, Corten K. Portal placement for endoscopic surgery in the deep gluteal area: a cadaveric study. J Hip Preserv Surg. 2020;7(1):147–52.

Endoscopy of the Medial and Anterior Hip

6

Tun Hing Lui, Alessio Giai Via, Filippo Randelli, Gennaro Pipino, Manuel Mazzoleni, Alberto Fioruzzi, Nicola Maffulli, Jin Zhang, Mingjin Zhong, Feng Chao, and Lu XueMin

Abstract

Internal snapping hip is a common clinical condition and is usually asymptomatic, but in few cases, mostly in athletes and professionals who participate in activities requiring extreme ranges of hip motion, the snap may become painful (internal snapping hip syndrome—ISHS). Traditionally, the ISHS pathogenesis was described as a snapping of the tendon over the anterior femoral head or the iliopectineal ridge, but currently the pathological mechanism is considered multifactorial. Most patients respond well to conservative treatment, but in recalcitrant cases, surgery may be indicated. Arthroscopic iliopsoas fractional lengthening can be performed in the central compartment, peripheral compartment or at the tendon's insertion on lesser trochanter. Better results have been reported with endoscopic iliopsoas tendon release compared with open techniques, which may be related to the treatment of concomitant intra-articular pathologies. Furthermore, endoscopic treatment showed fewer complications, decreased failure rate, and postoperative pain. Sub-spine impingement is an extra-capsular cause of femoroacetabular impingement (FAI) resulting in diminished

The corresponding author of section 6.1 is Alessio Giai Via, E-mail: alessiogiaivia@hotmail.it
The corresponding author of section 6.2 is Zhang Jin, E-mail: eiolia@163.com
The corresponding author of section 6.3 is Mingjin Zhong, E-mail: sportsmedzhong@sina.com
The corresponding author of section 6.4 is Mingjin Zhong, E-mail: sportsmedzhong@sina.com
The corresponding author of section 6.5 is Feng Chao, E-mail: chaofeng_jst@163.com

T. H. Lui (✉)
Department of Orthopaedics and Traumatology, North District Hospital, Hong Kong, China

The Second Affiliated Hospital, Shenzhen University, Shenzhen, China

A. Giai Via
Department of Orthopaedic Surgery and Traumatology, San Camillo-Forlanini Hospital, Rome, Italy
e-mail: agiaivia@unisa.it

F. Randelli · A. Fioruzzi
Hip Department (CAD), Gaetano Pini - CTO Orthopedic Institute, University of Milan, Milan, Italy
e-mail: filippo.randelli@asst-pini-cto.it; alberto.fioruzzi@asst-pini-cto.it

G. Pipino
Department of Orthopaedic Surgery and Traumatology, Villa Regina Hospital, Bologna, Italy

UCM Malta, Campus of Lugano, Lugano, Switzerland

Department of Orthopedics and Physiotherapy, UCM University, Warrensburg, MO, USA
e-mail: gennaro.pipino@ucm.edu.mt

M. Mazzoleni
Department of Life Health & Environmental Sciences, Unit of Orthopaedics and Traumatology, University of L'Aquila, L'Aquila, Italy
e-mail: manuel.mazzoleni@asst-pini-cto.it

N. Maffulli
Centre for Sports and Exercise Medicine, Barts and the London School of Medicine and Dentistry, Mile End Hospital, Queen Mary University of London, London, UK

Institute of Science and Technology in Medicine, Keele University School of Medicine, Stoke on Trent, UK
e-mail: n.maffulli@qmul.ac.uk

J. Zhang · F. Chao · L. XueMin
Beijing Jishuitan Hospital, Beijing, China

M. Zhong
Department of Sports Medicine, Health Science Center, The First Affiliated Hospital of Shenzhen University, Shenzhen, Guangdong Province, China

Shenzhen Second People's Hospital, Shenzhen, Guangdong Province, China

© The Author(s), under exclusive license to Springer Nature Singapore Pte Ltd. 2021
T. H. Lui (ed.), *Endoscopy of the Hip and Knee*, https://doi.org/10.1007/978-981-16-3488-8_6

hip range of motion and groin pain during hip flexion-based activities. Arthroscopic resection of the deformed AIIS, decompression of the sub-spine region, and treatment of concomitant FAI usually result in good clinical outcome. Calcific tendinitis of the rectus femoris (CTRF) is another underreported condition because it is usually self-limiting. Endoscopic treatment of CTRF is indicated for symptomatic cases recalcitrant to conservative treatment. Recently, arthroscopically assisted reduction of developmental dislocation of the hip (DDH) via medial approach has been developed with advantage of minimally invasive surgery. In this chapter, the endoscopic techniques are outlined.

Keywords

Hip · Arthroscopy · Endoscopy · Internal snapping hip syndrome · Iliopsoas · Tendinopathy · Iliopsoas release · Femoroacetabular impingement · Extra-articular impingement · Anterior inferior iliac spine · Calcific tendonitis · Rectus femoris · Developmental dislocation of hip · Arthroscopic reduction

6.1 Endoscopic Ilio-Psoas Release for Internal Snapping Hip

Alessio Giai Via
agiaivia@unisa.it

Filippo Randelli
filippo.randelli@asst-pini-cto.it

Gennaro Pipino
gennaro.pipino@ucm.edu.mt

Manuel Mazzoleni
manuel.mazzoleni@asst-pini-cto.it

Alberto Fioruzzi
alberto.fioruzzi@asst-pini-cto.it

Nicola Maffulli
n.maffulli@qmul.ac.uk

6.1.1 Introduction

Internal snapping hip (ISH) is a common disorder characterized by an audible click or snap at the groin. The prevalence is estimated about 5–10% in the general population, with a higher incidence in females [1]. The prevalence is higher in selected populations such as runners, football players, ballet dancers, and in young adults involved in sports and physically demanding activities that require large hip range of motion [2]. The prevalence of snapping or cracking sensation is up to 90% in ballet dancers [3]. Snapping hip is usually asymptomatic but, when the snap becomes painful, this condition is called snapping hip syndrome (SHS).

ISH was originally described by Nunziata and Blumenfeld in 1951 [4]. Its etiopathogenesis is traditionally ascribed to the snapping of the iliopsoas tendon (IPT) over the anterior femoral head or the iliopectineal eminence. The condition is relatively common, but few studies have been performed. Recent advances in imaging and arthroscopy gave new pulse to the understanding of hip disorders, and the interest in iliopsoas tendon's pathologies grew up. Furthermore, improvements in hip arthroscopy and endoscopy allow hip surgeons to treat periarticular pathologies with satisfactory results and minimize the complication rate.

In this chapter, the pathogenesis, diagnosis, and treatment of internal snapping hip syndrome (ISHS) are reviewed, focusing on endoscopic surgical techniques.

6.1.2 Anatomy and Function of the Iliopsoas Tendon

The iliopsoas (IP) muscle is represented by the union of the iliacus and psoas muscles. The muscle bundles are directed downwards, under the inguinal ligament, and through the lacuna musculorum, having close relationships with the anterosuperior labrum and the anterior hip joint capsule. The distal insertion of the tendon lies on the lesser trochanter. The iliopsoas muscle has an inverted teardrop-shaped insertion engaging the entire posterior surface of the lesser trochanter, and extending to the femoral shaft. The superior margin of the iliopsoas insertion is in close relation with the inferior joint capsule of the hip [5].

Two anatomical considerations are important to understand the pathogenesis and treatment of ISHS. Anatomical variations of the IPT have been described, which may contribute to snapping syndrome. The most common anatomic variation is the presence of multiple iliopsoas tendons. In an anatomical cadaveric study a bifid tendon was identified in 64.2% of cases, three tendons in 7.5% of cases, while a single tendon was found only in 28.3% of cases [6]. Crompton et al. found a prevalence of a bifid iliopsoas tendon of 26% on MR imaging in 87 hips in children [7]. An incidence of multiple iliopsoas tendons of 18% during endoscopic transcapsular release has been reported [8]. An accessory iliopsoas muscle, which originates from the middle third of the inner lip of the iliac crest and covered by a separate distinguishable fascia, has been exceptionally described [9]. It inserts along with the iliopsoas on the lesser trochanter and can cause compression of the femoral nerve from the L4 nerve root. The second important anatomic consideration is that the iliopsoas muscle has a progressive muscle insertion on the lesser trochanter. An anatomic study showed that the muscle-tendon unit (MTU), defined as the ratio between the circumference of the muscle belly and tendon, is 60% and 40% at the hip labrum, 47% and 53% at the joint capsule, and 40% and 60% near the lesser trochanter [10]. Therefore, many authors suggest to perform transcapsular iliopsoas tenotomy at the level of the acetabular labrum in order to preserve the muscular portion as much as possible.

The iliopsoas muscle is not only an important hip flexor and lumbar stabilizer, but it also plays a significant role as a dynamic hip stabilizer. The primary function of the IP muscle is hip flexion from 45° to 60° of flexion. Secondarily, the tendon is a stabilizer of the femoral head within the acetabulum from 0° to 15° of hip flexion [11]. When injured, it can be a source of snapping and/or discomfort, and due to its anatomic relation to hip structures, tightness or contracture can be symptomatic. Chronic IPT pathologies can also contribute to atraumatic hip microinstability [12].

6.1.3 Pathogenesis of Internal Snapping Hip

ISHS is traditionally considered to be caused by the iliopsoas tendon snapping over the anterior femoral head or the iliopectineal eminence. The snap occurs when the hip is moved from combined flexion, abduction, and external rotation (FABER position) back to neutral adduction and internal rotation. This explains why the patient usually feels the snap while climbing stairs or when getting out of a car, and its higher incidence in athletes and dancers.

A recent virtual model analysis elucidates the pathogenesis of ISH [13]. The authors showed that the majority of tendon movements occur over the anterior femoral head. With the ongoing hip abduction and external rotation, the IPT gradually moves from the medial to the lateral portion of the anterior femoral head. Upon return to neutral, the tendon tends to remain hooked in this lateral position, causing subsequently a sudden movement of the tendon and the snap. Females were slightly more prone to increased peak tendon movement as compared to males. Furthermore, it was interestingly confirmed that the iliopsoas snapping was associated with female sex, and some anatomic variations of the proximal femur, such as an increased femoral anteversion and a lower ischiofemoral distance [14]. This is the reason why IPT pathologies have been recently associated with hip dysplasia and posterior hip impingement [15].

However, this is not the only pathogenetic mechanism involved, because the pathogenesis is currently considered multifactorial. A bifid IPT can produce a snapping [16, 17]. Given the complex anatomic relationship between the IPT and the hip joint, many different structures are involved in the snap, and may be a source of pain. There is a positive correlation between symptomatic snapping and the presence of labral cysts and tears. This is common in patients with borderline hip dysplasia, as they have a larger labrum compared to normal hips and an increased femoral anteversion [18]. However, further dynamic studies are required to elucidate whether snapping becomes symptomatic in the presence of labral pathology or labral pathology can occur in patients with increased and recurrent psoas tendon movement.

A particular type of ISHS has been reported to occur after total hip arthroplasty, which is a common complication with an incidence about 5%. The pathogenesis is multifactorial, and it is usually related to the implantation of large cups and femoral heads, an excessive retroversion of the acetabulum (Fig. 6.1), anterior osteophytosis, extravasated cement, excessive off-set or leg length discrepancy (>1 cm) [1, 19].

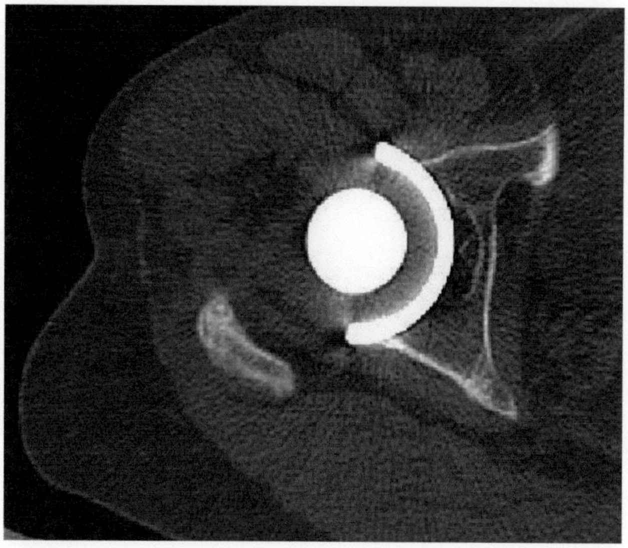

Fig. 6.1 The iliopsoas tendon, which runs close to the anterior hip joint capsule, may move on the surface of an excessive retroverted acetabular cup and become painful. The cup appears oversized and too retroverted, and the patient reported persistent groin pain

6.1.4 Clinical Evaluation and Investigation

A careful history and physical examination is important. The patient is usually able to locate the site of the snap, to report when it occurs, and to reproduce it voluntarily. Clinical examination may reveal focal tenderness over the iliopsoas tendon, pain on active straight leg raise, discomfort in the sitting position, a positive C-sign, positive FADIR and/or FABER test [2]. The hip range of motion (ROM) should be evaluated and a reduction of hip internal rotation or externally rotated hip flexion may reveal a misunderstood femoroacetabular impingement (FAI) (Fig. 6.2). A difference in the iliopsoas muscles strength between the affected and contralateral hip can be appreciated (Fig. 6.3). However, none of these tests is specific. The iliopsoas test is helpful to assess IP pathologies (Fig. 6.4). It is performed with the patient supine. The pain or weakness is assessed when the hip is flexed against resistance in abduction and external rotation.

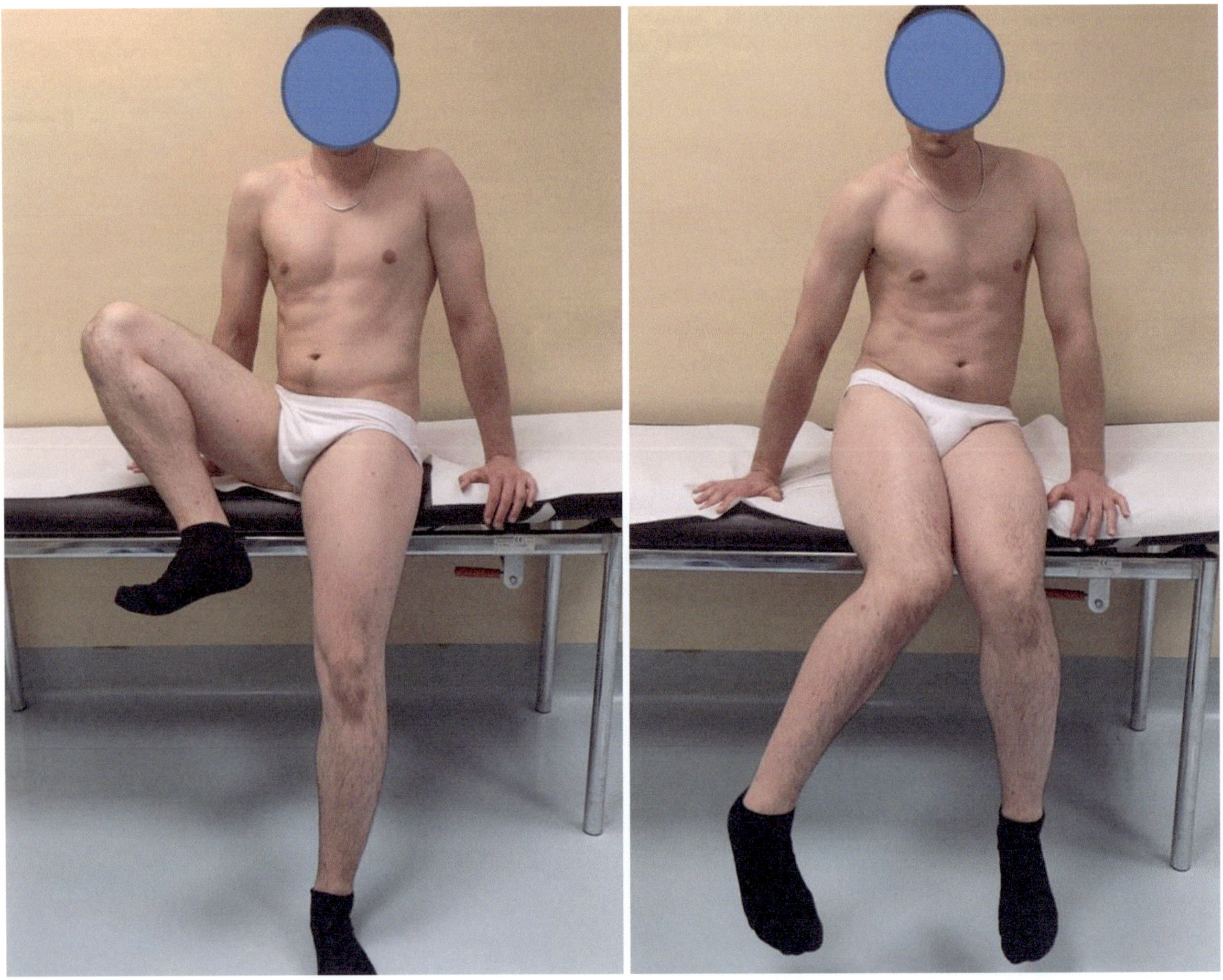

Fig. 6.2 When we ask the patients to actively flex the hip, external rotation may be observed. This is a common sign of FAI, which can be associated in many cases of ISHS. The internal rotation may be reduced in case of CAM or mixed femoroacetabular impingement

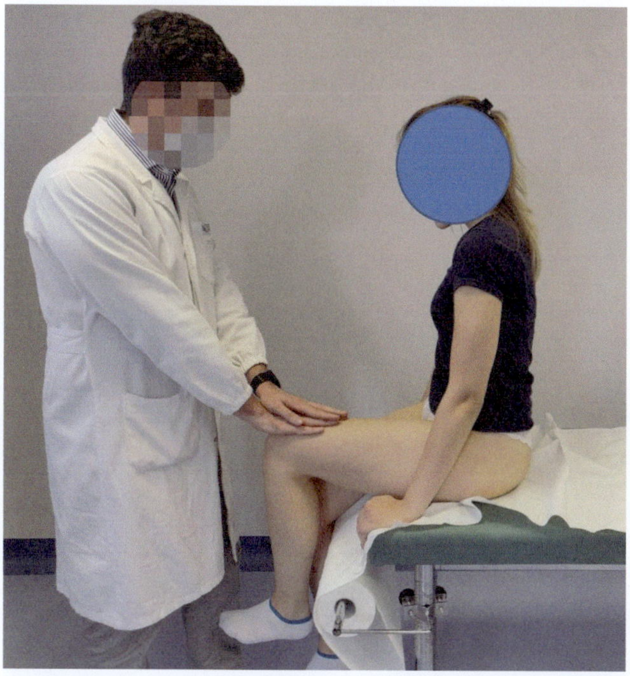

Fig. 6.3 A weakness of the iliopsoas on flexion of the hip against resistance, compared to the controlateral side, may suggest an iliopsoas tendinopathy

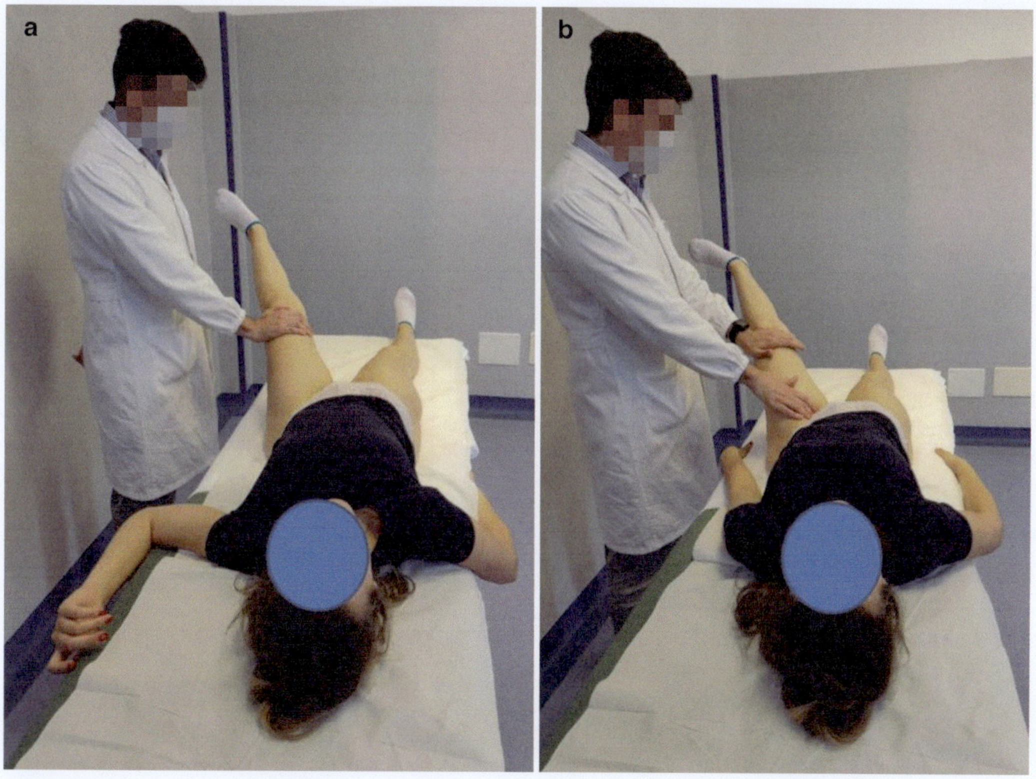

Fig. 6.4 (**a**) The iliopsoas test. The test is positive if pain or weakness is assessed during hip flexion with the hip in slight abduction, external rotation, and the knee extended. (**b**) Palpation of the iliopsoas tendon at the groin usually exacerbates the pain

The Thomas test and the Stinchfield test can also be useful (Fig. 6.5). However, the reproduction of the audible snap is the most sensitive clinical test (Fig. 6.6).

The diagnosis of ISHS is usually clinical, but imaging is necessary to rule out other pathologies and confirm the diagnosis. Anteroposterior radiographs of the pelvis and cross

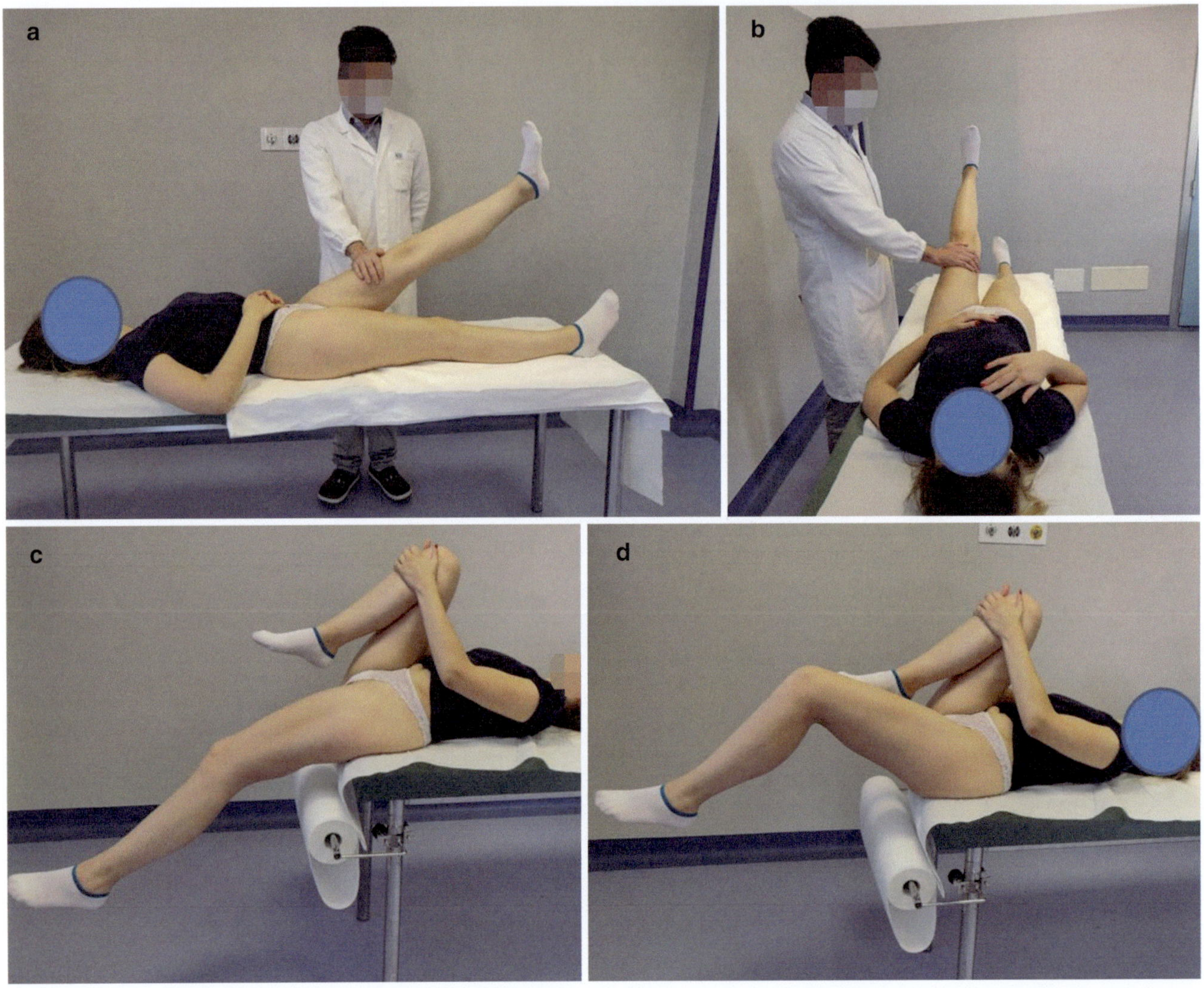

Fig. 6.5 (**a**, **b**) The Stinchfield test. The patient lies supine. With the hip flexed at 30°, ask the patient to fully flex the hip, while the examiner applies an opposing force. Pain in the anterior groin indicates a positive test. (**c**, **d**) The Thomas test is used to measure the flexibility of the hip flexors, in particular the retraction of the iliopsoas muscle, the tensor fascia latae, and iliotibial band. The Thomas test is negative when the subject's lower back and the sacrum are able to remain on the table. The hip can make a 10° posterior tilt or a 10° hip extension. The knee must be able to flex to 90°. The test is positive when the patient is unable to maintain the lower back and sacrum against the table, the hip has a large posterior tilt or hip extension greater than 15°, or when the knee is unable to flex than 80°

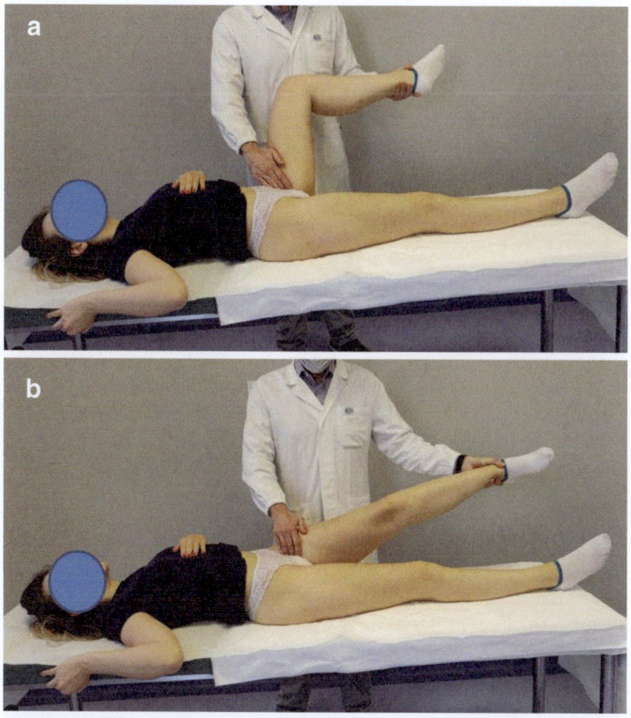

Fig. 6.6 The snap can be reproduced with the patient supine, bringing the hip from (**a**) a flexed, abducted, and externally rotated position (FABER position) to extended, adducted, internally rotated (**b**) or neutral position. The snap can be also appreciated at the groin of the patient under the examiner's finger. The reproduction of the audible snap is the most sensitive clinical test

table view of the hip are important to study the anatomy of the hip, as the snap may be associated with acetabular anteversion, coxa vara, FAI, and developmental dysplasia of the hip (DDH) [20]. Ultrasound scan (US) is commonly performed. The FABER position increases the sonographic tendon exposure and allows a complete evaluation of the distal iliopsoas complex [21]. Dynamic US examination is usually successful in demonstrating the snapping phenomenon. US also allows image-guided iliopsoas peritendinous injections, which are very useful in confirming the diagnosis and treatment [22]. MRI can show inflammation or signal changes in the IP tendon suspicious for tendon pathology, and it is useful to detect labral and cartilage injuries, as ISHS is frequently associated with intra-articular pathologies [23].

Diagnostic intra-articular injection is very useful in distinguishing whether the pain is intra- or extra-articular in origin. A negative test can rule out intra-articular pathologies and suggests the existence of an extra-articular cause such as the iliopsoas tendinopathy.

6.1.5 Treatment of Internal Snapping Hip Syndrome

6.1.5.1 Conservative Management

The management of ISHS is first conservative, which is focused on relieving pain and stretching exercises. Several treatments have been proposed such as rest and lifestyle modification, reduction of sporting activity, cryotherapy, NSAIDs, local ultrasound-guided corticosteroid injections, and physical therapies (laser therapy, extracorporeal shock wave therapy—ESWT) [24]. Physiotherapy is focused on iliopsoas tendon stretching, myofascial release, core stability and pelvic stabilizer exercises. As a high iliopsoas muscle activation and a gluteus medius weakness have been found in many patients, Philippon et al. proposed a rehabilitative protocol based on stretching exercises and gluteus medius strengthening [25]. The results of conservative treatment are heterogeneous. Good outcomes have been reported from 36% up to 100% of cases in a selected population of professional dancers [26]. However, no gold standard treatments and standardized protocols are available for conservative treatment of ISHS. Conservative treatment should be usually prolonged for 6 months, after which surgery may be indicated in refractory cases.

6.1.5.2 Surgical Management

Surgical treatment consists in the IPT lengthening or tenotomy, which can be performed both open and endoscopically. Arthroscopic or endoscopic release of the IPT has been recently described as a minimally invasive solution with favorable short-term outcomes [27], being less invasive and more effective compared to the open surgery techniques [28], with lower snapping recurrence (5.1% vs 21.7%) and better groin pain relief (89.1% vs 85.6%) [26]. Lower complication rates have been reported (4.2% vs 21.1%), including persistent hip pain, sensory deficit, post-operatory bleeding, superficial infection, and subjective weakness [26, 29, 30]. Other potential advantages of arthroscopic treatment over open surgery include fewer wound complications, shorter hospital stays, and quicker return to function [29].

Endoscopic iliopsoas release can be performed at the level of the lesser trochanter through an additional portal or by a transcapsular approach (Fig. 6.7). The endoscopic release of the iliopsoas tendon at the lesser trochanter was described by Byrd et al. in 2005 [31]. Nine patients were treated with good results and without any complications and recurrence. However, the MTU at the level of the lesser tro-

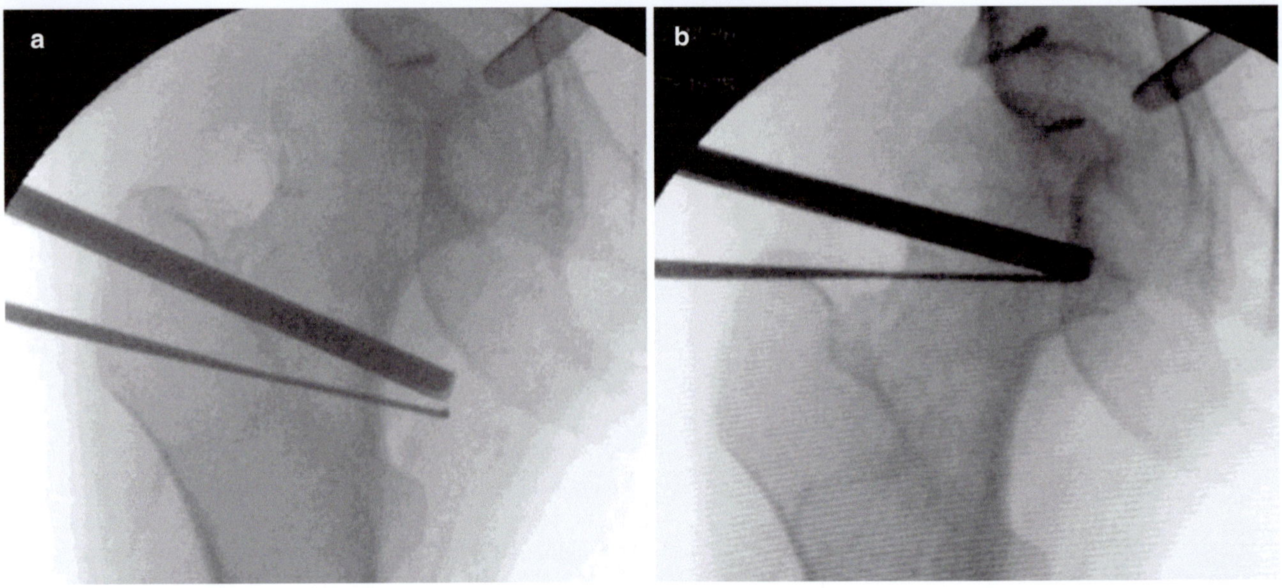

Fig. 6.7 Endoscopic iliopsoas release of the iliopsoas tendon can be performed at the level of the lesser trochanter by an additional portal (**a**) or at the level of the capsular joint or labrum by a transcapsular approach without the need of an accessory working portal (**b**)

chanter consists in 40% of muscle and 60% of tendon, and a tenotomy at this level would result in a significant loss of muscle function. Brandenburg showed a significantly reduced hip flexion strength (19% in the seated position) and iliopsoas muscle atrophy with a 25% volume loss after tenotomy compared to contralateral hips [32]. Flanum et al. reported on 6 patients who underwent endoscopic IPT release at the level of the lesser trochanter, and all patients experienced hip flexor weakness after surgery [33]. An interesting MRI study evaluates the changes of the hip muscles in patients after arthroscopic iliopsoas tenotomy, showing that 85% of patients developed atrophy of the iliacus muscle, 75% of the psoas muscle. According to the grade, 55% of patients had a grade 4 atrophy, 10% a grade 3, and 20% a grade 2. Surprisingly, 25% of patients showed also atrophy of the ipsilateral gluteus maximus, probably consequently to the loss of strength of the antagonist muscles, and less frequently of quadratus femoris and vastus lateralis [34]. However, no significant differences in hip function were reported at long-term follow-up.

To reduce the loss of strength, many authors suggest the IPT release through a transcapsular approach. The release can be performed at the level of the labrum, where the MTU consists of 60% muscle and 40% tendon, or at the femoral neck, where the MTU is about 50%–50%. The release can be easily performed through the standard anterolateral and mid-anterior arthroscopic portals. The IPT is usually identified behind the anterior capsule at 3 or 9 o'clock at the right and left hip, respectively. It is exposed after capsulotomy, and the release is performed using a shaver or a radiofrequency hook probe (Fig. 6.8).

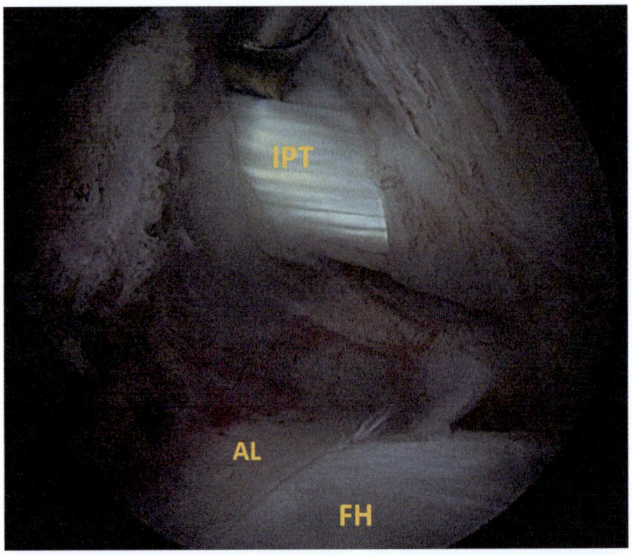

Fig. 6.8 Transcapsular release of the iliopsoas tendon. The IPT runs just beyond the medial joint capsule, at 3 o'clock. After capsulotomy, the IPT can be easily identified. The tendon release can be performed with a shaver or a radiofrequency hook probe. It is very important to perform the release from a medial to a lateral direction, in order to not put at risk the medial neurovascular bundle. *IPT* iliopsoas tendon, *FH* femoral head, *AL* acetabular labrum

Contreras et al. made a prospective study to determine whether arthroscopic surgery through the central compartment of the hip was effective in the management of ISHS [35]. All the 7 patients experienced resolution of the snapping postoperatively persisting at 2 years follow-up. Hwang et al. reported good to excellent results in 22/25 patients treated with a transcapsular release of iliopsoas tendon. The mean improvement of the Harris Hip Score (HHS) was from 65 to 84 points. Two patients experienced recurrent snap but only one had a revision surgery. No other complication has been reported [36]. A statistical significant improvement of the outcome score was also reported by Ilizaliturri et al. at 2 years follow-up in 14 patients, with only one recurrence of snapping and no complications [37]. A recent systematic review of the literature, including 7 studies, reported good outcomes in 82% to 100% of patients after endoscopic approach, and a recurrence rate of the snap between 0% and 18% [38].

Given the complex anatomic relationship between the iliopsoas tendon and the anterior surface of the hip, intra-articular hip pathologies such as FAI syndrome, labral tears, and cartilage lesions can be associated with ISHS in more than 50% of the patients [39]. The possibility to address and treat intra-articular pathologies is another advantage of endoscopic transcapsular techniques, potentially leading to superior outcomes. In a recent study on a selected population of competitive athletes, the intra-operative findings showed labral tears in 98% of patients and chondral damage in 83% of the cases. Mardones et al. [39] reported on 15 patients treated arthroscopically for FAI syndrome and iliopsoas tendinopathy. The IPT release was performed through the central compartment at the level of the labrum with statistically significant improvement of PROMs and pain relief. Two patients reported a recurrence of pain one year after surgery, and they were treated conservatively. No other complications were reported. The authors concluded that arthroscopic iliopsoas tendon release was effective and safe, and that failure in diagnosing and treating IPT pathologies may be the reason of poor results after hip arthroscopy and revision surgery. One year later, Perets et al. [40] compared a group of competitive athletes who underwent hip arthroscopy for treatment of iliopsoas tendinopathy and FAI to a control group treated for FAI syndrome only. The iliopsoas release was performed at the level of the labrum, and the procedure was called iliopsoas fractional lengthening. Favorable improvements in PROMs and VAS, high satisfaction, and high rate of symptom resolution were reported at 2 years follow-up. Most patients were able to return to sports and maintain or improve their competitive levels, and no differences were found with patients not requiring IPT release. More than 80% of patients experienced resolution of painful internal snapping and pain at 5 years follow-up [41]. Only 2 patients underwent secondary arthroscopy for recurrent painful snapping (snapping recurrence rate of 3.5%).

6.1.6 Contraindications for Iliopsoas Tenotomy

Endoscopic IPT release is not without risk, and formal contraindications exist. As the iliopsoas muscle is an important active stabilizer of the hip, iliopsoas tenotomy is not indicated in patients with hip dysplasia, increased femoral anteversion, and hypermobility. Micro-instability, early joint degeneration, subluxation, and hip dislocation have been reported after hip arthroscopy and iliopsoas tenotomy in patients affected by hip dysplasia, mostly if excessive acetabular rim trimming, a large capsulotomy, or ligamentum teres resection was performed [42–44].

6.1.7 Conclusion

Internal snapping hip is a common condition, but only few patients are symptomatic and require treatments. Careful clinical examination and accurate diagnosis are mandatory. Most patients respond well to conservative treatments, while those with ISHS refractory to conservative management are candidates to surgery. Endoscopic techniques provide better outcomes, less complications, faster recovery, and better cosmetic results than open surgery. Concerns have been raised regarding patients developing hip flexion weakness after release of the iliopsoas tendon, and patients should be informed about this possible complication. However, existing data are insufficient to conclude whether hip flexion weakness is a clinical downside of endoscopic iliopsoas release, which warrants further clinical research. Finally, there are no level I studies published in literature, and the gold standard treatment for ISHS is still not defined.

6.2 Endoscopic Ilio-Psoas Fractional Lengthening for Internal Snapping Hip or Iliopsoas Impingement

Jin Zhang

6.2.1 Iliopsoas Tendon-Muscle Complex

The iliopsoas tendon-muscle complex is a deep muscle group of lower limbs, which is divided into three components: the iliacus, psoas major, and psoas minor.

The psoas major is a long fusiform muscle, originating from the vertebral bodies, transverse processes, and intervertebral disks of T12 to L5, lying anterior to the hip joint, and eventually inserts directly on the lesser trochanter. The tendon of psoas major originates from the center of the muscle, above the level of the inguinal ligament. It has a characteristic rotation: As the tendon courses distally, it rotates clockwise (right hip) and migrates posteriorly within the muscle. After this rotation, the main tendon spreads out to cover the lesser trochanter of the femur.

The iliacus is a shorter, flat, and triangular fan-shaped muscle, which is composed of medial and lateral bundles, originating from the superior two-thirds of the iliac fossa, ventral lip of the iliac crest and sacral ala. And there is a smaller bundle called the ilio-infratrochanteric muscle, in a deeper position under the iliopsoas tendon. It has been observed ran along the anterolateral edge of the iliacus, inserted under the lesser trochanter.

At the level of the L5 to S2 vertebrae, the psoas major and iliacus converge downward to form the iliopsoas muscle. Innervation of the iliopsoas musculotendinous unit is, respectively, from the ventral rami of L1 to L3 and femoral nerve (L1 to L2) [45–49].

Anatomic variability of the iliopsoas musculotendinous unit has been reported in some researches [47, 48]. In a study of 14 cadavers, Tatu and colleagues [47] show that the iliopsoas tendon is made up of 2 tendinous structures: the psoas major and iliacus tendons. The medial iliacus muscle bundle was observed to insert onto the iliacus tendon, then iliacus tendon converges with more medial psoas major tendon. The lateral iliacus muscle bundle courses distally and inserts on the anterior surface of the lesser trochanter and infratrochanteric ridge without any tendinous attachments. Conversely, a cadaveric and MRI study by Polster and coworkers [50] showed that the medial iliacus bundle directly inserted into the psoas major tendon, and the medial-most fibers of the lateral iliacus bundle inserted on a distinct thin intramuscular tendon [51]. Furthermore, Philippon and colleagues [48] studied 53 cadavers, demonstrated at the level of the hip joint the prevalence of a single-, double-, and triple-banded iliopsoas tendon was 28.3%, 64.2%, and 7.5%, respectively. Although controversy exists regarding the number of tendons and the difference of the musculotendinous complex components, the current literature evidences the challenges of the traditional well-accepted concept that the iliopsoas tendon consists of a single common conjoint tendon.

The iliopsoas bursa (aka iliopectineal bursa) is located between the iliopsoas tendon-muscle complex and the bony pelvis and proximal femur surfaces [45]. It is the largest bursa in the human body, typically extending from the iliopectineal eminence to the lower portion of the femoral head, with an average length of 5–6 cm and width of 3 cm. Normally, the iliopsoas bursa is collapsed. It could reduce tendon friction of the hip joint during joint movement [52]. However, the communication of the bursa, through a congenital defect between the iliofemoral and pubofemoral ligaments, is reported variable. Some studies have observed a direct communication between the joint and bursa in 15% of patients, which can be congenital or acquired [52–54]. It is important to consider this communication during diagnostic injections, because the anesthetic drug can flow between the intra-articular and bursal compartments, confounding the test results.

The iliopsoas unit plays an important role in many activities of daily living. It has the function as the primary hip flexor and may assist in tilting the pelvis anteriorly. Besides, it also has important function, as a core muscle attached to the spine, in femoral external rotation and with lateral bending, flexion, and balance of the trunk. The iliacus and psoas major have been shown their individual and task-specific activation patterns. The iliacus is important for stabilizing the pelvis and for early rapid hip flexion while running. The psoas major is important for sitting in an erect position and anterior stability of the spine. Variable contribution of each muscle is observed during sit-ups depending on the angle of hip flexion [45, 55–57].

The psoas minor is a long slender muscle, separated from the psoas major and iliacus muscles. It is located in front of the major psoas, originates from the vertebra of T12 and L1, and only present in 60% to 65% of individuals [46]. Distally, it merges with the iliac fascia and psoas major tendon. In Donald and colleagues' 32 hips study [58], 100% of the tendon of the psoas minor firmly blended into the iliac fascia, 90.5% attached distally to bone and fascia. The attachment to both the iliac fascia and the bony pelvis may assist in partially controlling the position and mechanical stability of the underlying iliopsoas as it crosses the femoral head, through adjusting the tension in the iliac fascia or through other pathomechanisms.

The blood supply of the iliopsoas muscle is from the common iliac artery, and the most important artery among them is the external iliac artery. Then, the external iliac vein collects blood from the iliopsoas muscle, which is the continuation of the femoral vein. The lymphatic system that involves is the external iliac lymphatic plexus, which finally merges into the common iliac plexus.

6.2.2 Internal Snapping Hip

Iliopsoas snapping (IS), also known as coxa saltans, is a dysfunction of the iliopsoas complex, which has been subclassified, as the clinical terminology evolved, into two types eventually: external and internal. The internal hip snapping is a disorder characterized by audible or palpable snapping of the iliopsoas during hip movement, with or without pain. In a long period of time, could be months or even years, symptoms will develop and increase. It most commonly occurs as the movement of the iliopsoas complex tendon over the anterior capsule of the femoral head, involving the iliopectineal eminence (muscle pulley), or the presence of exostoses of the lesser trochanter [46, 59].

Symptomatic snapping most commonly occurs with activities or sports that require significant hip range of motion, such as dance, soccer, hockey, weightlifting, and football. Incidence of the disease is observed more commonly in girls and women than in boys and men. A history of acute trauma has been associated with the development of snapping in up to 50% of cases. Although the real prevalence of this disorder is unclear, symptomatic snapping has been observed in up to 58% of elite ballet dancers, and most of them had bilateral involvement. External hip rotation and abduction at or over 90° is the movement that provokes snapping. Even so, the prevalence of asymptomatic snapping in the general population has been shown to be as high as 40%. Therefore, it is important to carefully assess the symptoms before proceeding with a treatment plan [49, 55, 59–61].

6.2.2.1 Snapping Mechanism

In 1951, Nunziata and Blumenfeld [62] first described the mechanism of internal hip snapping—that snapping is occurred as the iliopsoas tendon over the iliopectineal eminence of the pelvis when the femur is moved from the flexion position and extended. Since then, many researchers have confirmed this mechanism using dynamic US, as the primary source of iliopsoas snapping. Number of studies reported a sudden jerking movement and audible or palpable snapping sensation of the iliopsoas over the iliopectineal eminence as the hip moved from a position of flexion, abduction, and external rotation (FABER) to extension and neutral, especially at 30° to 45° of flexion [63].

Along with the deep-going of the research, alternative mechanisms have been proposed. Several studies propose that abnormalities of the soft tissue could be linked to snapping, such as an accessory iliopsoas tendinous slip, a paralabral cyst, or stenosing tenosynovitis [63]. And others have shown that the iliopsoas snapping occurs over a bony prominence other than the iliopectineal eminence, such as the lesser trochanter or the femoral head [55].

More recently, some investigators found that a sudden flipping of the psoas tendon over the iliacus muscle may be the reason of snapping occurring [16, 49]. In these studies, part of the iliopsoas muscle suddenly interposed between the psoas tendon and the superior pubic rami, when the hip was in a flexed, abducted, and externally rotated position. Therefore, while the hip is brought back to the neutral position, part of the medial iliacus muscle became trapped as the tendon followed a medial displacement and posterior rotation movement to its original position. The trapped iliacus is suddenly released laterally, resulting in an audible snap of the tendon against the pubic bone [16].

These literatures are contrary to the initial mechanism described by Nunziata and Blumenfeld, the iliopectineal eminence was located in the medial of the psoas tendon, and clearly not related with the internal hip snapping phenomena [62]. Overall, the certain mechanism of snapping remains controversial and the consensus is also lacking, but fortunately, it explored the possibility of several potential causes for this disorder.

6.2.2.2 History and Physical Examination

The diagnosis of iliopsoas snapping begins with a thorough, accurate history. Patients often report painful snapping with hip movement during sporting or recreational activities, and they can usually point out the painful area, even re-create the snap. The position of pain is generally present in the groin, sometimes may radiate into the thigh or top of the knee. It could be unilateral or bilateral [59, 63]. If accompanied by weakness or pain, it may be caused by tendonitis or bursitis [60].

Some patients may have pre-existing asymptomatic snapping, which becomes painful just after repetitive training activities at high flexion angles of hip. Symptoms can also occur during daily activities, such as climbing stairs or standing from a sitting position [55].

Physical examination should include a complete musculoskeletal evaluation of the hip and focuses on specialty tests specific for the suspected diagnosis. The most commonly described method of physical examination for detecting

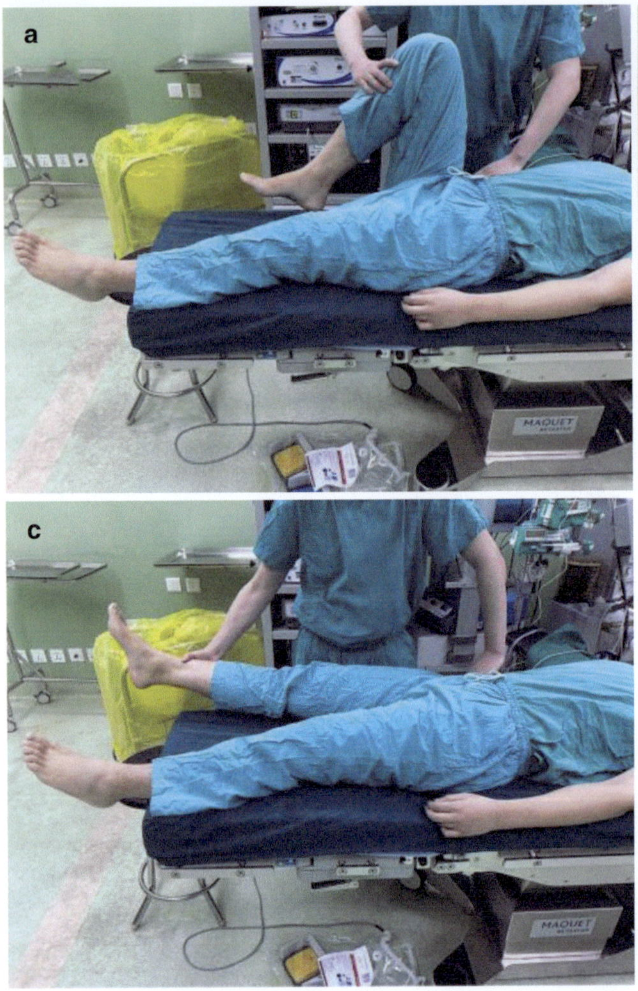

Fig. 6.9 The "active iliopsoas snapping test" for internal snapping of the iliopsoas. The patient actively moves the hip from flexion (**a**) to abduction and external rotation (**b**), and then to extension and neutral (**c**). A palpable clunk or pop is often felt with the examiner's hand placed over the hip

internal hip snapping is the "active iliopsoas snapping test." This test is performed by having the patient actively move the hip from the FABER position to extension and neutral, with the patient supine (Fig. 6.9) [38, 55, 64].

The operator should place his hand on the inguinal area to palpate the iliopsoas snapping, which typically occurs with the hip at 30–45° of flexion. Iliopsoas strength is assessed by resisted hip flexion in the sitting position. During palpation, the operator may evoke a groin pain, but does not always reappear snapping.

For a differential diagnosis, the "bicycle test" may help to understand if the snapping is the external type. The test is performed in lateral decubitus, by making patient actively extending the leg of the non-supporting side, like bicycle riding movement. If the noise or an abnormal sliding movement is felt on the great trochanter, it usually means positive. Besides, note that snapping accompanied with the inter-articular pathology (such as labral pathology) may confound the physical exam findings, because it has seen in almost half of the patients [46]. However, intra-articular injection of local anesthetic can be helpful in distinguishing labral tears from other pathologic lesions [60].

6.2.2.3 Imaging

Although iliopsoas snapping is typically diagnosed with a thorough history and physical examination, imaging studies are valuable for confirming the diagnosis and identifying concomitant abnormality. Radiographic evaluation should begin with anteroposterior (AP) pelvis and lateral hip radiographs to look for the presence of acute or chronic osseous abnormalities, and to find radiographic signs of femoroacetabular impingement (FAI) or other hip pathology. If a cam deformity is quite large anteriorly, the iliopsoas can snap over the femoral head. But this plain radiograph actually has little use to confirm the diagnosis most of the time. Dynamic US has a more successful application in the analysis of iliopsoas tendon movement during provocative maneuvers, especially in cases wherein the source of snapping is uncertain. US can also use in identifying hip tissue changes, such as joint effusions and synovitis, rectus femoris tendinopathy, iliopsoas bursitis and tendonitis, and muscle tears [49, 63, 64]. MRI has good contrast resolution for soft tissues, thus may reveal indirect evidence of snapping. Aside from iliopsoas tendinitis and bursitis, MRI can also be used in diagnosing associated chondral and labral abnormality, which are present in 67% to 100% of patients exhibiting painful iliopsoas snapping. Moreover, US-guided injections of the iliopsoas bursa are useful in evaluation of iliopsoas snapping as well. Comparing the changes between pre- and postinjection, if the patient experiences pain relief, the diagnosis of painful snapping is supported [60, 64, 65].

6.2.2.4 Surgical Treatment

The treatment is needed only when pain is present upon snapping. Conservative methods are recommended in current literature. Most of the patients find relief with rest, activity modification, physical therapy, nonsteroidal anti-inflammatory drugs (NSAIDs), and corticosteroid injections [59].

Surgical treatment is uncommon, considered in patients who have failed at least 3 months of a dedicated conservative program. The goal of surgical treatment is to lengthen the iliopsoas musculotendinous unit to prevent snapping and mechanical overpressurization of the underlying bursa [66]. Generally, arthroscopic release of the IP tendon is performed in conjunction with other procedures to treat related labral tears and FAI.

Various techniques have been developed to lengthen or completely release the iliopsoas tendon [38]. Historically, open surgery has been used. Nunziata and Blumenfeld [62] firstly treated internal snapping of the hip by surgical release in 1951. However, as clinical experience is accumulated, these procedures have been found increased morbidity and inferior results compared with arthroscopic techniques. In a systematic review of 11 studies, Khan and colleagues [67] demonstrated that the complication rate of open procedures is 21%, compared with 2.3% in arthroscopic therapy. Furthermore, patients undergoing open procedures had more severe postoperative pain, and higher recurrent snapping rate that occurred in 23% of open compared with 0% of arthroscopic surgeries. In addition to lower complications and recurrent snapping, the arthroscopic approach can be used to diagnose and treat concomitant intra-articular abnormality during the procedure. Treatment of related intra-articular abnormalities combined with iliopsoas snapping may improve patient-reported outcomes (PROs) relative to open procedures. Currently, however, there are no direct comparative studies evaluating arthroscopic versus open release for iliopsoas lengthening.

Arthroscopic release of the iliopsoas tendon has been described at three different anatomic regions: in the central compartment, in the peripheral compartment, and at the lesser trochanter. At these levels, the ratio of tendon to muscle is 40%/60%, 53%/47%, and 60%/40%, respectively.

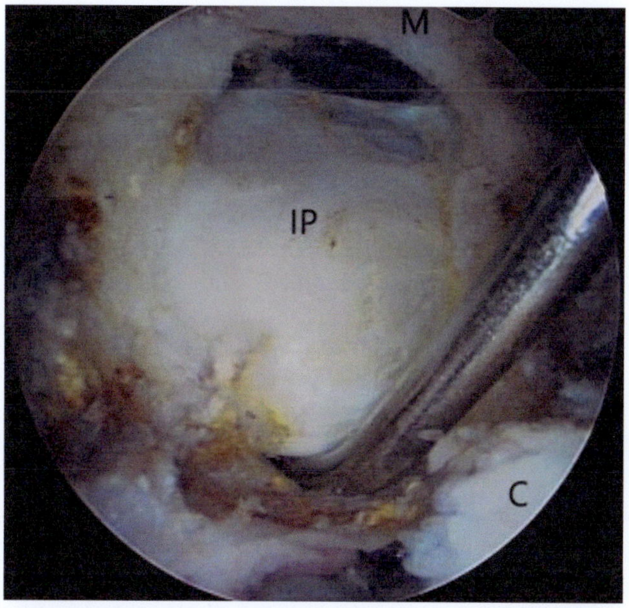

Fig. 6.10 Arthroscopic hip joint examination of preoperation. *IP* iliopsoas tendon, *M* muscular portion, *C* capsule

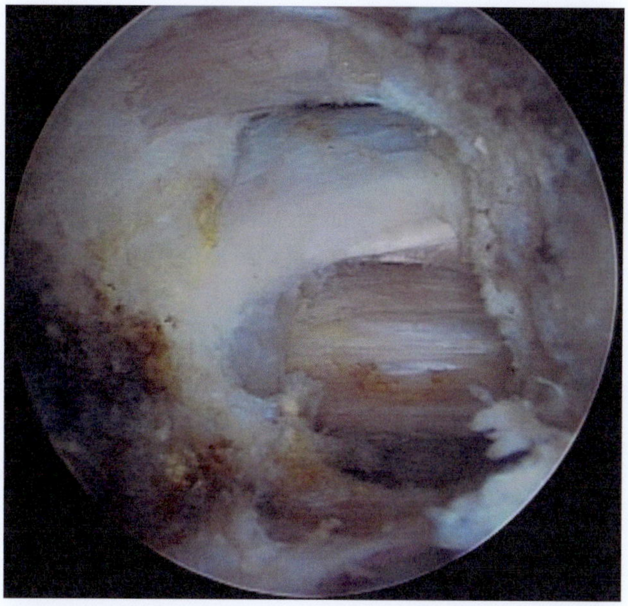

Fig. 6.11 The iliopsoas tendon image after arthroscopic iliopsoas release

To release the iliopsoas tendon in the central compartment, a 70° arthroscope is placed in the anterolateral portal for visualization with traction applied, and a beaver blade is used to extend the interportal capsulotomy medially to expose the IP tendon. We could see the iliopsoas tendon located at the 3 o' clock position on the acetabulum, anterior to the iliopsoas notch. Then the tendon can be released with the blade or the electrocautery device, while taking care to leave the muscle intact, causing recession-type fractional lengthening of the tendon (Figs. 6.10 and 6.11).

In peripheral compartment release of the iliopsoas tendon, traction is released for convenient visualization, and the hip is flexed 30°. A 30° arthroscope is placed in the anterolateral portal and pointed anteriorly toward the capsule. The iliopsoas tendon can be identified through a small (1 cm) transverse capsulotomy lateral to the medial synovial fold and anterior to the zona orbicularis. The tendon can be divided by an electrocautery device or beaver blade.

At the lesser trochanter release of the iliopsoas tendon, the hip need to be flexed 30° and rotated externally until the lesser trochanter is parallel to the coronal plane of the body and maximally visualized with fluoroscopy. A spinal needle is then pushed anteriorly perpendicular to the femur until it reaches the lesser trochanter, where a cannula is placed. The second portal is made similarly to the first one at intervals of 5–7 cm. Subsequently, a 30° arthroscope is placed in the proximal portal, and an electrocautery device is inserted via the distal portal to clear any soft tissues and release the iliopsoas tendon at its insertion on the lesser trochanter.

Series studies evaluating these techniques universally report good PROs, low recurrence rates, and less complications. In a systematic review of arthroscopic iliopsoas tenotomy by Kyle and coworkers in 2021, the overall cases, including the level of the labrum and the lesser trochanter, reported success rate of the procedure in resolving snapping hips [68]. The study by Ilizaliturri and colleagues [37] found some favorable results with iliopsoas tendon release, either at the lesser trochanter or in the central compartment, but there are no significant differences between the two techniques. Although outcomes are generally good, transient postoperative weakness and atrophy of the iliopsoas have been observed on MRI. Even so, complete resolution of the weakness commonly occurs by 3–6 months. There is no significant difference in post-operative hip flexion strength among three different levels of tendon release.

6.2.2.5 Complications of Iliopsoas Release

The most common adverse effect of iliopsoas release is hip flexor weakness. If the tendon is over released or the surrounding area is damaged, the hip flexor strength may be declined. Other complications for tendon release include infection, heterotopic ossification, muscle atrophy, continued symptoms, or nerve damage [59]. No major complications were reported [68]. To minimize the risk for weakness in hip flexion, the procedure should leave intact a maximum amount of the muscular portion, while releasing enough of the tendinous portion [69].

The postoperative persistence of painful snapping also has been observed, which may be related to multiple causes, such as undetected anatomic variability of iliopsoas, scar tissue formation of the tenotomy site or capsule, tightness of the muscular portion, and other subtle concomitant pathologies during the procedure.

Several further studies have evaluated predictive variables of worse clinical outcomes. In a level IV case series by Bitar and coworkers [69], patients with postoperative recurrent snapping after iliopsoas lengthening in the central compartment showed little improvement in PROs and lower satisfaction compared with those with resolution of snapping. Fabricant and colleagues [70] studied the association between femoral anteversion and clinical outcomes after arthroscopic lengthening. They hypothesized that patients with increased femoral anteversion (>25°) may lead to inferior clinical outcomes at greater risk, because the iliopsoas may act as an important dynamic stabilizer of the hip joint. In summary, deeper research is necessary to determine the best technique of iliopsoas release and further predictors of functional outcome and PROs.

6.2.3 Iliopsoas Impingement

Iliopsoas impingement (IPI) was firstly described by Heyworth and colleagues in 2007 [71], as a pathomechanical process that the excessively tight iliopsoas tendon impinges on the underlying labrum, resulting in characteristic abnormal labral anteriorly, such as tears or inflammation. In this initial report, 7 of 24 revision hip arthroscopy cases present this phenomenon, but each of them observed free of impingement from the tendon, after arthroscopy iliopsoas release. Another study by Domb and coworkers [72] supported that the tendon release could decrease compression on the labrum. Investigators also further defined the pathophysiologic mechanism of this phenomenon. 25 patients were identified who had anterior labral tears at the 3 o'clock position (right hip), but lack of relative bony abnormalities. Interestingly, the location of labral abnormality corresponds

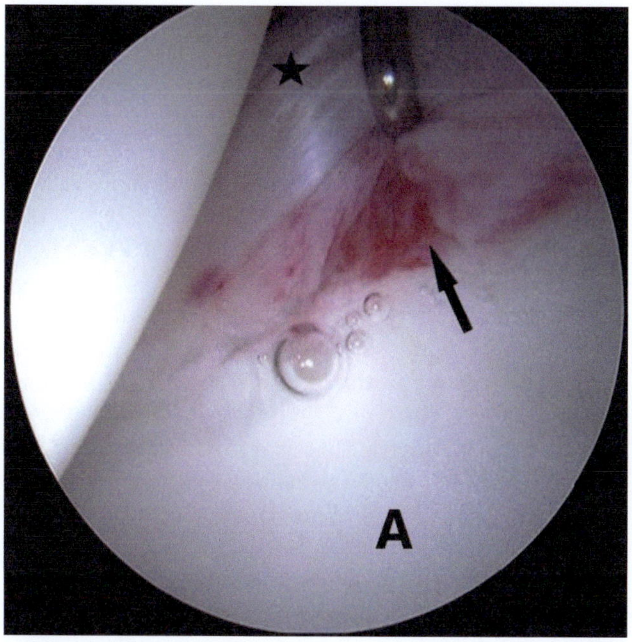

Fig. 6.12 Arthroscopic view from the posterolateral portal of a labral tear at the 3 o'clock position (*arrow*) in a patient with IPI. The iliopsoas notch, anterior labrum (*star*), and anterior acetabulum (*A*) are well visualized from this portal

to the iliopsoas notch (Fig. 6.12), just underlying the iliopsoas tendon. This is a significant difference from the 1–2 o'clock position injury caused by femoroacetabular impingement.

Sometimes, the labrum appeared inflammatory without obvious tearing, known as the "IPI sign." Furthermore, adjacent tendinitis and scarring of the tendon to the anterior capsule were observed in some patients. The investigators also discovered that the labral injury was possibly caused by a repetitive traction injury from adhesions of the tendon to the adjacent capsulolabral complex. Similar to the observations of Heyworth and colleagues, Domb and coworkers found releasing the tendon decreased compression on the underlying labrum in all cases. In a cadaveric study by Yoshio and colleagues [11], maximal pressure underneath the iliopsoas tendon is observed at the joint level during hip extension, what supports the possibility that excessive tension from the iliopsoas probably results in labral injury.

6.2.3.1 Etiology

Iliopsoas impingement occurs frequently in young active women participating in regular sports. The pain becomes worse with athletic activities and activities of daily living, such as active hip flexion, prolonged sitting, and getting out of a car. A total hip arthroplasty (THA) is traditionally reported as a cause of iliopsoas impingement as well, which may be associated with excess retroversion, an oversized acetabular fossa, or excess stem anteversion. Osteoarthritis of hip can also cause this impact phenomenon, probably because the iliopsoas rubs against the anterior bony process, which brings about abnormal mechanical stress within the tendon [9].

6.2.3.2 Diagnosis

Iliopsoas impingement has similar clinical presentation with traditional labral pathology of FAI, showing insidious onset of hip pain with typically "C-sign" distribution (from groin area to posterior greater trochanter). Snapping is also observed in IPI, though is less common, but has been reported in up to 17% of cases. These atypical symptoms may be a challenge to diagnosis accurately, suggesting that this pattern of impingement should be suspected if there is an absence of bony impingement with radiographic evidence of anterior labral pathology [9, 73].

Physical examination is not specific, but can also provide help of the diagnosis of IPI. Patients typically have a positive impingement test (flexion, adduction, and internal rotation), scour sign (flexion, adduction, and axial compression), discomfort in the sitting position, and focal tenderness with manual compression over the iliopsoas at the anterior joint line. Approximately half of the patients have pain with FABER and resisted straight-leg raise testing [55].

Intra-articular injections have shown variable results with some studies reporting transient improvement in 50% of patients, whereas other studies report improved symptoms in all patients undergoing injection. Some studies found that patients with chondral defects have greater relief after an intra-articular injection. If a negative result is seen, it is usually due to existence of extra-articular cause, like iliopsoas impingement.

US-guided iliopsoas peritendinous injection is a technique that has both diagnostic and therapeutic implications. After the injection, more than half of patients were reported immediate relief, and about 40% of patients remained pain free for up to 1 year [9].

Plain film radiographs are used for exclusion of other sources of pain, may show signs of FAI or frank dysplasia. However, the most pertinent radiographic finding is an anterior labral tear at or near the 3 o'clock position (right hip) or 9 o'clock position (left hip) seen on MRI.

6.2.3.3 Surgical Management

Surgical management of IPI focuses on lengthening of the iliopsoas tendon and treatment of concurrent labral abnormality, which performed after conservative regimen fails. Several studies have demonstrated favorable results with this treatment. In the study with average of 21 months follow-up by Domb and colleagues [72], after arthroscopic tendon lengthening and either labral debridement or repair, 95% of patients reported their physical ability improvement, and none reported worse. HHS and hip outcome scores were demonstrated significant improvements at final follow-up, compared with preoperative scores. Cascio and colleagues [74] also noted the HHS improved from a mean of 70 preoperatively to 94 postoperatively; however, one of these cases required revision surgery at 18 months to repair unaddressed labral tear.

The research by Nelsone and Keene [75] reported good to excellent results (modified HHS ≥ 80 points) in 23 of 30 IPI patients undergoing tendon release. However, some adverse effects were reported, such as avascular necrosis (3.33%), progressive degenerative joint disease (3.33%), trochanteric bursitis (6.67%), or recurrent painful iliopsoas snapping (10%). 2 of 3 patients with recurrent snapping were performed a revision surgery of iliopsoas release at the lesser trochanter and demonstrated good to excellent outcomes after 1 year of the surgery. Although these reports are encouraging, it is necessary to determine the optimal treatment for IPI studies with future long-term follow-up.

6.2.4 Arthroscopic Iliopsoas Fractional Lengthening

Arthroscopic iliopsoas fractional lengthening (IFL) is useful for painful internal snapping syndrome or IPI, which is commonly accompanied by FAI and acetabular labral injury. After the procedure, most of the cases had good short to mid-term follow-up results and significant improvement in PROs.

Surgical management of IPI is typically performed arthroscopically in 1 of 3 levels: in the central compartment, in the peripheral compartment, and at the tendon's insertion on lesser trochanter. The advantage of accessing the iliopsoas tendon from the central compartment is that it allows the simultaneous resolvent of associated intra-articular pathology, and it leaves the muscular portion intact. Therefore, it helps to preserve hip flexion strength.

6.2.4.1 Indications and Contraindications [76]

Indications

- Painful internal hip snapping—diagnosed clinically.
- IPI—diagnosed by clinical pain and/or tenderness around the iliopsoas musculotendinous unit and arthroscopic finding of an IPI lesion.

Contraindications

- No IPI symptoms and/or no painful internal hip snapping.
- Athletes required kicking or sprinting activities.

6.2.4.2 Step-by-Step Description of Procedure

Step 1: Patient Preparation and Portals

The procedure is performed with the patient in the supine position on a traction table. After applying manual traction, access to the joint is gained through a standard anterolateral, mid-anterior, and distal anterolateral accessory portals (Fig. 6.13).

The capsulotomy is performed from the 2 to 9 o'clock position (right hip), connecting anterolateral and mid-anterior portals. It is important to ensure that the operator performed enough capsulotomy, to obtain proper visualization and free movement of the instruments.

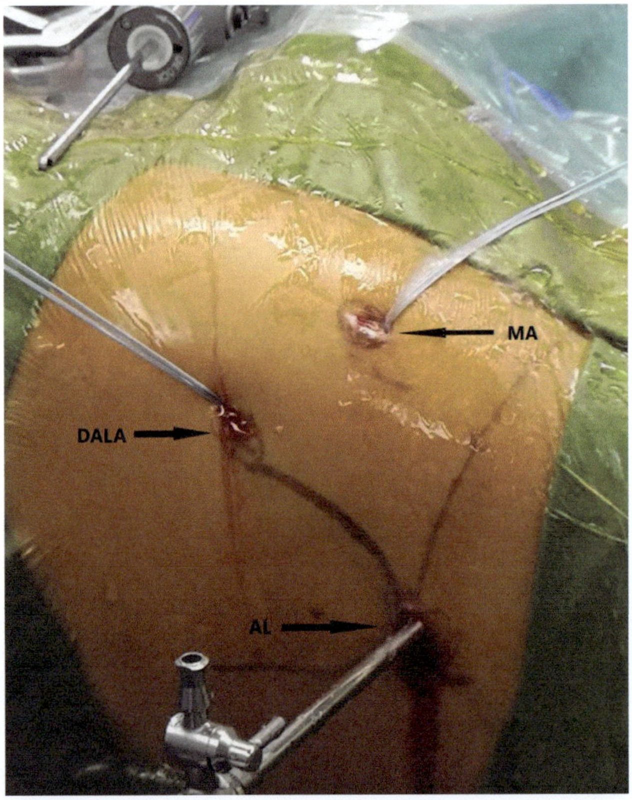

Fig. 6.13 Hip arthroscopy portals in the right hip. The patient's head is to the right. *AL* anterolateral portal, *MA* mid-anterior portal, and *DALA* distal anterolateral accessory portal

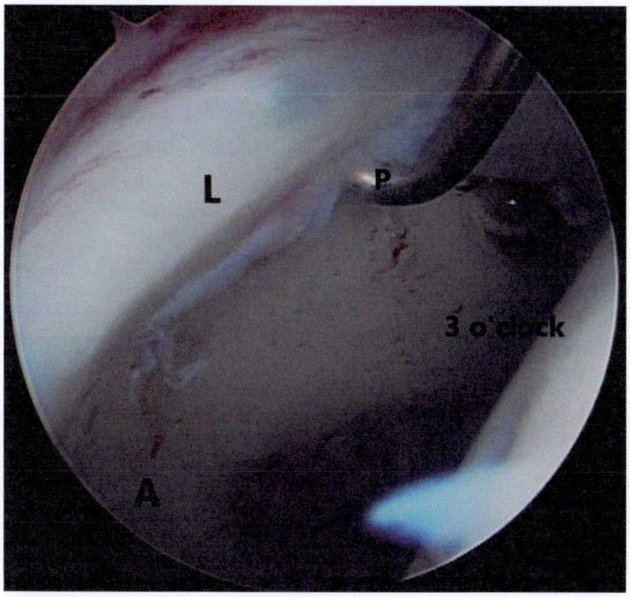

Fig. 6.14 View from the anterolateral portal in the right hip with a 30° arthroscope and the probe (P) coming from the mid-anterior portal. The asterisk indicates the iliopsoas impingement sign. *L* labrum, and *A* acetabulum

Step 2: Diagnostic arthroscopy

As we know, painful internal snapping hip usually presents with other pathologies, such as FAI and labral tears, thus we should examine systematically for other lesions, such as ligamentum teres tears, synovitis, loose bodies, labral tears, FAI, articular cartilage damage. The "IPI sign" is defined as labral injury at 2 o'clock to 3 o'clock area (right hip) (Fig. 6.14).

Step 3: Capsular Management

It is important to preserve capsular tissue, especially in patients with borderline dysplasia and/or laxity [77, 78].

The shaver is used to expose the junction between the capsule and the labrum. The surgeon should remove only synovial tissue, but not capsular tissue. Radiofrequency ablation is used to create space between the capsule and labrum, exposing the acetabular rim. A traction stitch can be used to hold the capsule in place during bone preparation and labral treatment, for better visualization and protection of the capsule.

Step 4: Attention of Concomitant Procedures

If concomitant procedures are required, for instance, acetabular rim trimming, acetabuloplasty, labral repair or reconstruction, and femoroplasty in conjunction with IFL, we should perform IFL at the end of the hip arthroscopy, just after other procedures. This process can help to minimize the risk of intra-abdominal fluid extravasation.

Step 5: IP Tendon Visualization

As proper visualization is critical for this procedure, fractional lengthening of the iliopsoas tendon should be performed through the central compartment at the level of the joint line. At this level, the proportion of iliopsoas tendon to muscle is approximately 50%/50%. Traction must still be applied during the procedure. A curved Beaver Blade is carefully used to extend the capsulotomy medially to the 3 o'clock position (right hip), but remember don't go beyond that.

A shaver can be used to debride the iliopsoas bursa in some cases when need to improve visualization of the iliopsoas tendon. Once identified the iliopsoas tendon, the curved Beaver Blade can be used to transversely section the iliopsoas tendon under direct visualization. Be sure to leave the muscular portion intact in the operating process (Fig. 6.15).

Step 6: Address Anatomical Variants [48]

Anatomical variants of the iliopsoas unit are more common than previously thought. It is imperative to be conscious of the possibility that more than 1 tendon may be present and require release, therefore the surgeons should spend sufficient time searching for additional tendons to prevent the clinical failure of surgical management.

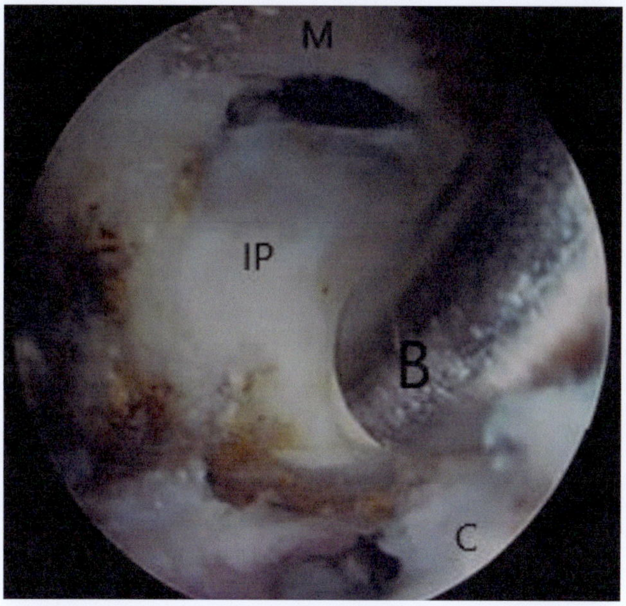

Fig. 6.15 View from the anterolateral portal in the right hip with a 30° arthroscope, the curved Beaver Blade (B) is used to transversely incise the iliopsoas (IP) tendon while leaving the muscular portion (M) intact, coming from the mid-anterior portal. *C* capsule

Step 7: Capsular Closure [77, 79]
In recent years, the function of capsular has got further understanding. It is generally believed that the joint capsular plays a primary role of stabilization in hip movement, especially in extreme translation and rotation movements. However, there is no unified consensus on this issue, literatures of repair of the capsular at the end of surgical procedure still have been controversial. Although lacking of clarity in the literature, many researchers still recommend the execution of the capsular suture. We believe that the restoration of capsular anatomy is critical for achieving good outcomes.

The patient is placed in approximately 30° to 40° of hip flexion, while close or plicate the capsule. 3–6 polyglactin resorbable sutures were placed starting medially and proceeding laterally. After all sutures are placed in the proper position, the operator can begin to tie. Then, after tying, gently bring the hip of the patient into extension position to ensure that there is no disruption of the repaired joint capsule.

Appropriate capsular preservation and management are even more important in patients indicated for IFL than for arthroscopic management of FAI and labral tears, as the setting of ligamentous laxity or borderline acetabular dysplasia associated with iliopsoas impingement.

6.2.4.3 Summary

IFL treatment of patients with iliopsoas impingement and painful internal snapping showed significant improvement in PROs between the preoperative and latest follow-up evaluations. In addition, most of the patients reported good to excellent results. However, capsular management and anatomical variants should pay great attention. All in all, overall clinical outcomes from this procedure were favorable based on recent studies.

6.3 Endoscopic Management of Anterior Inferior Iliac Spine/Sub-spine Impingement

Mingjin Zhong

6.3.1 Introduction

- The anterior inferior iliac spine (AIIS) is a bony eminence just above and anteromedial to the superolateral corner of the acetabular rim. It is the origin of the direct head of the rectus femoris and the ilio-capsularis muscles [80–84].
- Recently, many surgeons are investigating the various extra-articular causes of femoroacetabular impingement (FAI), in which the role of abnormal morphology of the AIIS and the bony sub-spine region is gaining particular attention [81].
- Arthroscopic AIIS/sub-spine decompression is demonstrated to be technically reproducible and excellent clinical outcomes can be guaranteed at short-term follow-up [83–85].

6.3.2 Indications

- Pain on palpation of the anterior inferior iliac spine
- Limitation in flexion and internal rotation of the hip
- Positive sub-spinal impingement test
- A prominent AIIS deformity on radiographs
- With or without intra-articular pathologies (such as FAI, labrum lesion)

6.3.3 Contraindications

- Infection
- Arthrofibrosis
- Excessive obesity
- Other contraindications of hip arthroscopic surgery

6.3.4 Author Preferred Technique

6.3.4.1 Pre-operative Planning

- Suspect AIIS/sub-spinal impingement should be suspected in patients with limited flexion and internal rotation of the hip.
- Low lying AIIS that is close to the acetabulum can be appreciated in anteroposterior radiograph of the pelvis (Fig. 6.16). Three-dimensional (3D) CT reconstruction views can offer comprehensive assessment of pelvic anat-

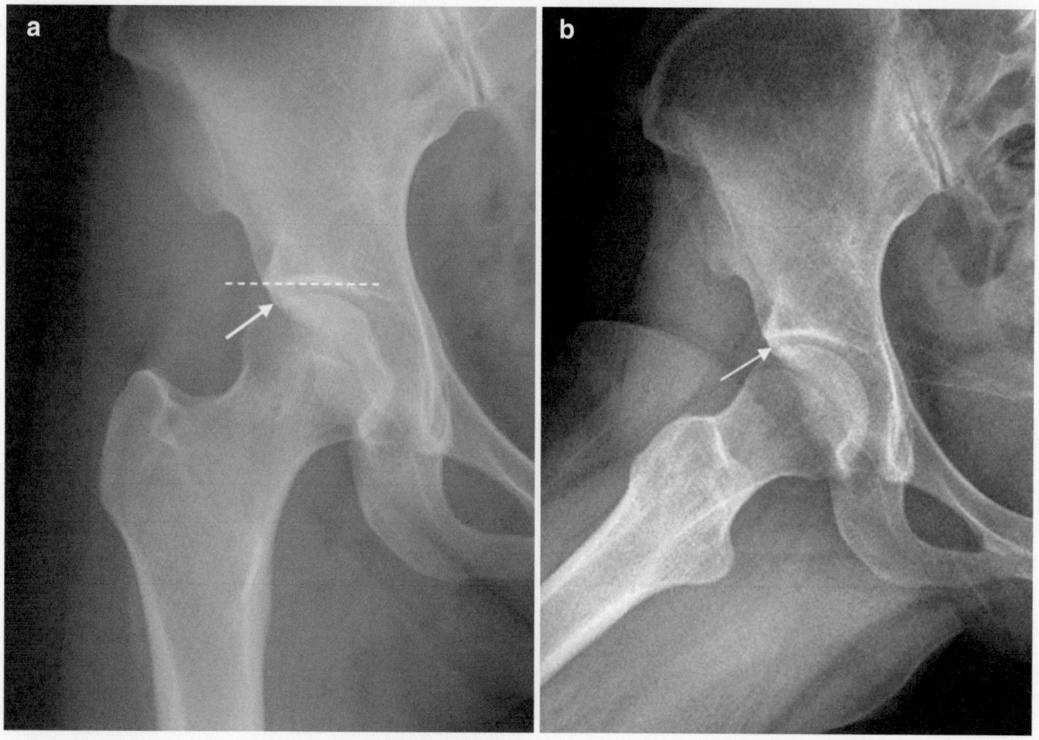

Fig. 6.16 X-ray radiographs of the left hip show a prominent AIIS (arrow), extending caudally to the level of the anterosuperior acetabular rim. (**a**) Anteroposterior position; (**b**) Frog position

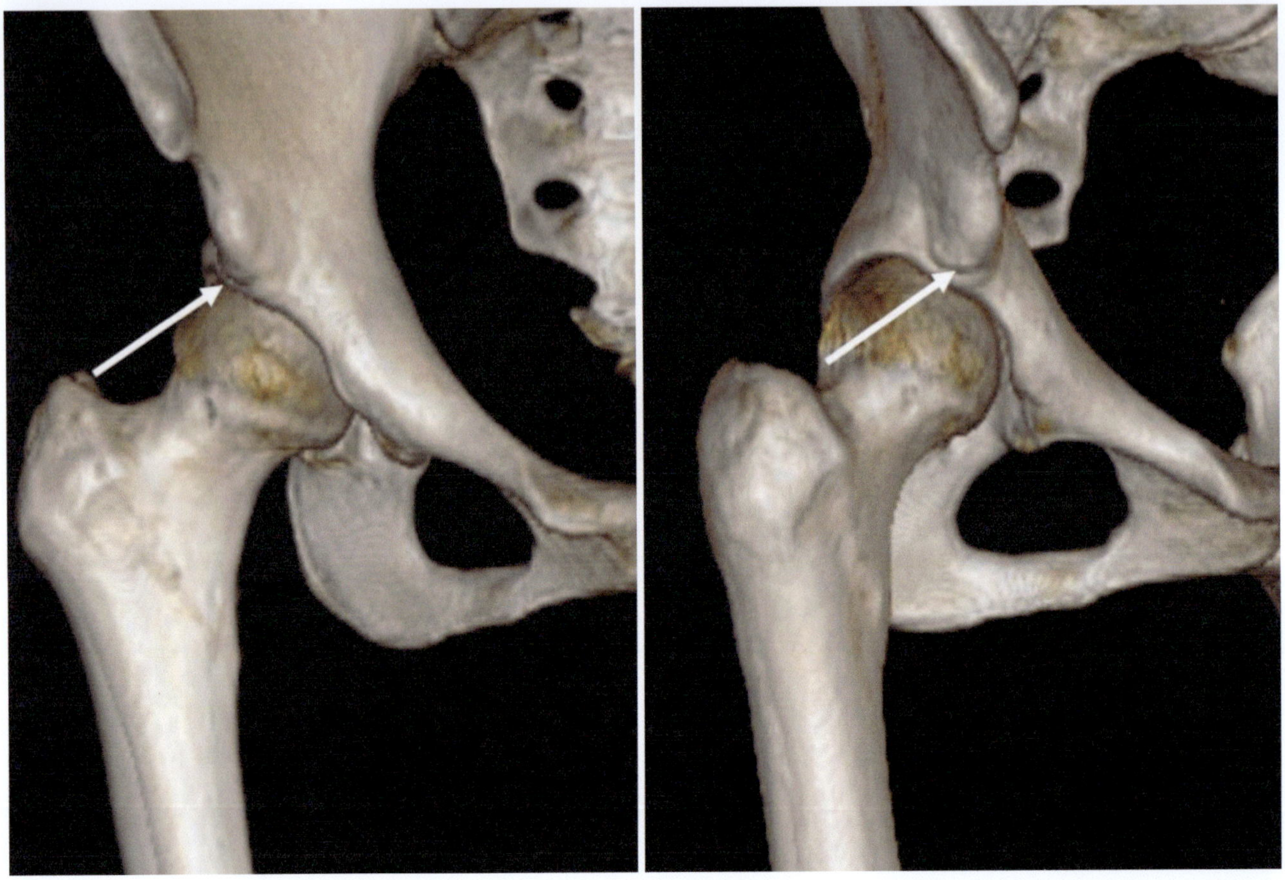

Fig. 6.17 3D CT reconstruction views show the prominent AIIS (arrow) extending caudally to the level of the anterosuperior acetabular rim

omy and help to confirm the diagnosis of low lying AIIS/ sub-spinal impingement (Fig. 6.17).

6.3.4.2 Patient Positioning

- The patient is positioned supine in a traction table after general anesthesia. Standard preparation of hip arthroscopy is performed by fixing the ankles on the traction frame with sponge padding of the perineal column of the table in order to avoid perineal injury by traction (Fig. 6.18).
- Key bony landmarks are identified, including the AIIS and the greater trochanter (Fig. 6.19).
- After sterilization and draping of the operative area, the operated hip is distracted with 10 kg weight. Hip arthroscopy can be started after the hip joint space is distracted to 8–10 mm (Fig. 6.20).

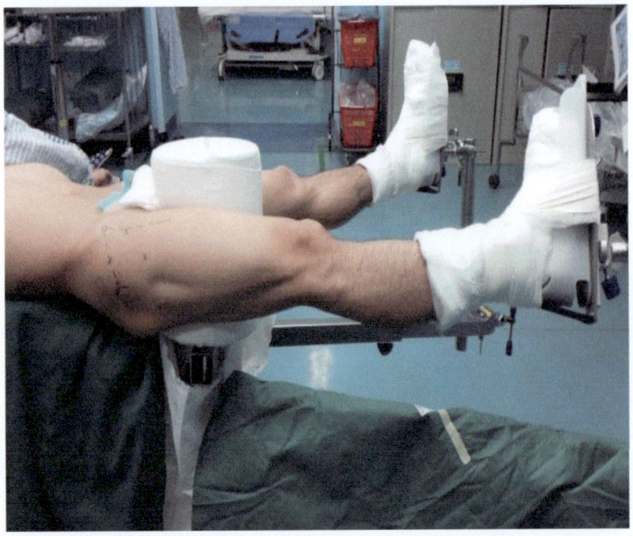

Fig. 6.18 Preparation and portal placement. (**a**) The patient is positioned supine on the traction table. The operated hip is positioned in neutral extension, approximately neutral abduction, and 15° of internal rotation

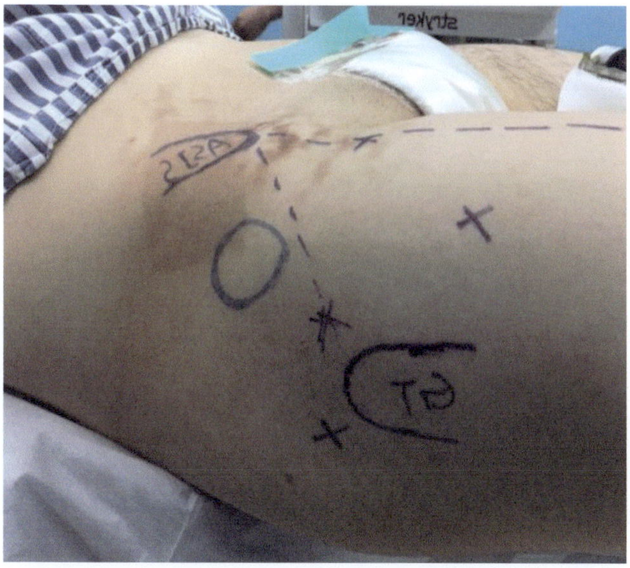

Fig. 6.19 Mark the bone anatomy with a marker pen

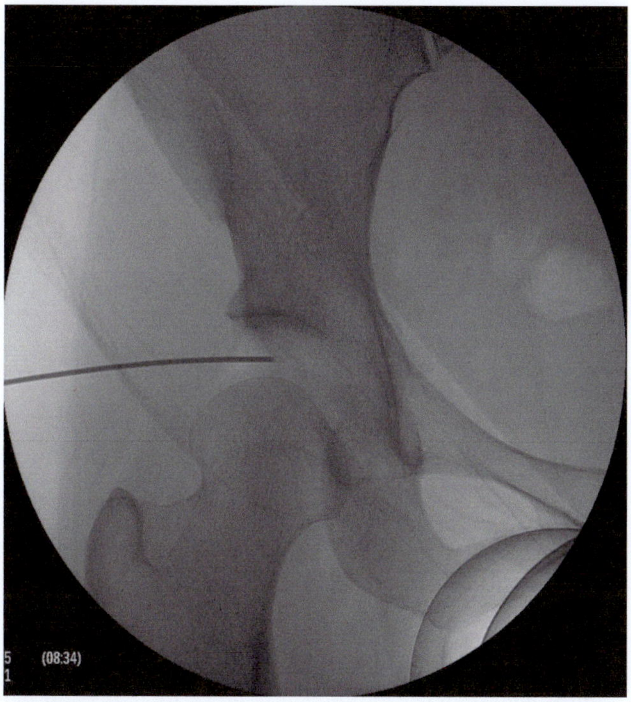

Fig. 6.20 The hip joint space is distracted to 8–10 mm to facilitate the hip arthroscopic surgery

6.3.5 Portal Design

- ***Anterolateral portal (AL)***: The portal is located at the midpoint of the line joining the anterior superior iliac spine (ASIS) and the tip of the greater trochanter. The AL portal is the most commonly used hip arthroscopy portal. The only important anatomical structure at risk is the superior gluteal nerve. This nerve, after exiting from the sciatic fossa, runs laterally and anteriorly and passes through the deep surface of the gluteal medius.
- ***Anterior portal (AP)***: The portal is located at the intersection point between a longitudinal line through the ASIS and a transverse line through the tip of the greater trochanter.
- This is an uncommonly used hip arthroscopy portal.
- ***Mid-anterior auxiliary portal (MAP):*** An imaginary line joining the anterolateral and anterior portals forms the bottom edge of an inverted equilateral triangle. The mid-anterior auxiliary portal is located at the apex of this inverted triangle. It can be shifted 1–2 cm medially according to the patient's height and muscle conditions. A portal is created at the intermuscular plane between the sartorius and the tensor fascia lata muscle to reduce injury to the muscles which can facilitate postoperative rehabilitation. This portal is the most commonly used working portal (Fig. 6.21).
- ***Creation of hip arthroscopy portals***: The anterolateral portal is the first portal to be established. Under fluoroscopic guidance, the puncture needle is inserted via the portal and advanced 45° from proximal to distal and 30° from the midline. The puncture needle penetrates the lateral hip joint capsule. After confirming the proper position of the needle inside the hip joint, the guide wire is inserted along the puncture needle and the puncture needle is removed leaving the guide wire in situ. After that, a 5 mm-diameter hollow core guide rod is inserted along the guide wire to enter the hip joint cavity. Arthroscopic puncture cannula is then inserted along the guide rod into the hip joint cavity. With the anterolateral portal as the viewing portal, the mid-anterior auxiliary portal is established under arthroscopic guidance.

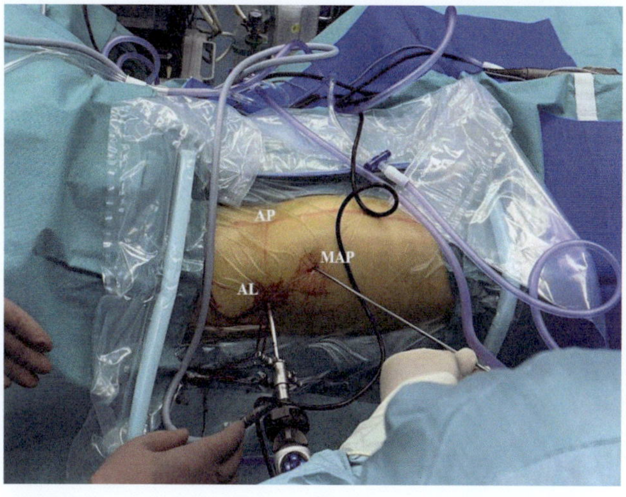

Fig. 6.21 The commonly used portals of hip arthroscopy. *AP* anterior portal, *AL* anterolateral portal, *MAP* mid-anterior auxiliary portal

- Interportal capsulotomy between these two portals is performed with an arthroscopic blade to facilitate instrument maneuverability.

6.3.6 Step-by-Step Description of the Technique

- ***Find arthroscopic signs of impingement:*** The hip joint is evaluated thoroughly with a 70° scope. The typical arthroscopic findings associated with sub-spine impingement include bruising or tearing of the labrum facing the protruding AIIS and an adjacent wave sign at the corresponding chondro-labral junction (Fig. 6.22).
- ***Expose the AIIS***: The AIIS can be exposed by partial labral elevation from the acetabular rim and capsular stripping proximally to the origin of the direct head of the rectus femoris. The direct head of the rectus femoris tendon at the rostral edge of the AIIS should be preserved. The AIIS is then fully exposed by means of an extra-long 5.5-mm full-radius shaver and a radiofrequency ablator (Fig. 6.23).
- ***Assess protruding AIIS***: The morphology of the sub-spine region can be classified into four types [85]. Type 1 (normal type): a smoothly concave or flat surface extended from the base of the AIIS to the acetabular rim; Type 2 (hypertrophy type): convex sub-spine region extended to and stopped at the level of the acetabular rim; Type 3 (prominence type): discrete prominence of the sub-spine region of variable size which is distinctly separated from the acetabular rim and extends antero-inferiorly and Type 4 (combined type): hypertrophy and prominence of the sub-spine region which extends distally below the level of the acetabular rim.

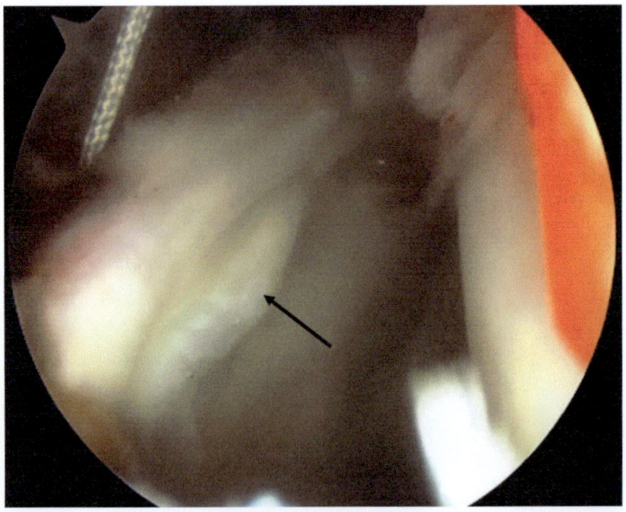

Fig. 6.22 The labral wave sign. The surgeon can demonstrate the sign by applying pressure on the acetabular labrum and the "wave" is elicited in the acetabular articular cartilage adjacent to the labrum (black arrow)

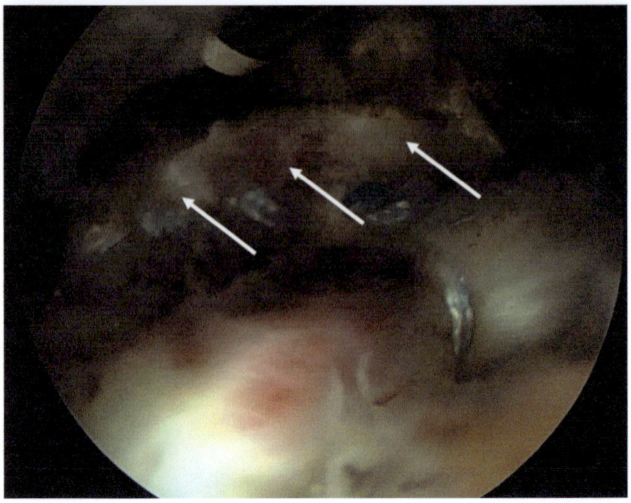

Fig. 6.23 Intra-operative arthroscopic image shows full exposure of the AIIS (white arrow)

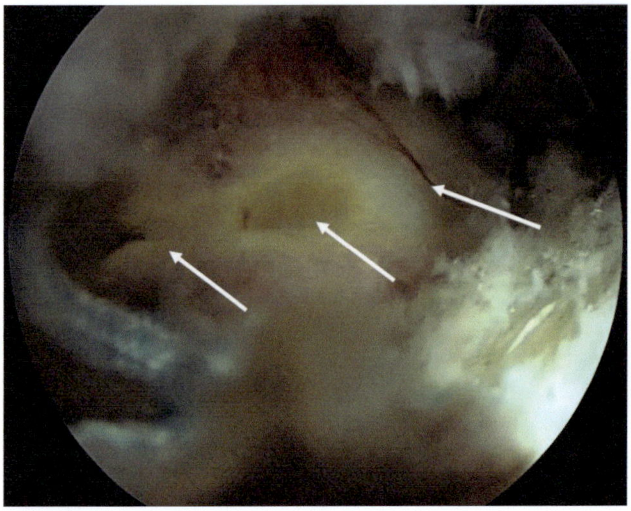

Fig. 6.24 Intra-operative arthroscopic view showed the completed AIIS decompression (arrows)

- ***Burring***: Endoscopic AIIS decompression is performed with an arthroscopic 5.5-mm round burr to achieve a minimum of 11-mm (2 burr widths) clearance between the most anteroinferior prominent point of the AIIS and the acetabular rim (Fig. 6.24). During the osteoplasty, the acetabular rim and the rectus femoris tendon origin must be preserved. A false profile fluoroscopic view can confirm adequacy of the AIIS decompression and dynamic assessment by hip flexion can ensure adequate decompression for good clinical outcome. Labral repair and femoral osteoplasty if indicated can be performed during the same operation settings [86, 87].
- Labral repair is needed in order to optimize the stability and sealing mechanism of the hip joint. The labrum is repaired with suture anchors by a labral cuff repair tech-

nique (Fig. 6.25). The capsule, which has been stripped from the acetabular rim, can be repaired back using suture anchors. In most cases, the significant caudal extension of the inferior border of the AIIS is easily accessed arthroscopically and extended re-contouring can be performed.

- The extent of bone resection should be titrated with intra-operative fluoroscopic monitoring and optimal resection can be evaluated with postoperative CT scan (Fig. 6.26).

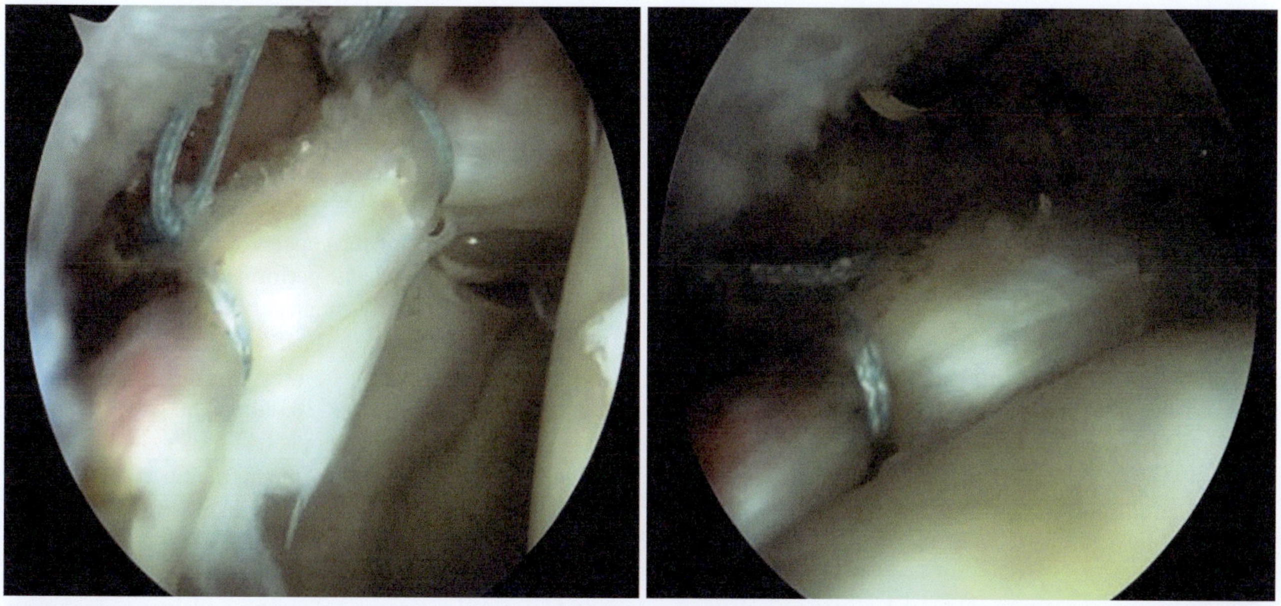

Fig. 6.25 Labral "cuff" repair preserves the free body of the labrum; Cuff repair following release of distraction with an optimal sealing mechanism

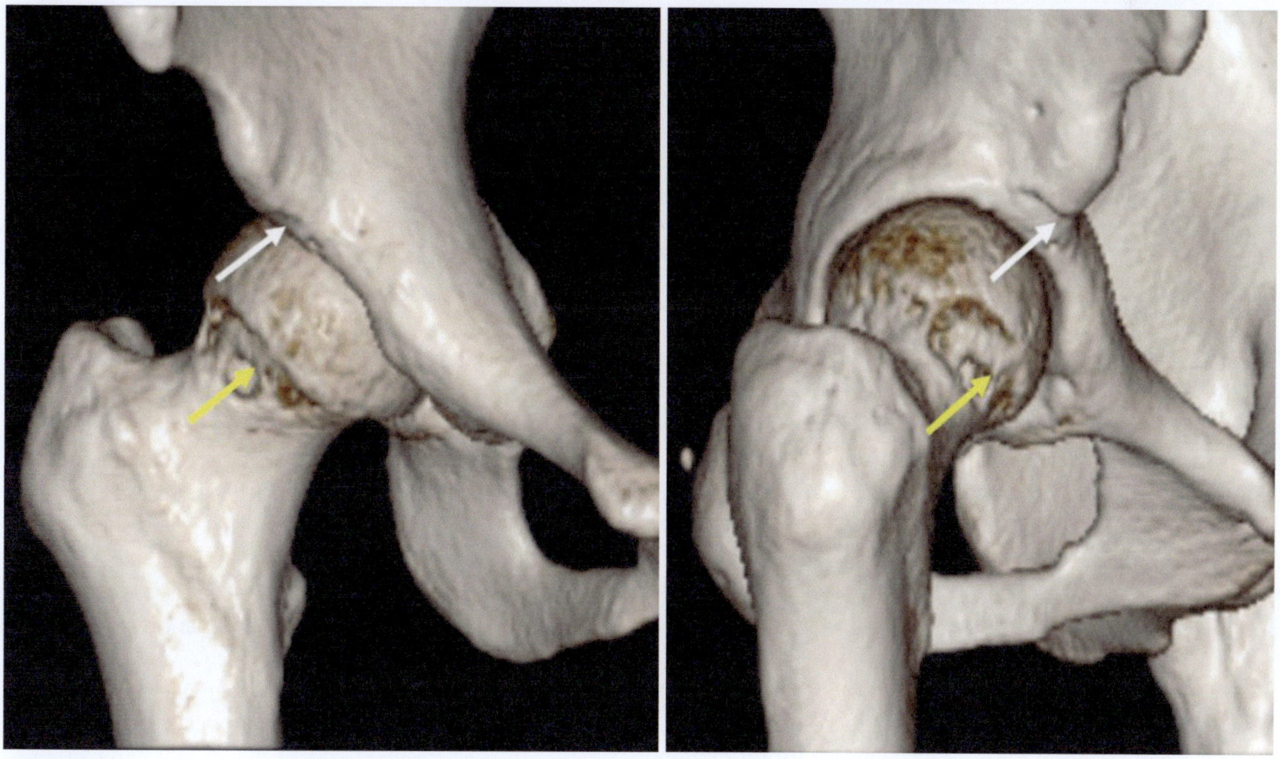

Fig. 6.26 The arrows show the sites of decompression of the low AIIS (white arrow) and Cam deformity (yellow arrow)

6.3.7 Complications and Management

- **Distraction-related injuries:** Distraction-related injuries are the most frequently reported complication of hip arthroscopy. These complications are usually associated with prolonged surgery and/or use of excessive traction force, and almost always present as transient nerve palsies in the form of neurapraxia.

Recommendations

- Continuous traction more than 2 h should be avoided. Intermittent release of the traction is recommended for prolonged surgery
  - In most situations, the traction force should be limited to less than 22.7 kg (50 lbs)
  - "Trial of traction" can reduce the total traction time

- **Compression-related injuries:** These injuries are associated with the compressive force applied by the perineal post, which is used to provide countertraction

Recommendations

- The perineal post and foot plate/boot must be heavily padded.
  - The perineal post should be at least 9 cm in diameter, and should be placed against the medial thigh rather than the groin crease.
  - The lateral force vector exerted by the post should not be excessive, especially in women.

- **Heterotopic ossification:** Heterotopic ossification (HO) after hip arthroscopy was usually without known reasons. It is theorized that surgical trauma to the gluteal muscles and the bone debris generated during bone resection might trigger the formation of heterotopic bone [88–91].

Recommendations

- The hip joint should be thoroughly irrigated to remove the bone debris after completion of the arthroscopic procedures.
  - In these cases, pharmacological prophylaxis [indomethacin (75 mg daily for 4 days) followed by naproxen (500 mg twice daily for 30 days)] should be administered, unless contraindicated.

6.3.8 Postoperative Care

- Weight bearing as pain tolerated with crutches for 2 weeks.
- Non-weight bearing for 4 weeks is necessary for labrum or cartilage repair.
- Early range-of-motion exercises are instructed to avoid soft-tissue adhesions and facilitate early recovery.
- Restoration of passive motion range should be restored and followed by active mobilization exercise and finally muscle strengthening exercise.

6.3.9 Outcome

- Study has reported complete symptoms relief, rapid return to sport activities and excellent clinical outcomes upon 2-year follow-up in all patients after arthroscopic AIIS decompression [84–86].
- However, in most of the reports, arthroscopic AIIS/sub-spine decompression was performed together with other FAI surgery, the improvements in clinical outcome cannot be totally attributed to the AIIS/sub-spine decompression surgery [81–83].
- In a retrospective study of 163 hips (150 patients) undergone concomitant arthroscopic FAI surgery and AIIS/sub-spine decompression, the mean modified Harris Hip Score (mHHS) improved from 63.1 (range 21–90) to 85.3 (37–1 00) and the SF1 2 score from 70.4 (34–93) to 81 0.3 (31 to 99) after an average postoperative follow-up period of 11.1 months. No rectus femoris avulsions or long-term muscle strength deficits were noted [80].

6.3.10 Summary

- Abnormal morphology of the AIIS region is usually the result of malunion of avulsed AIIS apophysis or avulsion fracture of the origin of the direct head of rectus femoris. This abnormal AIIS/sub-spine region is a known source of extra-articular hip impingement resulting in chronic groin pain and restriction of hip motion.
- In contrast to open AIIS decompression, arthroscopic AIIS/sub-spine decompression is particularly valuable in patients with combined intra- and extra-articular sources of hip dysfunction, because all pathologies can be addressed with the same arthroscopic approach.
- Arthroscopic AIIS/sub-spine decompression has been demonstrated to be technically reproducible and can relieve clinical symptoms of FAI and restore hip joint function.
- The arthroscopic technique used to manage the AIIS/sub-spine impingement is depended on the type and extent of the abnormal bony morphology and the presence of any associated intra-articular pathology.
- Further studies are necessary to evaluate the true therapeutic effect of isolated AIIS/sub-spine decompression rather than as a component of the overall surgical management of symptomatic FAI.

6.4 Endoscopic Removal of Calcific Tendinitis of the Rectus Femoris

Mingjin Zhong

6.4.1 Introduction

- Calcific tendinitis is a common pathological condition resulted from deposition of calcium hydroxyapatite crystals in the muscles, tendons, and periarticular regions [92–94].
- Although the pathogenesis is still unclear, calcific tendinitis is likely to be a multifactorial disease with traumatic, genetic, and local metabolic factors as contributing components [95–97].
- The supraspinatus tendon of the rotator cuff is the commonest structure to be affected by calcific tendinitis. Although the hip region is also commonly involved by calcific tendinitis, calcific tendinitis of the rectus femoris (CTRF) is rarely occurred (Fig. 6.27).
- Calcific tendinitis can be asymptomatic and may even resolve spontaneously. Conservative treatment of rest, heat/cold, physiotherapy, nonsteroidal anti-inflammatory drugs, or extracorporeal shock wave therapy is the first line of treatment. Invasive treatment modalities including local steroid or anesthetic injections, open or endoscopic debridement of the calcific lesions are indicated when the pain is not relieved by conservative treatment [98].
- Arthroscopic resection of intractable CTRF is a minimally invasive approach that can accelerate the postoperative recovery [99–101].

6.4.2 Indications

- Acute or chronic pain affecting hip motion and daily activities.
- Conservative therapy fails.

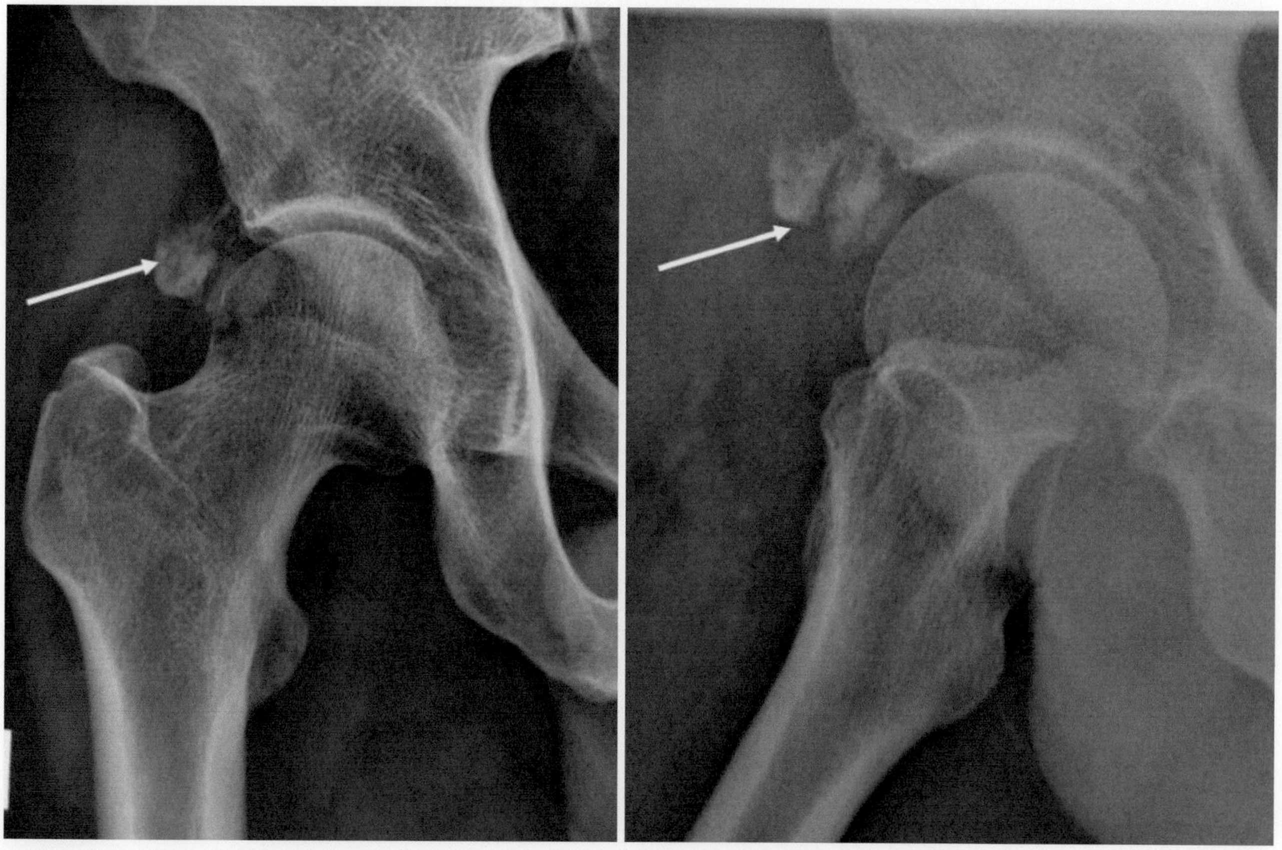

Fig. 6.27 The anteroposterior view shows a well-formed round radio-opacity (white arrow) in close proximity to the anterosuperior acetabular rim

6.4.3 Contraindications

- Infection
- Other contraindications of arthroscopic surgery

6.4.4 Author Preferred Technique

6.4.4.1 Pre-operative Planning

- In general, arthroscopic procedures for CTRF follow the same standard quality and safety measures of hip arthroscopy [99].
- Computed tomography (CT) and magnetic resonance imaging (MRI) are important preoperative investigations. CT can help the surgeon to evaluate the bony involvement of the CTRF and MRI can demonstrate soft-tissue edema. These investigations can raise the accuracy of diagnosis and detect and evaluate any concomitant intra-articular pathology.

6.4.4.2 Patient Positioning

- The operation is performed under general anesthesia and the patient is positioned supine on a traction table with the operated lower extremity in 15° of abduction and neutral rotation without traction. Both ankles are fixed on the traction frame. The perineal column is heavily padded with sponge pad to prevent traction injury and perineal injury. The surface bony landmarks of anterior superior iliac spine and greater trochanter and the femoral pulse are outlined on the skin to facilitate subsequent safe portal placement (Fig. 6.28).
- After standing sterilization and draping of the operative area, a C-arm image intensifier is centered over the operative hip (Fig. 6.29). The calcific lesion is located by a spinal needle under fluoroscopic guidance. The correct placement of the needle toward the lesion can also be guided by direct arthroscopic visualization.

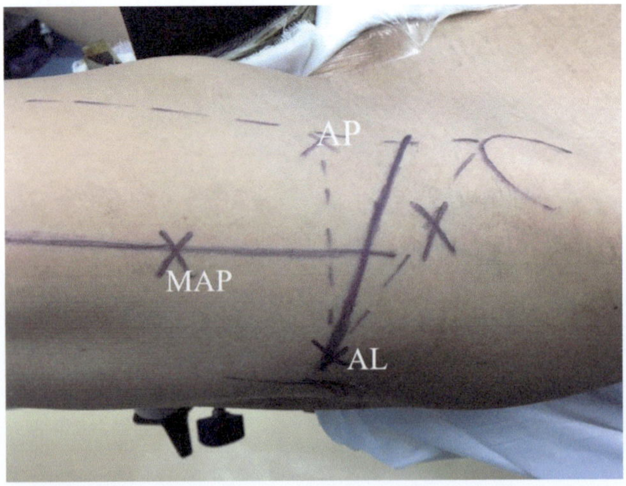

Fig. 6.28 Bony landmarks and the commonly used portals of hip arthroscopy were outlined. *AP* anterior portal, *AL* anterolateral portal, *MAP* mid-anterior auxiliary portal

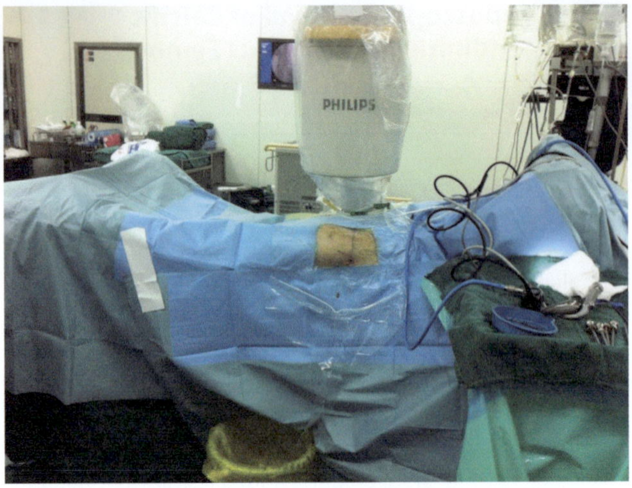

Fig. 6.29 C-arm image intensifier is centered over the operative hip

6.4.4.3 Portal Design

- The anterolateral portal (AL) is established first. Under the fluoroscopic guidance, the puncture needle is inserted via the portal and advanced 45° from proximal to distal and 30° from the midline. The puncture needle penetrates the lateral hip joint capsule. After confirming the proper position of the needle inside the hip joint by fluoroscopy, the guide wire is inserted along the puncture needle into the hip joint and the puncture needle is removed leaving the guide wire in situ. After that, a 5 mm-diameter hollow core guide rod is inserted along the guide wire into the joint cavity. Subsequently, a nitinol wire is inserted through the needle and a cannula trocar is assembled over the needle wire (Fig. 6.30). A 70° arthroscope is inserted through this portal.
- ***Mid-anterior auxiliary portal (MAP):*** An imaginary line joining the anterolateral and anterior portals forms the bottom edge of an inverted equilateral triangle. The mid-anterior auxiliary portal is located at the apex of this inverted triangle. It can be shifted 1–2 cm medially according to the patient's height and muscle conditions. A portal is created at the intermuscular plane between the sartorius and the tensor fascia lata muscle to reduce injury to the muscles which can facilitate postoperative rehabilitation. This portal is the most commonly used working portal (Fig. 6.31).
- In some cases, we can make the direct visualization portals toward the calcific lesion. Commonly, a spinal needle is inserted via a proximal accessory hip arthroscopy portal toward the calcific lesion under fluoroscopic guidance

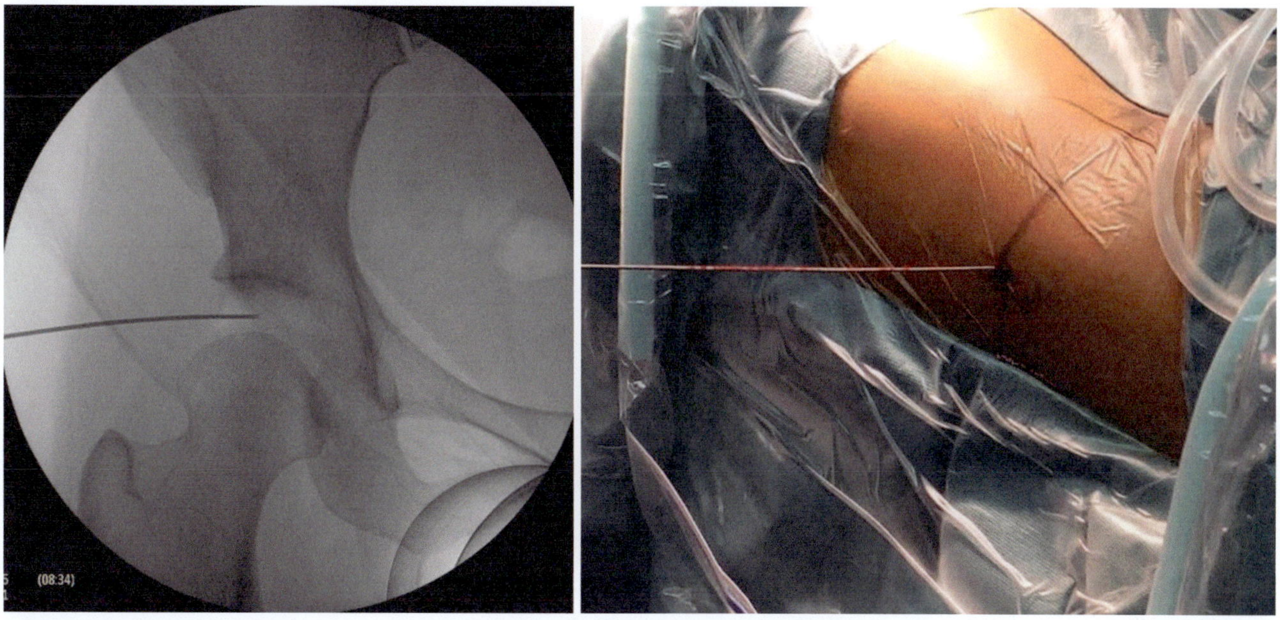

Fig. 6.30 Establishment of the anterolateral portal of hip arthroscopy

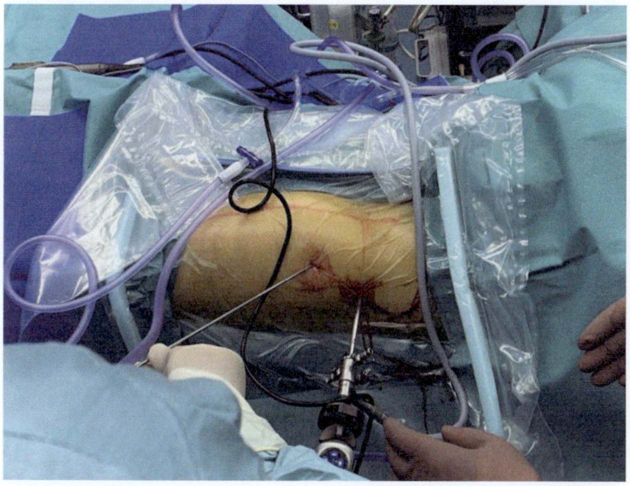

Fig. 6.31 Establishment of the mid-anterior auxiliary portal of the hip joint

and direct arthroscopic visualization. The proximal accessory portal is placed 3–4 cm proximal to the first portal aiming toward the calcific lesion under fluoroscopic and arthroscopic guidance.

6.4.4.4 Step-by-Step Description of the Technique

- The hip joint is evaluated for any concomitant intra-articular pathology with the AL portal as the viewing portal and intra-articular debridement is also performed if indicated.
- After that, superolateral paralabral sulcus is explored. The calcific lesion can be easily identified as a large calcific bulging sign in a superficial region. Sometimes, it is difficult to see any protuberance on the outer surface of the capsule side and intra-operative fluoroscopy is helpful for localization of the calcific deposits.

- The surrounding soft tissue should be resected by means of an arthroscopic shaver and radiofrequency ablator in order to define the extent of the calcific lesion (Fig. 6.32).
- With a longitudinal cut over the degenerated tendon, white, soft, toothpaste-like material spurted out, which is then completely removed with blunt instruments

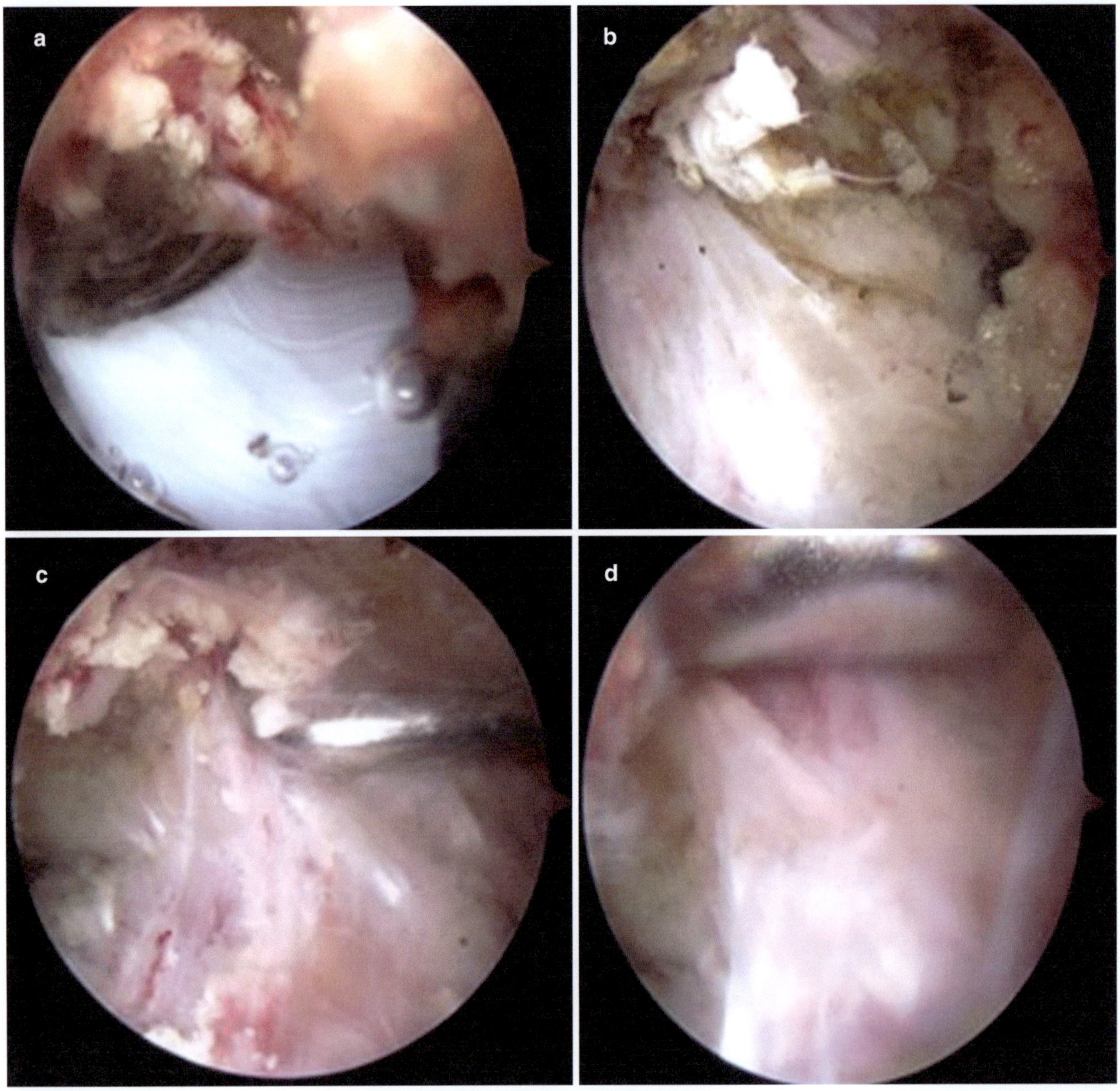

Fig. 6.32 Endoscopic view of the calcified lesion with the anterolateral portal as the viewing portal. The direct head of the rectus femoris was probed to reveal the white, soft, toothpaste-like material (**a**, **b**). Using the motorized shaver, the calcific material was removed (**c**, **d**)

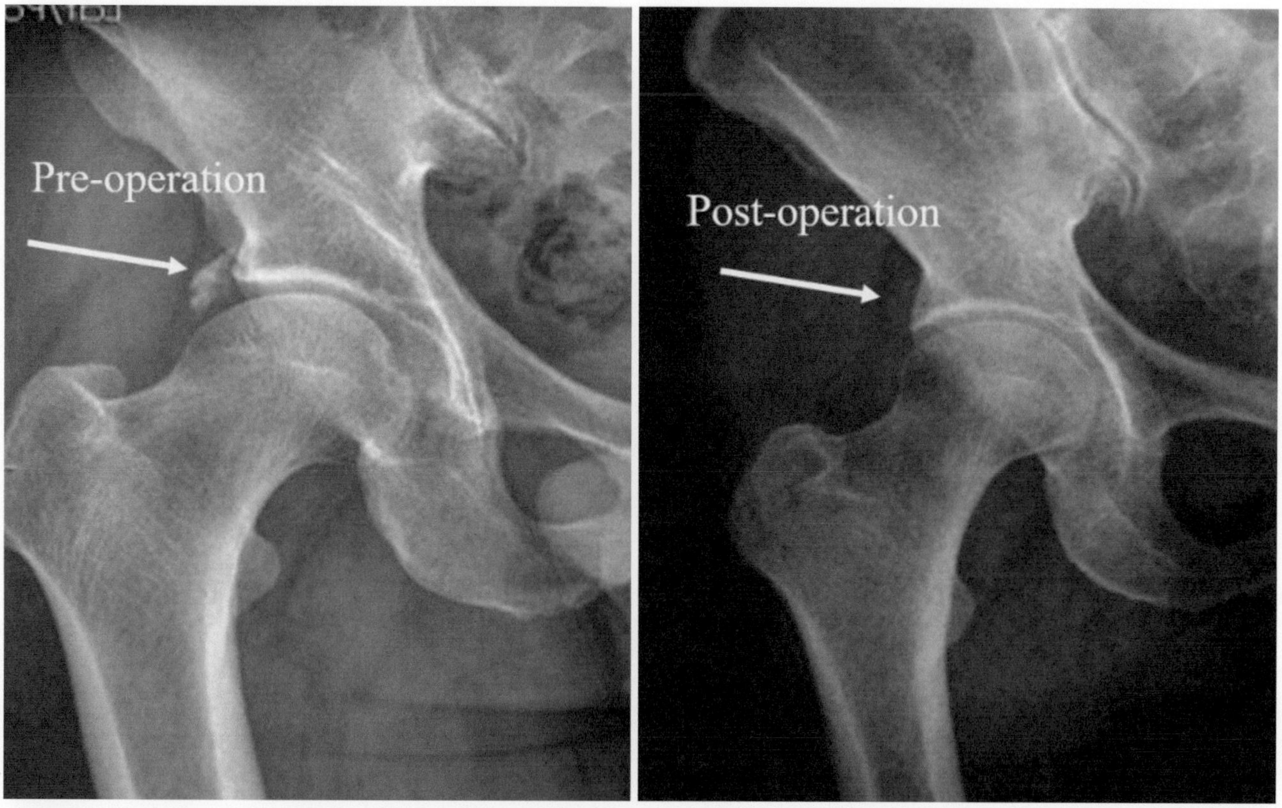

Fig. 6.33 Postoperative anteroposterior radiograph of the hip joint showed complete removal of the calcific lesion

(Fig. 6.33). Arthroscopic debridement of the tendon with an arthroscopic shaver should be done cautiously in order to preserve integrity of the reflected head of rectus femoris and minimize the risk of tendon rupture.

- In order to achieve complete resection of the calcific lesions, the burr can be switched between the working portals by using a slotted metal cannula.
- Finally, anteroposterior and lateral fluoroscopic views should be checked again to ensure complete resection of the lesion. The specimen is sent for histological examination to confirm the presence of hydroxyapatite crystals. A non-absorbable suture anchor is used to stabilize the labrum back to the acetabular rim.

6.4.4.5 Complications and Management

- Lateral portal placement in the hip safe zones under fluoroscopic control minimizes neurovascular risks.
- Strictly following the technical steps is the key to achieve complete and accurate resection of the lesion.
- Gentle soft-tissue handling can reduce the risk of recurrence of the calcific lesion.
- After controlling the bleeding, drain is inserted.
- Postoperative heterotopic ossification prophylaxis should be prescribed to the patient.

6.4.4.6 Postoperative Care

- Starting on postoperative day 1, the patient is mobilized as pain tolerated.
- Naproxen is prescribed as heterotopic ossification prophylaxis with the regime of 500 mg twice per day for three weeks starting within 24 h after surgery.

6.4.4.7 Outcome

- There are only few reports of endoscopic management of calcific tendinitis around the hip [92, 94, 96, 97].
- Peng et al. [92] reported 3 patients with chronically painful calcific tendinitis in the reflected head of the rectus femoris that were effectively treated by arthroscopic surgery with satisfactory outcomes.
- Yang et al. [100] described a patient with intractable calcific tendinitis of the deep part of the rectus femoris. There was a rapid relief of pain and a significant improvement in the visual analogue pain scale (VAS) from 9 to 1 after the arthroscopic surgery. On postoperative week 3, the patient was symptom free and return to daily activities without limp.

6.4.5 Summary

- Although uncommon, calcific tendinitis should be on the list of differential diagnosis of acute or chronic hip pain.
- Endoscopic treatment of calcific tendinitis combined with arthroscopic treatment of concomitant intra-articular pathologies of the hip joint is an effective minimally invasive approach to treat patients with symptoms recalcitrant to conservative treatment.
- It is important to emphasize that the longitudinal incision in the capsule fibers and rectus femoris reflected head tendon fibers should be small, partial thickness and a sparing single opening. Transverse incision should be avoided as this may lead to tissue retraction and prevent the tendon from healing.
- Postoperative heterotopic ossification prophylaxis should be given to the patient.

6.5 Arthroscopically Assisted Reduction of Developmental Dislocation of the Hip

Feng Chao and Lu XueMin

6.5.1 Introduction

- Developmental dislocation of the hip (DDH) is one of the most common hip abnormalities in children and infants [102, 103].
- Clinically, the early identification and therapy for DDH are crucial for avoiding risks of disability [104]. For the infants and young children, the therapeutic strategy employing a Pavlik harness before sixth months of the life has been proven to be effective for most patients [105, 106].
- However, the patients in the developing countries often delay or miss the optimal treating period. Also, there are some patients who failed close reduction.
- For the infants and young children who miss or fail the early treatment opportunities, open-reduction of the hip joint must be conducted. The optimal methods and incision approaches of open-reduction are still controversial [107].
- In the recent years, the arthroscopic reduction technique, as a minimally invasive surgical approach for open-reduction, has been extensively conducted for DDH treatment [108, 109].

6.5.2 Indications

- DDH,
- In patients 6 months to 2 years of age,
- Miss or fail the early Pavlik harness treatment opportunities,
- Persistent dislocation or subluxation, soft-tissue interposition, or reducible but unstable reductions other than in extreme positions of abduction.

6.5.3 Contraindications

- Patients age younger than 6 months or older than 2 years,
- Congenital dislocations,
- Hip infections,
- Immune system disorders,
- History of previous hip surgery.

6.5.4 Author's Preferred Technique

6.5.4.1 Pre-operative Planning

- The hip is graded on radiographs according to the Tönnis classification. Subluxated or dislocated hip is candidate for the procedure.
- Required instruments: 2.7 mm or 4.0 mm, 30° arthroscope, lightweight camera, shaver system with 3.0-mm full-radius blades, surgical instrument set, such as probes, baskets, graspers, and curettes, and an arthroscopic radiofrequency system.

6.5.4.2 Adductor, Iliopsoas Tendon Release and Close Reduction

- The patient is placed supine on the operating table,
- The medial approach as described by Ferguson is in the plane between the adductor brevis and the adductor magnus [110].
- The adductor longus and iliopsoas tendons are released routinely through the same incision.
- Arthrography is performed after close reduction. Safe zone angle and the medialization ratio on the arthrogram were compared before and after closed reduction of the hip joint.
- Close reduction is considered failed if persistent subluxation due to soft-tissue interposition or unstable reductions happens.

6.5.4.3 Portal Design, Step-by-Step Description of the Technique

- Through the same medial approach a single-portal arthroscopic-assisted reduction technique is performed,
- A 0.5 cm small incision was made through the capsule to create the capsular portal.
- After assessing the intra-articular structures, the hypertrophic ligamentum teres and acetabular pulvinar are resected, and transverse acetabular ligament (TAL) is released (Fig. 6.34).
- A limited release of the capsule is performed prior to reduction of the hip,

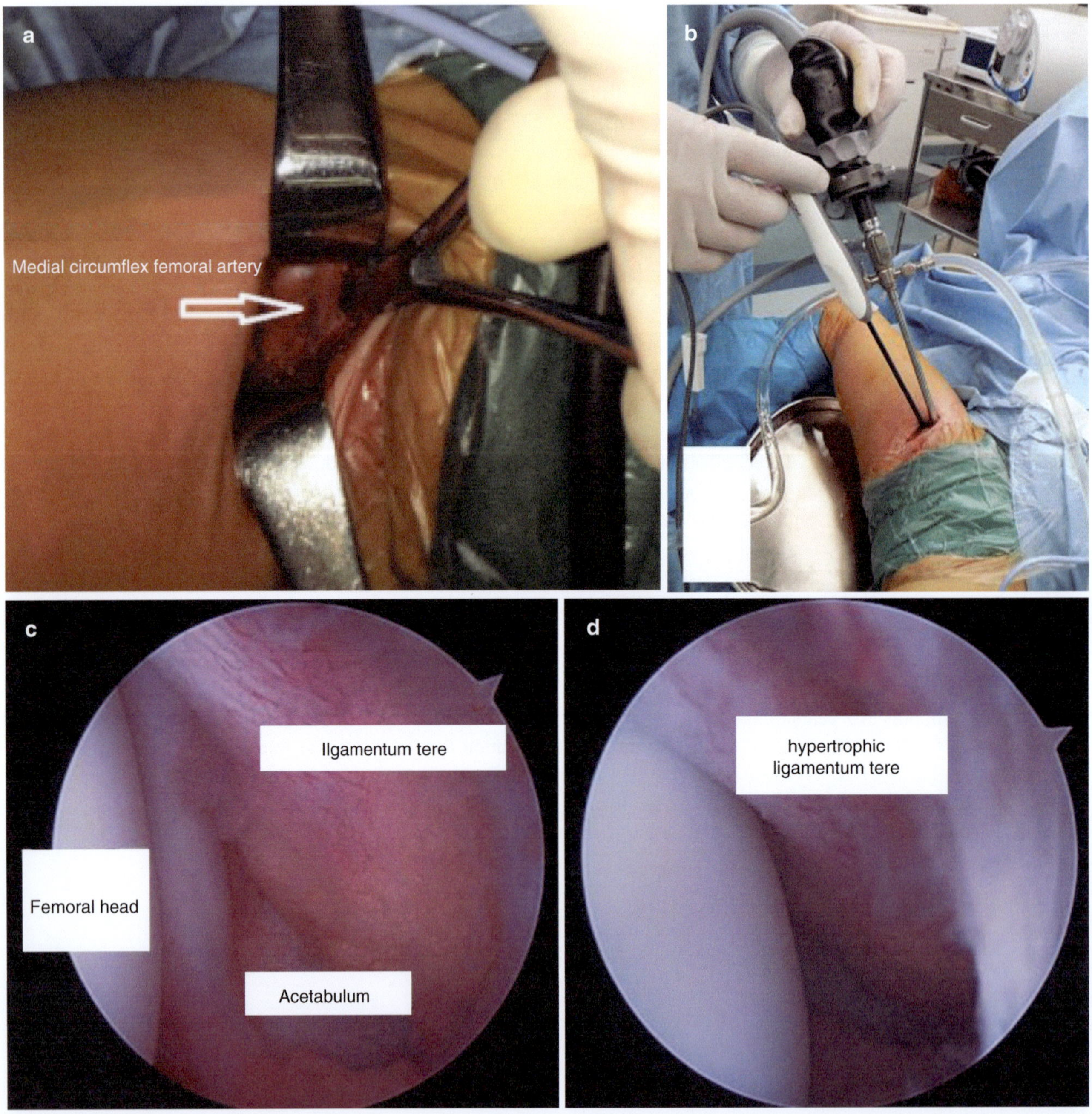

Fig. 6.34 The specific surgery procedures and the clear-up procedures of fibrous adipose tissue at the bottom of acetabulum. (**a**) Cut off or adductor muscle and iliopsoas muscle to illustrate the medial circumflex femoral artery. (**b**) Using the single approach, the arthroscope and plasma knife could be inserted through the same portal. (**c**, **d**) The hypertrophic ligamentum teres blocks closed reduction of the hip joint. (**e**, **f**) For the inverted acetabular labrum, 2/3 of which is cut open with preservation of the integrity of the remaining 1/3 that is attached to the bony acetabular rim. (**g**, **h**) The fibrous adipose tissues at the bottom of acetabulum is resected and the transverse acetabular ligament (TAL) is released

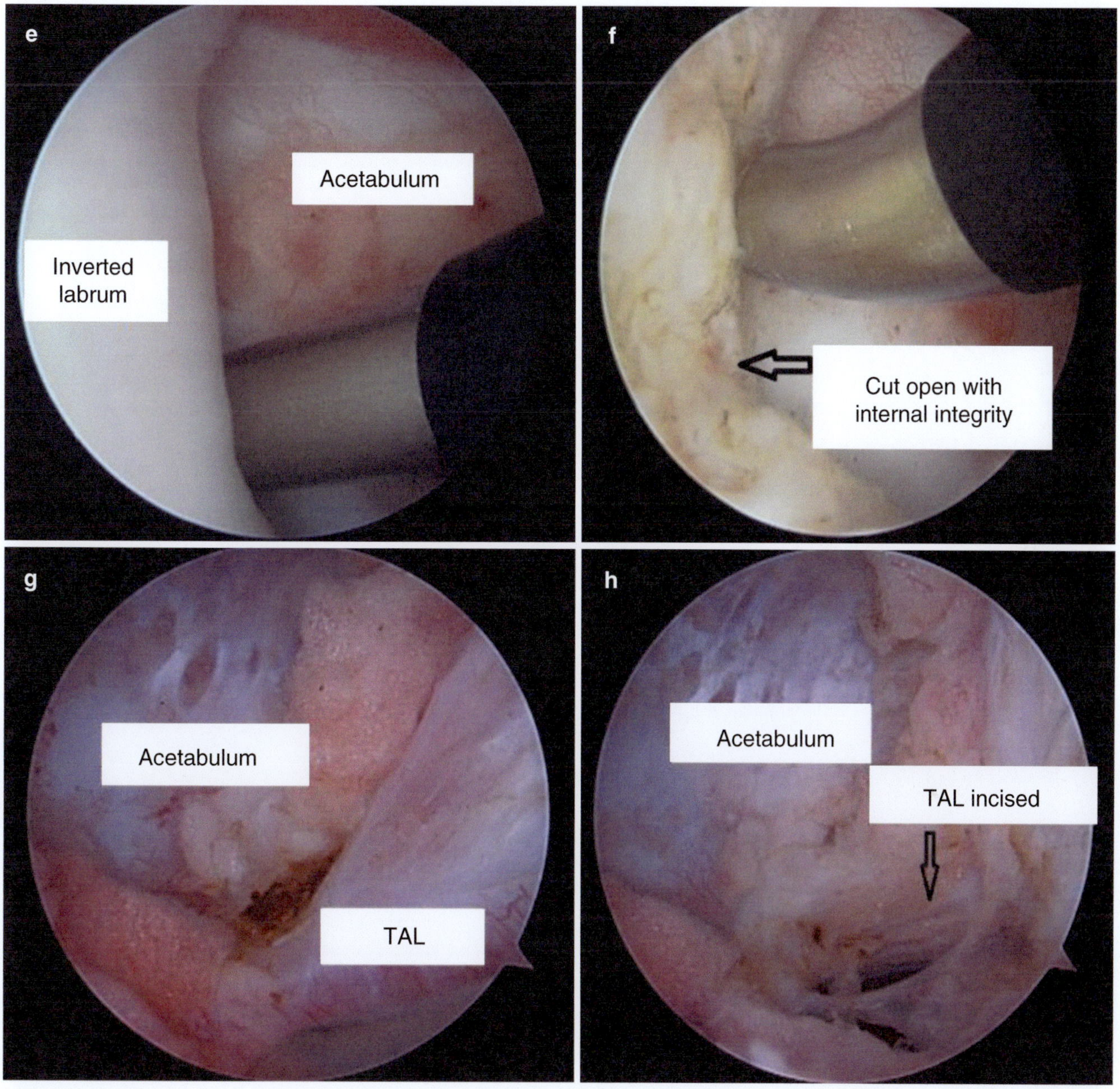

Fig. 6.34 (continued)

- Arthrography is performed after reduction of the hip joint.
- Safe zone angle and the medialization ratio on the arthrogram before the arthroscopically assisted hip reduction are compared to that after the reduction.
- Acetabular index is compared at 2 time points: before operation and at the latest follow-up.

6.5.4.4 Complications

- Femoral head avascular necrosis (AVN),
- Redislocation,
- Limited range of motion,
- Infection.

6.5.4.5 Postoperative Care

- The reduced hip is immobilized with bilateral hip spica cast in human position, and the cast is changed 6–8 weeks later (Fig. 6.35). Bilateral hip spica cast in human position maintains the hips in 95° flexion, neutral rotation and 60°–70° abduction. We switch the human position to the second-stage cast which maintains the hips in 60°–70° flexion, neutral rotation and 40°–50° abduction.

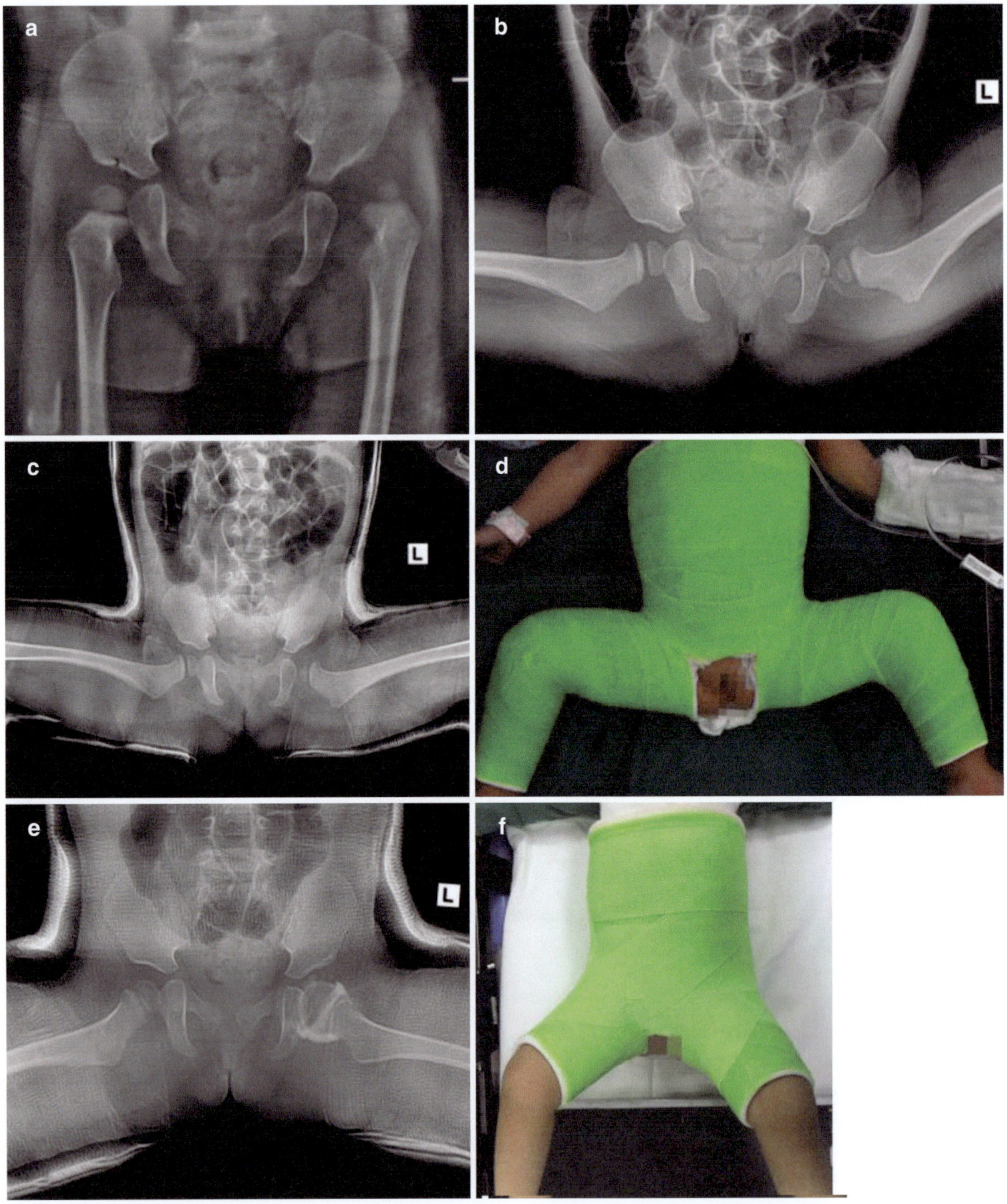

Fig. 6.35 A 14-month-old female child. (**a**) Unilateral left side dislocation. (**b**) Radiograph after arthroscopically assisted reduction confirmed congruent reduction of the left hip. (**c, d**) The first-stage frog cast external fixation after the arthroscopic procedure. (**e, f**) The second-stage frog cast external fixation after the arthroscopy clearance. (**g**) Radiograph taken at two and a half years after the operation confirmed the hip remained congruently reduced and the development is comparable to the contralateral hip

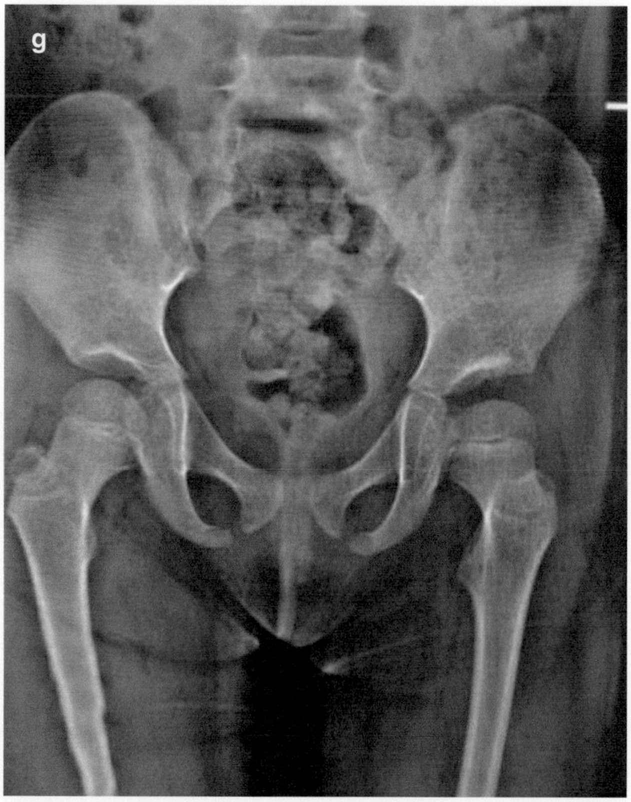

Fig. 6.35 (continued)

6.5.4.6 Outcomes

- Between January 2014 and December 2016, we had performed single portal arthroscopically assisted hip reduction in 13 hips [12 patients with a median age of 14 months (10 to 20 months)]. The reduction was confirmed on arthrography.
- Safe zone angle increased from 18.50° ± 3.78° to 61.88 ± 6.51°immediately after arthroscopic reduction ($p < 0.01$); and the medialization ratio on the arthrogram increased from 62.43 ± 19.81% to 103.57 ± 16.26% immediately after arthroscopic reduction ($p < 0.05$).
- With a median follow-up of 26 months (18 to 36 months), all 13 hips remained stable.
- The mean acetabular index decreased from 40.63 ± 4.95° to 29.36 ± 4.95° at the latest follow-up ($p < 0.01$).
- Kalamchi-MacEwen type I avascular necrosis was developed in 1 case and residual dysplasia was observed in 2 hips.

6.5.5 Summary

- Single-portal arthroscopic-assisted reduction technique is safe and effective in the treatment of developmental dislocation of the hip in infants.

References

1. Yen YM, Lewis CL, Kim YJ. Understanding and treating the snapping hip. Sports Med Arthrosc. 2015;23:194–9. https://doi.org/10.1097/JSA.0000000000000095.
2. Giai Via A, Fioruzzi A, Randelli F. Diagnosis and management of snapping hip syndrome: a comprehensive review of literature. Rheumatology (Sunnyvale). 2017;7:4. https://doi.org/10.4172/2161-1149.1000228.
3. Winston P, Awan R, Cassidy JD, Bleakney RK. Clinical examination and ultrasound of self-reported snapping hip syndrome in elite ballet dancers. Am J Sports Med. 2006;35:118–26.
4. Nunziata A, Blumenfeld I. Cadera a resorte; a proposito de una Variedad. Prensa Med Argent. 1951;38:1997–2001.
5. Philippon MJ, Michalski MP, Campbell KJ, et al. Surgically relevant bony and soft tissue anatomy of the proximal femur. J Sports Med. 2014;2:2325967114535188.
6. Philippon MJ, Devitt BM, Campbell KJ, et al. Anatomic variance of the iliopsoas tendon. Am J Sports Med. 2014;42:807.
7. Crompton T, Lloyd C, Kokkinakis M, Norman-Taylor F. The prevalence of bifid iliopsoas tendon on MRI in children. J Child Orthop. 2014;8:333–6.
8. Ilizaliturri VM, Suarez-Ahedo C, Acua M. Internal snapping hip syndrome: incidence of multiple-tendon existence and outcome after endoscopic transcapsular release. Arthroscopy. 2015;31:1991–5.
9. Andronic O, Nakano N, Daivajna S, Board TN, Khanduja V. Non-arthroplasty iliopsoas impingement in athletes: a narrative literature review. Hip Int. 2019;29(5):460–7. https://doi.org/10.1177/1120700019831945.
10. Alpert JM, Kozanek M, Li G, Kelly BT, Asnis PD. Cross-sectional analysis of the iliopsoas tendon and its relationship to the acetabular labrum: an anatomic study. Am J Sports Med. 2009;37:1594–8.
11. Yoshio M, Murakami G, Sato T, Sato S, Noriyasu S. The function of the psoas major muscle: passive kinetics and morphological studies using donated cadavers. J Orthop Sci. 2002;7:199–207.
12. Bolia I, Chahla J, Locks R, Briggs K, Philippon MJ. Microinstability of the hip: a previously unrecognized pathology. Muscles Ligaments Tendons J. 2016;6(3):354–60.
13. Audenaert EA, Khanduja V, Claes P, Malviya A, Steenackers G. Mechanics of psoas tendon snapping. A virtual population study front. Bioeng Biotechnol. 2020;8:264. https://doi.org/10.3389/fbioe.2020.00264.
14. Gomez-Hoyos J, Schroder R, Reddy M, Palmer IJ, Martin HD. Femoral neck anteversion and lesser trochanteric retroversion in patients with ischiofemoral impingement: a case-control magnetic resonance imaging study. Arthroscopy. 2016;32:13–8. https://doi.org/10.1016/j.arthro.2015.06.034.
15. Ilizaliturri VM Jr, Villalobos FE Jr, Chaidez PA, Valero FS, Aguilera JM. Internal snapping hip syndrome: treatment by endoscopic release of the iliopsoas tendon. Arthroscopy. 2005;21(11):1375–80.
16. Deslandes M, Guillin R, Cardinal E, Hobden R, Bureau NJ. The snapping iliopsoas tendon: new mechanisms using dynamic sonography. AJR Am J Roentgenol. 2008;190(3):576–81.
17. Liebeskind B, Olinger K. Bifid iliopsoas tendon as a cause for internal snapping hip syndrome: a case report. J Clin Ultrasound. 2020;48(6):346–9.
18. Matthew J, Kraeutler MJ, Garabekyan T, Pascual-Garrido C, Mei-Dan O. Hip instability: a review of hip dysplasia and other contributing factors. Muscles Ligaments Tendons J. 2016;6(3):343–53.
19. Capogna BM, Shenoy K, Youm T, Stuchin SA. Tendon disorders after total hip arthroplasty: evaluation and management. J Arthroplasty. 2017;32:3249–55. https://doi.org/10.1016/j.arth.2017.04.015.
20. Saltychev M, Pernaa K, Seppänen M, Mäkelä K, Laimi K. Pelvic incidence and hip disorders. Acta Orthop. 2018;89(1):66–70.
21. Balius R, Pedret C, Blasi M, et al. Sonographic evaluation of the distal iliopsoas tendon using a new approach. J Ultrasound Med. 2014;33:2021–30.
22. Blankenbaker DG, De Smet AA, Keene JS. Sonography of the iliopsoas tendon and injection of the iliopsoas bursa for diagnosis and management of the painful snapping hip. Skelet Radiol. 2006;35(8):565–71.
23. Bakhsh W, Childs S, Kenney R, Schiffman S, Giordano B. Iliopsoas snapping hip: improving the diagnostic value of magnetic resonance imaging with a novel parameter. Skelet Radiol. 2019;48:889–96. https://doi.org/10.1007/s00256-018-3083-5.
24. Frizziero A, Vittadini F, Pignataro A, et al. Conservative management of tendinopathies around hip. Muscles Ligaments Tendons J. 2019;6:281–92.
25. Philippon MJ, Decker MJ, Giphart JE, et al. Rehabilitation exercise progression for the gluteus medius muscle with consideration for iliopsoas tendinitis: an in vivo electromyography study. Am J Sports Med. 2011;39:1777–85.
26. Laible C, Swanson D, Garofolo G, et al. Iliopsoas syndrome in dancers. Orthop J Sports Med. 2013;1:2325967113500638.
27. Gouveia K, Shah A, Kay J, et al. Iliopsoas tenotomy during hip arthroscopy: a systematic review of postoperative outcomes. Am J Sports Med. 2021;49(3):817–29. https://doi.org/10.1177/0363546520922551.
28. Longstaffe R, Hendrikx S, Naudie D, et al. Iliopsoas release: a systematic review of clinical efficacy and associated complications. Clin J Sport Med. 2021; https://doi.org/10.1097/JSM.0000000000000784.
29. Hoskins JS, Burd TA, Allen WC. Surgical correction of internal coxa saltans: a 20-year consecutive study. Am J Sports Med. 2004;32(4):998–1001.
30. Via AG, Basile A, Wainer M, Musa C, Padulo J, Mardones R. Endoscopic release of internal snapping hip: a review of literature. Muscles Ligaments Tendons J. 2016;6:372–7.
31. Byrd JW. Evaluation and management of the snapping iliopsoas tendon. Tech Orthop. 2005;20:45–51.
32. Brandenburg JB, Kapron JL, Wylie JD, et al. The functional and structural outcomes of arthroscopic iliopsoas release. Am J Sports Med. 2016;44(5):1286–91. https://doi.org/10.1177/0363546515626173.
33. Flanum ME, Keene JS, Blankenbaker DG, Desmet AA. Arthroscopic treatment of the painful "internal" snapping hip: results of a new endoscopic technique and imaging protocol. Am J Sports Med. 2007;35:770–9.
34. Hain KS, Blankenbaker DG, De Smet AA, Keene JS, Munoz del Rio A. MRI appearance and clinical significance of changes in the hip muscles and iliopsoas tendon after arthroscopic iliopsoas tenotomy in symptomatic patients. HSSJ. 2013;9:236–41.
35. Contreras ME, Dani WS, Endges WK, De Araujo LC, Berral FJ. Arthroscopic treatment of the snapping iliopsoas tendon through the central compartment of the hip: a pilot study. J Bone Joint Surg Br. 2010;92(6):777–80.
36. Hwang DS, Jung-Mo Hwang JM, Kim PS, et al. Arthroscopic treatment of symptomatic internal snapping hip with combined pathologies. Clin Orthop Surg. 2015;7:158–63.
37. Ilizaliturri VM, Buganza-Tepole M, Olivos-Meza A, Acuna M, Acosta-Rodriguez E. Central compartment release versus lesser trochanter release of the iliopsoas tendon for the treatment of internal snapping hip: a comparative study. Arthroscopy. 2014;30:790–5.
38. Potalivo G, Bugiantella W. Snapping hip syndrome: systematic review of surgical treatment. Hip Int. 2017;27:111–21. https://doi.org/10.5301/hipint.5000464.

39. Mardones R, Giai Via A, Tomic A, Rodriguez C, Salineros M, Somarriva M. Arthroscopic release of iliopsoas tendon in patients with femoroacetabular impingement: clinical results at mid-term follow-up. Muscles Ligaments Tendons J. 2016;6:378–83.
40. Perets I, Hartigan DE, Chaharbakhshi EO, Ashberg L, Mu B, Domb BG. Clinical outcomes and return to sport in competitive athletes undergoing arthroscopic iliopsoas fractional lengthening compared with a matched control group without iliopsoas fractional lengthening. Arthroscopy. 2018;34(2):456–63. https://doi.org/10.1016/j.arthro.2017.08.292.
41. Perets I, Chaharbakhshi EO, Mansor Y, et al. Midterm outcomes of iliopsoas fractional lengthening for internal snapping as a part of hip arthroscopy for femoroacetabular impingement and labral tear: a matched control study. Arthroscopy. 2019;35(5):1432–40. https://doi.org/10.1016/j.arthro.2018.11.050.
42. Mei-Dan O, McConkey MO, Brick M. Catastrophic failure of hip arthroscopy due to iatrogenic instability: Can partial division of the ligamentum teres and iliofemoral ligament cause subluxation? J Arthrosc Relat Surg. 2012;28:440–5.
43. Matsuda DK. Acute iatrogenic dislocation following hip impingement arthroscopic surgery. Arthrosc J Arthrosc Relat Surg. 2009;25:400–4.
44. Yoon SJ, Ko JH, Matsuda DK. Anterior dislocation of THA after Iliopsoas tenotomy in spinopelvic imbalance: a rare case report. BMC Musculoskelet Disord. 2020;21(1):723. https://doi.org/10.1186/s12891-020-03711-6.
45. Lifshitz L, Bar Sela S, Gal N, Martin R, Fleitman KM. Iliopsoas the hidden muscle: anatomy, diagnosis, and treatment. Curr Sports Med Rep. 2020;19(6):235–43.
46. Bordoni B, Varacallo M. Anatomy, bony pelvis and lower limb, iliopsoas muscle. 2021 Feb 7. In: StatPearls [Internet]. Treasure Island, FL: StatPearls Publishing; 2021.
47. Tatu L, Parratte B, Vuillier F, Diop M, Monnier G. Descriptive anatomy of the femoral portion of the iliopsoas muscle. Anatomical basis of anterior snapping of the hip. Surg Radiol Anat. 2001;23(6):371–4.
48. Philippon MJ, Devitt BM, Campbell KJ, Michalski MP, Espinoza C, Wijdicks CA, Laprade RF. Anatomic variance of the iliopsoas tendon. Am J Sports Med. 2014;42(4):807–11.
49. Guillin R, Cardinal E, Bureau NJ. Sonographic anatomy and dynamic study of the normal iliopsoas musculotendinous junction. Eur Radiol. 2009;19(4):995–1001.
50. Polster JM, Elgabaly M, Lee H, Klika A, Drake R, Barsoum W. MRI and gross anatomy of the iliopsoas tendon complex. Skelet Radiol. 2008;37(1):55–8.
51. Guillin R, Bertaud V, Garetier M, Fantino O, Polard JL, Lambotte JC. Ultrasound in total hip replacement: value of anterior acetabular cup visibility and contact with the iliopsoas tendon. J Ultrasound Med. 2018;37(6):1439–46.
52. Bianchi S, Martinoli C, Keller A, Bianchi-Zamorani MP. Giant iliopsoas bursitis: sonographic findings with magnetic resonance correlations. J Clin Ultrasound. 2002;30(7):437–41.
53. Loneragan R, Anderson J, Taylor J. Distended iliopsoas bursa: case reports and anatomical dissection. Australas Radiol. 1994;38(4):331–5.
54. Schaberg JE, Harper MC, Allen WC. The snapping hip syndrome. Am J Sports Med. 1984;12(5):361–5.
55. Anderson CN. Iliopsoas: pathology, diagnosis, and treatment. Clin Sports Med. 2016;35(3):419–33.
56. Mann RA, Moran GT, Dougherty SE. Comparative electromyography of the lower extremity in jogging, running, and sprinting. Am J Sports Med. 1986;14(6):501–10.
57. Andersson E, Oddsson L, Grundström H, Thorstensson A. The role of the psoas and iliacus muscles for stability and movement of the lumbar spine, pelvis and hip. Scand J Med Sci Sports. 1995;5(1):10–6.
58. Neumann DA, Garceau LR. A proposed novel function of the psoas minor revealed through cadaver dissection. Clin Anat. 2015;28(2):243–52.
59. Musick SR, Varacallo M. Snapping hip syndrome. 2020. In: StatPearls [Internet]. Treasure Island, FL: StatPearls Publishing; 2021.
60. Laible C, Swanson D, Garofolo G, Rose DJ. Iliopsoas syndrome in dancers. Orthop J Sports Med. 2013;1(3):2325967113500638.
61. Janzen DL, Partridge E, Logan PM, Connell DG, Duncan CP. The snapping hip: clinical and imaging findings in transient subluxation of the iliopsoas tendon. Can Assoc Radiol J. 1996;47(3):202–8.
62. Nunziata A, Blumenfeld I. Cadera a resorte; a propósito de una variedad [Snapping hip; note on a variety]. Prensa Med Argent. 1951;38(32):1997–2001. Undetermined Language
63. Winston P, Awan R, Cassidy JD, Bleakney RK. Clinical examination and ultrasound of self-reported snapping hip syndrome in elite ballet dancers. Am J Sports Med. 2007;35(1):118–26.
64. Yen YM, Lewis CL, Kim YJ. Understanding and treating the snapping hip. Sports Med Arthrosc Rev. 2015;23(4):194–9.
65. Piechota M, Maczuch J, Skupiński J, Kukawska-Sysio K, Wawrzynek W. Internal snapping hip syndrome in dynamic ultrasonography. J Ultrason. 2016;16(66):296–303.
66. Meghpara MB, Bheem R, Diulus SC, Rosinsky PJ, Shapira J, Maldonado DR, Lall AC, Domb BG. An iliopsoas impingement lesion in the absence of painful internal snapping may not require iliopsoas fractional lengthening. Am J Sports Med. 2020;48(11):2747–54.
67. Randelli F, Mazzoleni MG, Fioruzzi A, Giai Via A, Calvisi V, Ayeni OR. Surgical interventions for external snapping hip syndrome. Knee Surg Sports Traumatol Arthrosc. 2020. https://doi.org/10.1007/s00167-020-06305-w.
68. Gouveia K, Shah A, Kay J, Memon M, Simunovic N, Cakic JN, Ranawat AS, Ayeni OR. Iliopsoas tenotomy during hip arthroscopy: a systematic review of postoperative outcomes. Am J Sports Med. 2021;49(3):817–29.
69. El Bitar YF, Stake CE, Dunne KF, Botser IB, Domb BG. Arthroscopic iliopsoas fractional lengthening for internal snapping of the hip: clinical outcomes with a minimum 2-year follow-up. Am J Sports Med. 2014;42(7):1696–703. https://doi.org/10.1177/0363546514531037.
70. Fabricant PD, Bedi A, De La Torre K, Kelly BT. Clinical outcomes after arthroscopic psoas lengthening: the effect of femoral version. Arthroscopy. 2012;28(7):965–71.
71. Heyworth BE, Shindle MK, Voos JE, Rudzki JR, Kelly BT. Radiologic and intraoperative findings in revision hip arthroscopy. Arthroscopy. 2007;23(12):1295–302.
72. Domb BG, Shindle MK, McArthur B, Voos JE, Magennis EM, Kelly BT. Iliopsoas impingement: a newly identified cause of labral pathology in the hip. HSS J. 2011;7(2):145–50.
73. Degen RM. Extra-articular hip impingement: clinical presentation, radiographic findings and surgical treatment outcomes. Phys Sportsmed. 2019;47(3):262–9.
74. Cascio BM, King D, Yen YM. Psoas impingement causing labrum tear: a series from three tertiary hip arthroscopy centers. J La State Med Soc. 2013;165(2):88–93.
75. Nelson IR, Keene JS. Results of labral-level arthroscopic iliopsoas tenotomies for the treatment of labral impingement. Arthroscopy. 2014;30(6):688–94. https://doi.org/10.1016/j.arthro.2014.02.027.
76. Maldonado DR, Lall AC, Battaglia MR, Laseter JR, Chen JW, Domb BG. Arthroscopic iliopsoas fractional lengthening. JBJS Essent Surg Tech. 2018;8(4):e30.
77. Di Benedetto P, Zangari A, Mancuso F, Buttironi MM, Causero A. Capsular management in the arthroscopic treatment of the femoro-acetabular impingement in athletes: our experience. Acta Biomed. 2020;91(14-S):e2020023.

78. Economopoulos KJ, Chhabra A, Kweon C. Prospective randomized comparison of capsular management techniques during hip arthroscopy. Am J Sports Med. 2020;48(2):395–402.
79. Di Benedetto P, Zangari A, Giardini P, Mancuso F, Castriotta L, Causero A. Capsular closure after hip arthroscopy: our experience. Acta Biomed. 2020;91(4-S):92–7.
80. Carton P, Filan D. Anterior inferior iliac spine (AIIS) and subspine hip impingement. Muscles Ligaments Tendons J. 2016;6(3):324–36.
81. De Sa D, Alradwan H, Cargnelli S, et al. Extra-articular hip impingement: a systematic review examining operative treatment of psoas, subspine, ischiofemoral, and greater trochanteric/pelvic impingement. Arthroscopy. 2014;30:1026–41.
82. Hetsroni I, Larson CM, Dela Torre K, Zbeda RM, Magennis E, Kelly BT. Anterior inferior iliac spine deformity as an extra-articular source for hip impingement: a series of 10 patients treated with arthroscopic decompression. Arthroscopy. 2012;28(11):1644–53.
83. Sharfman ZT, Grundshtein A, Paret M, Amit L, Amar E, Rath E. Surgical technique: arthroscopic osteoplasty of anterior inferior iliac spine for femoroacetabular impingement. Arthrosc Tech. 2016;5(3):e601–6.
84. Perets I, Rybalko D, Mu BH, Friedman A, Morgenstern DR, Domb BG. Hip arthroscopy: extra-articular procedures. Hip Int. 2019;29(4):346–54.
85. Hetsroni I, Poultsides L, Bedi A, Larson CM, Kelly BT. Anterior inferior iliac spine morphology correlates with hip range of motion: a classification system and dynamic model. Clin Orthop Relat Res. 2013;471(8):2497–503.
86. Pan H, Kawanabe K, Akiyama H, Goto K, Onishi E, Nakamura T. Operative treatment of hip impingement caused by hypertrophy of the anterior inferior iliac spine. J Bone Joint Surg Br. 2008;90(5):677–9.
87. Amar E, Druckmann I, Flusser G, Safran MR, Salai M, Rath E. The anterior inferior iliac spine: size, position, and location. An anthropometric and sex survey. Arthroscopy. 2013;29(5):874–81.
88. Carton P, Foley M, Patterson K. The arthroscopic classification of sub-spine morphology in the hip. Arthroscopy. 2013;29(12):e195–6.
89. Hapa O, Bedi A, Gursan O, Akar MS, Güvencer M, Havitçioğlu H, et al. Anatomic footprint of the direct head of the rectus femoris origin: cadaveric study and clinical series of hips after arthroscopic anterior inferior iliac spine/subspine decompression. Arthroscopy. 2013;29(12):1932–40.
90. Morales-Avalos R, Leyva-Villegas J, Sanchez-Mejorada G, Mendez-Aguirre O. A new morphological classification of the anterior inferior iliac spine. relevance in subspine impingement. Int J Morphol. 2015;33(2):626–31.
91. Larson CM, Kelly BT, Stone RM. Making a case for anterior inferior iliac spine/subspine hip impingement: three representative case reports and proposed concept. Arthroscopy. 2011;27:1732–7.
92. Peng X, Feng Y, Chen G, Yang L. Arthroscopic treatment of chronically painful calcific tendinitis of the rectus femoris. Eur J Med Res. 2013;18(1):49.
93. Uhthoff HK, Sarkar K, Maynard JA. Calcifying tendinitis: a new concept of its pathogenesis. Clin Orthop Relat Res. 1976;118:164–8.
94. Yun HH, Park JH, Park JW, Lee JW. Calcific tendinitis of the rectus femoris. Orthopedics. 2009;32:490.
95. Pope TL Jr, Keats TE. Case report 773: calcific tendinitis of the origin of the medial and lateral heads of the rectus femoris muscle and the anterior iliac spine (AIIS). Skelet Radiol. 1992;21:271–2.
96. Zini R, Panascì M, Papalia R, Franceschi F, Vasta S, Denaro V. Rectus femoris tendon calcification: arthroscopic excision in 6 top amateur athletes. Orthop J Sports Med. 2014;2(12):2325967114561585.
97. Pierannunzii L, Tramontana F, Gallazzi M. Case report: calcific tendinitis of the rectus femoris: a rare cause of snapping hip. Clin Orthop Relat Res. 2010;468(10):2814–8.
98. Comba F, Piuzzi NS, Zanotti G, Buttaro M, Piccaluga F. Endoscopic surgical removal of calcific tendinitis of the rectus femoris: surgical technique. Arthrosc Tech. 2015;4(4):e365–9.
99. Schmitz CC, Haas H, Muller-Stromberg J. Endoscopic treatment of calcinosis circumscripta of the hip joint: a report of 2 cases of arthroscopic removal of a calcific deposition between the labrum and capsule. Arthroscopy. 2010;26:1135–8.
100. Yang JH, Oh KJ. Endoscopic treatment of calcific tendinitis of the rectus femoris in a patient with intractable pain. J Orthop Sci. 2013;18(6):1046–9.
101. Kandemir U, Bharam S, Philippon MJ, Fu FH. Endoscopic treatment of calcific tendinitis of gluteus medius and minimus. Arthroscopy. 2003;19:E4.
102. Thanacharoenpanich S, Boyle MJ, Murphy RF, et al. Periacetabular osteotomy for developmental hip dysplasia with labral tears: is arthrotomy or arthroscopy required? J Hip Preserv Surg. 2018;5:23–33.
103. Qu Y, Jiang T, Zhao H, et al. Mid-term results of metal-on-metal hip resurfacing for treatment of osteoarthritis secondary to developmental dysplasia of the hip: a 8-years of follow up. Med Sci Monit. 2016;20:2363–8.
104. Eastwood DM. Neonatal hip screening. Lancet. 2003;361:595–7.
105. Zhao L, Yan H, Yang C, et al. Medium-term results following arthroscopic reduction in walking-age children with developmental hip dysplasia after failed closed reduction. J Orthop Surg Res. 2017;12:135.
106. Cashman JP, Round J, Taylor G, et al. The natural history of development dysplasia of the hip after early supervised treatment in the Pavlik harness. a prospective longitudinal follow-up. J Bone Joint Surg Br. 2002;84:418–25.
107. Senaran H, Bowen JR, Harcke HT. Avascular necrosis rate in early reduction after failed Pavlik harness treatment of developmental dysplasia of the hip. J Pediatr Orthop. 2007;27:192–7.
108. Eberhardt O, Fernandez FF, Wirth T. Arthroscopic reduction of the dislocated hip in infants. J Bone Joint Surg Br. 2012;94:842–7.
109. Ozturk H, Bulut O, Tezeren G, et al. Hip arthroscopy for developmental dislocation. Orthopedics. 2007;30:600.
110. Ferguson AB Jr. Treatment of congenital dislocation of the hip in infancy using the medial approach. In: Tachdjian MO, editor. Congenital dislocation of the hip. New York, NY: Churchill Livingstone; 1982. p. 283.

7 Bone Endoscopy and Endoscopic Bony Procedures Around the Hip

Tun Hing Lui, Chunbao Li, Shanxing Zhang, Qingfeng Yin, and Soshi Uchida

Abstract

Bone endoscopy of the hip can be applied to femoroacetabular impingement, osteonecrosis of the femoral head, and hip dysplasia. The concept of femoroacetabular impingement (FAI) has been popularized as a mechanical cause of hip pain and development of osteoarthritis in the hip. Bony correction with hip arthroscopy has been increasingly used as a minimally invasive means of addressing symptomatic FAI with pain relief and function improvement. Osteonecrosis of the femoral head (ONFH) is a common disease affecting young and middle aged population. Core decompression is an effective and classical procedure for early stage ONFH. With the advancement of hip arthroscopy, endoscopically assisted core decompression with expanded intra-operative visualization demonstrates a more accurate procedure and more promising outcome than traditional method. Patients with hip dysplasia have a higher incidence of acetabular labral tear and hip instability, predisposing them to osteoarthritis. An open surgical approach such as periacetabular osteotomy is commonly used for hip dysplasia. In fact, many high-demand athletes, especially hypermobile athletes, elect against a traditional open approach because it requires longer recovery times and has cosmetic issues. A new surgical technique of endoscopic shelf acetabuloplasty has been developed which is less invasive and can concurrently address the capsular, labral, and bony pathologies arthroscopically. In this chapter, the endoscopic techniques are outlined.

Keywords

Femoroacetabular impingement · Hip arthroscopy Labral tear · Cam · Pincer · Osteonecrosis of the femoral head · Core decompression · Hip dysplasia · Endoscopic shelf acetabuloplasty · Labral preservation · Shoelace capsular plication

The corresponding author of section 7.1 is Chunbao Li, E-mail: lichunbao301@163.com
The corresponding author of section 7.2 is Qingfeng Yin, E-mail: Geoffreyin84@gmail.com
The corresponding author of section 7.3 is Soshi Uchida, E-mail: soushi@med.uoeh-u.ac.jp

T. H. Lui (✉)
Department of Orthopaedics and Traumatology, North District Hospital, Hong Kong, China

The Second Affiliated Hospital, Shenzhen University, Shenzhen, China

C. Li
The PLA General Hospital, Beijing, China

S. Zhang
The First Affiliated Hospital of Zhejiang Chinese Medical University, Zhejiang, China

Q. Yin
The Second Hospital of Shandong University, Jinan, Shandong, China

S. Uchida
Department of Orthopaedic Surgery and Sports Medicine, Wakamatsu Hospital of the University of Occupational and Environmental Health, Fukuoka, Japan
e-mail: soushi@med.uoeh-u.ac.jp

© The Author(s), under exclusive license to Springer Nature Singapore Pte Ltd. 2021
T. H. Lui (ed.), *Endoscopy of the Hip and Knee*, https://doi.org/10.1007/978-981-16-3488-8_7

7.1 Arthroscopic Management of Femoroacetabular Impingement

Chunbao Li and Shanxing Zhang

7.1.1 Introduction

- The concept of femoroacetabular impingement (FAI) has been popularized as a mechanical cause of hip pain and development of osteoarthritis in the hip. It has been defined as a dynamic impingement between the anterior femoral head–neck junction and anterior acetabular rim, causing chondral and labral damages as a consequence of repetitive hip motion [1, 2].
- Impingement can result from structural abnormalities including reduced anterolateral femoral head–neck offset and over-coverage of the anterosuperior acetabular rim. Based on the osseous deformities present, two distinct types of FAI have been identified, cam and pincer, but these morphological variations are not mutually exclusive [3, 4].
- Nonoperative treatment is critical in distinguishing the patients in whom the area of damage to the joint may heal from those who may remain symptomatic. Currently, the keys are to avoid the aggravating activity for a time, work on maintaining muscle strength, and judiciously use anti-inflammatory drugs or intra-articular injections of hyaluronic acid and steroid [5–7].
- Surgical management of FAI is necessary for the patients who have no response to nonoperative treatments. Open surgeries such as surgical dislocation of hip or anterior mini-arthrotomy and hip arthroscopy have their own advantages and disadvantages. The mini-anterior approach increases visualization of the femoral head–neck junction and allows for shorter recovery times without the morbidity of a surgical dislocation and trochanteric osteotomy. These advantages come at the cost of limited access to posterior pathology and decreased global visualization of the socket and femoral head.
- Hip arthroscopy has been increasingly used as a minimally invasive mean of addressing symptomatic FAI to give pain relieve and function improvement [8]. Labral repair or debridement, acetabulum trimming, and femoral head–neck osteoplasty are the major procedures to settle the labral tear and prevent from abnormal contacting of the acetabular rim against the femoral neck.

7.1.2 Indications

Patients who had medical history, physical examination, and radiographic findings consistent with FAI; failed conservative treatment for more than 3 months.

7.1.3 Contra-Indications

- Joint space of hip in AP view X-ray is less than 2 mm.
- Severe developmental dysplasia of the hip (DDH) defined as lateral center edge (LCE) angle is less than 20°. Extreme caution should be exercised on hips with borderline DDH (BDDH), the LCE of which is between 20° and 25°.
- Negative response to blocking test of intra-articular injection.
- Low extremities cannot bear distraction.
- Hips with stiffness, infection, or severe inflammation.

7.1.4 Author's Preferred Technique

7.1.4.1 Pre-operative Planning

- Imaging tests such as X-rays, non-arthrographic 3T MR imaging, CT scanning, and three-dimensional (3D) reconstruction imaging should be performed before hip arthroscopy. Radiographic evaluation of FAI begins with an AP pelvis radiograph including anteroposterior pelvic view and Dunn view [9]. The LCE angle and joint space width at its lowest point are measured from the anteroposterior pelvic view; and alpha angle and off-set in millimeters (mm) are measured from the Dunn view [10]. Cam impingement is defined as an alpha angle >50° and/or an off-set of less than 7.2 mm. Pincer impingement is defined as an LCE angle >39°, or the presence of the crossover sign, coxa profunda, or protrusio acetabuli [6]. MRI is performed as evaluation of the labrum and cartilage in patients with clinically suspected FAI [11]. Routine CT scanning and 3D-reconstruction imaging are performed to specifically localize the pincer or cam morphology.
- Ultrasound-guided blocking test by hip intra-articular injection of 4 ml 1% lidocaine and 4 ml 10% ropivacaine will be performed on all FAI patients before surgery.
- Pre-operative skin preparation will be well done by removing all the hairs at the perineum.
- Patients will be taught to do exercises such as ankle pump, isometric contraction of the gluteus, quadriceps, waist

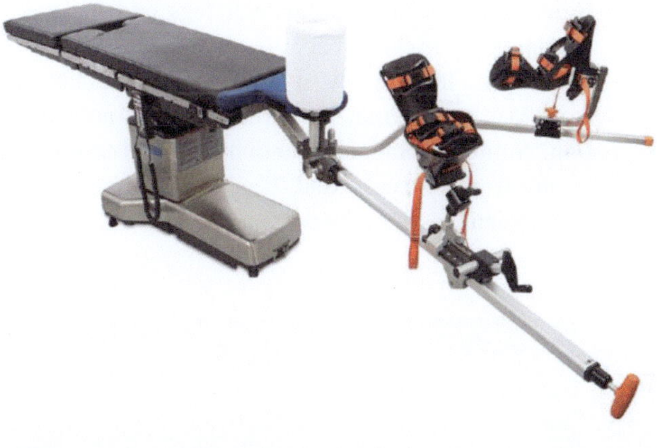

Fig. 7.1 Hip arthroscopy tables of Smith & Nephew

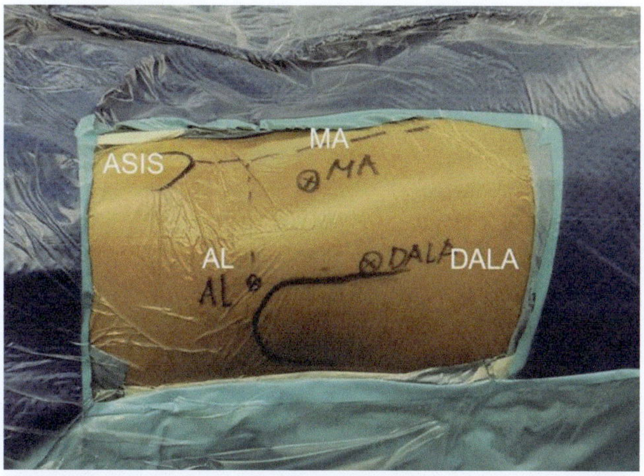

Fig. 7.2 The portals of right hip during hip arthroscopy for femoralacetabular impingement: anterolateral (AL) portal, modified mid-anterior (MA) portal, and modified distal anterolateral approach (DALA). *ASIS* anterior superior iliac spine

and back muscles, as well as partial weight-bearing walking using crutches.

- Standard operating room tables and fracture tables are normally enough for hip arthroscopic surgery for FAI. Commercial hip arthroscopy tables and/or table attachments designed specifically may make the procedure convenient and give well protection on nerves and perineum (Fig. 7.1).

7.1.4.2 Patient and Medical Team Positioning

- The patient is positioned in the supine position with both legs in well-padded traction boots.
- The perineal post should be as large and soft as possible, generally not less than 12 cm in diameter.
- Gross traction is applied to both legs to ensure that the patient's groin is in full contact with the perineal post. It is also critical to check the genitalia, particularly in male patients, to avoid direct compression during the traction process.
- The surgery is usually performed under general anesthesia with full pharmacological relaxation.

7.1.4.3 Portal Design

Most of the time, anterolateral (AL) portal, modified mid-anterior (MA) portal, and modified distal anterolateral approach (DALA) will be established to perform during hip arthroscopy for FAI (Fig. 7.2)

- The AL portal is placed at the level of the tip of the greater trochanter and anterior edge of the greater trochanter.
- Modified mid-anterior (MA) portal is placed as the anterior portal approximately 4–5 cm distal and 4–5 cm anterior to the anterior AL portal.
- The modified DALA portal is placed at 5–7 cm distal to the AL portal along the anterior edge of the femur. The lines between these 3 portals will form a triangle.

7.1.4.4 Step-by-Step Description of Technique

- Before prepare and drape the hip, working of traction should be checked. Mild traction is used to fix the contralateral leg and fine traction is used on the operating leg to make the hip be distracted approximately 8–10 mm. Once successful distraction is confirmed by fluoroscopy, the traction is released until the joint is radiographically reduced.
- When prepare and drape the hip, it is critical to expose the area proximal to the anterior superior iliac spine ASIS, medial to the line with the ASIS and approximately 20 cm distal to the tip of the greater trochanter to ensure access to all standard and accessory hip portals.
- The traction is reapplied and start time of traction is confirmed with nurses and anesthetist and tracked throughout the case.
- The anterolateral para-trochanteric portal is established first. It is critical to make the slope tip of the spinal needle face to the femoral head and aim toward two-thirds of the way from acetabulum to femoral head, checked by fluoroscopy.
- The inner stylet of the spinal needle is removed next, a guidewire is placed through the spinal needle, a small incision is made, and cannulated guide rod is introduced along the guidewire. Then an arthroscopic cannula can be placed through along the guide rod.

- We initially perform a dry hip arthroscopy to avoid bubble formation or "blood blindness" and to confirm that the initial portal is placed in such a way as to allow adequate visualization of the anterior capsule.
- If the joint space is still not enough for entry of the scope even under the maximum traction, the "outside-in" technique could be selected.

– Release the traction of bilateral legs and make the operating hip in flexion at 30°.

– Assisted by fluoroscopy, spinal needle was punctured from MA portal to lateral portion of head–neck junction. Similar technique mentioned above is used to establish this access and head–neck junction and labrum can be seen with camera (Fig. 7.3).

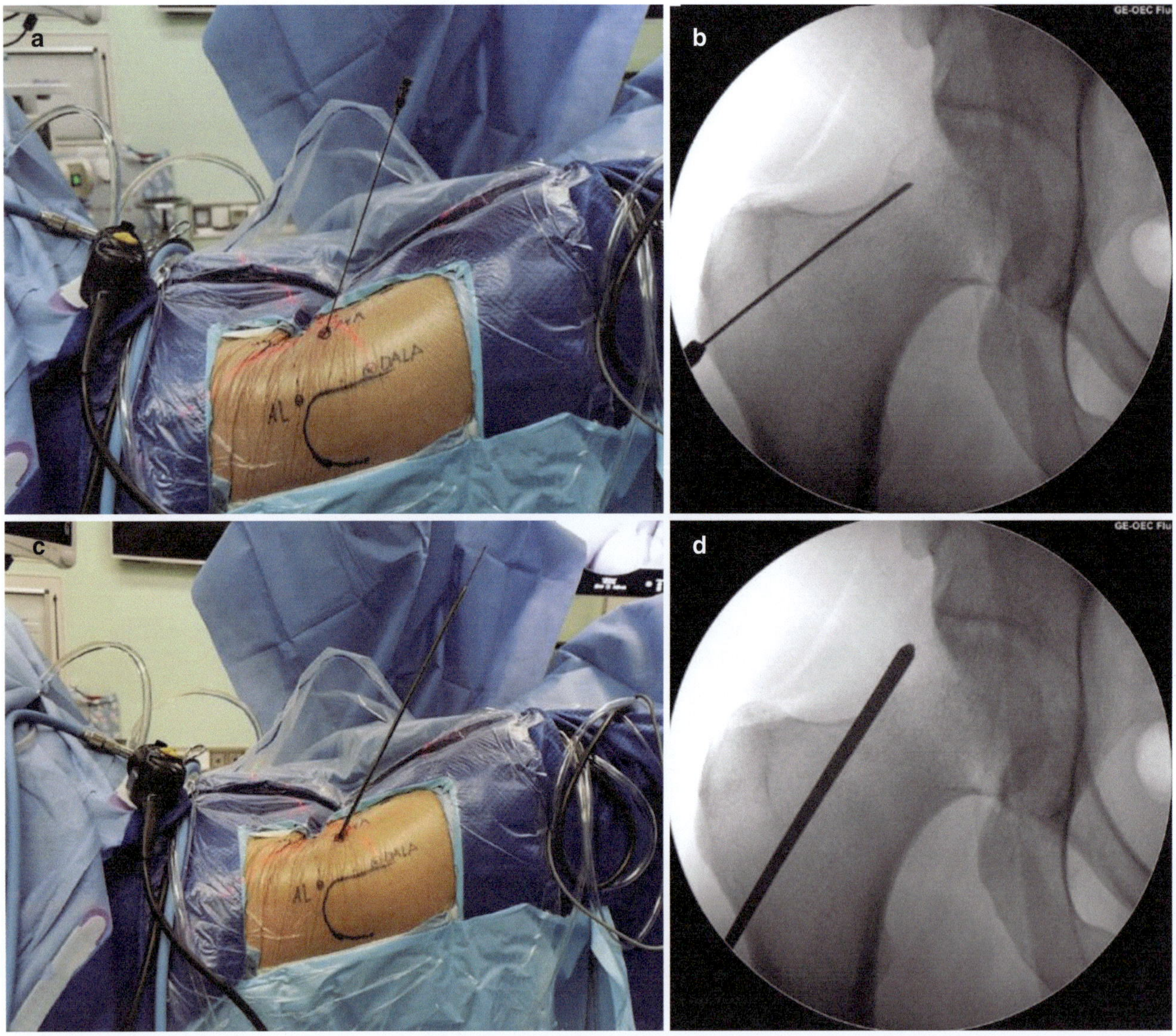

Fig. 7.3 The step-by-step of the establishment of modified mid-anterior (MA) access on right hip using "outside-in" technique. (**b**), (**d**), and (**f**) are fluoroscopy records of steps (**a**), (**c**), and (**e**), respectively

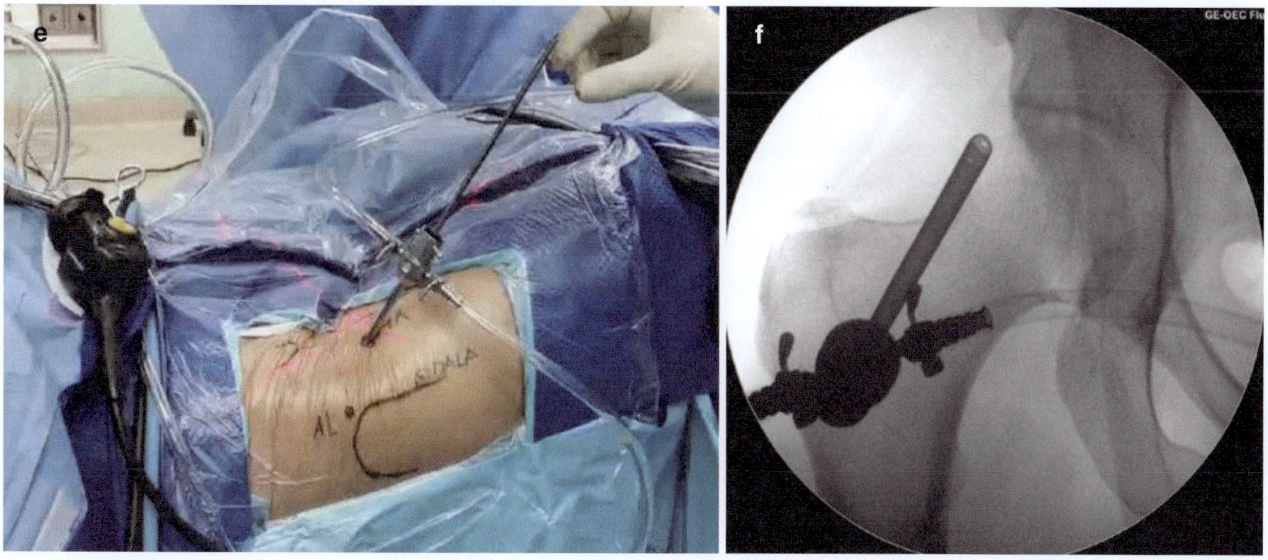

Fig. 7.3 (continued)

- Put the camera to the lateral side of head–neck junction, then a triangle region formed by lateral labrum, capsule, and femoral head could be seen (Fig. 7.4).
- Then fully extend the hip and slowly increase the traction force on the operative leg. The space of joint could be seen slowly increased under the camera. Traction will be stopped until the joint space is enough for the management of center compartment, normally 8–10 mm. Then the AL access could be established by the spinal needle under direct vision of arthroscopy

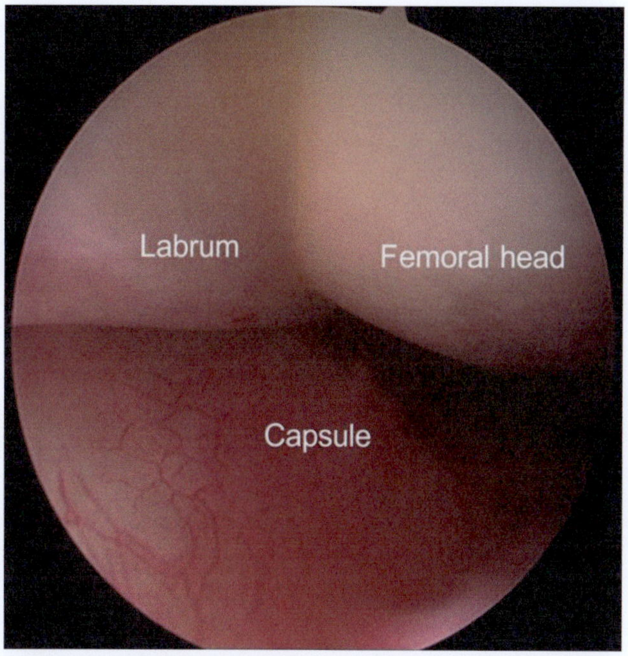

Fig. 7.4 Triangle region formed by lateral labrum, capsule, and femoral head, viewing from modified mid-anterior (MA) portal

and followed by routine manipulations (Fig. 7.5). The most advantage of this "outside-in" technique is that all those important steps are performed under camera that can ensure an appropriate but not undue distraction of the hip. Furthermore, establishing the AL access under direct vision with camera can effectively prevent injury to the labrum and cartilage.

– To reduce radiological exposure of patients and surgeons, senior author invents a slotted cannulated guide rod to facilitate the establishment access of MA access. Firstly, make a small incision of skin at MA portal and bluntly separate the tissue on the anterior capsule with vessel forceps. Then put the slotted cannulated guide rod in the access and use the tip of the rod as a probe to easily find the expected location of puncture on the capsule. Finally, insert the spinal needle into capsule along the chute of the slotted cannulated guide rod (Fig. 7.6).

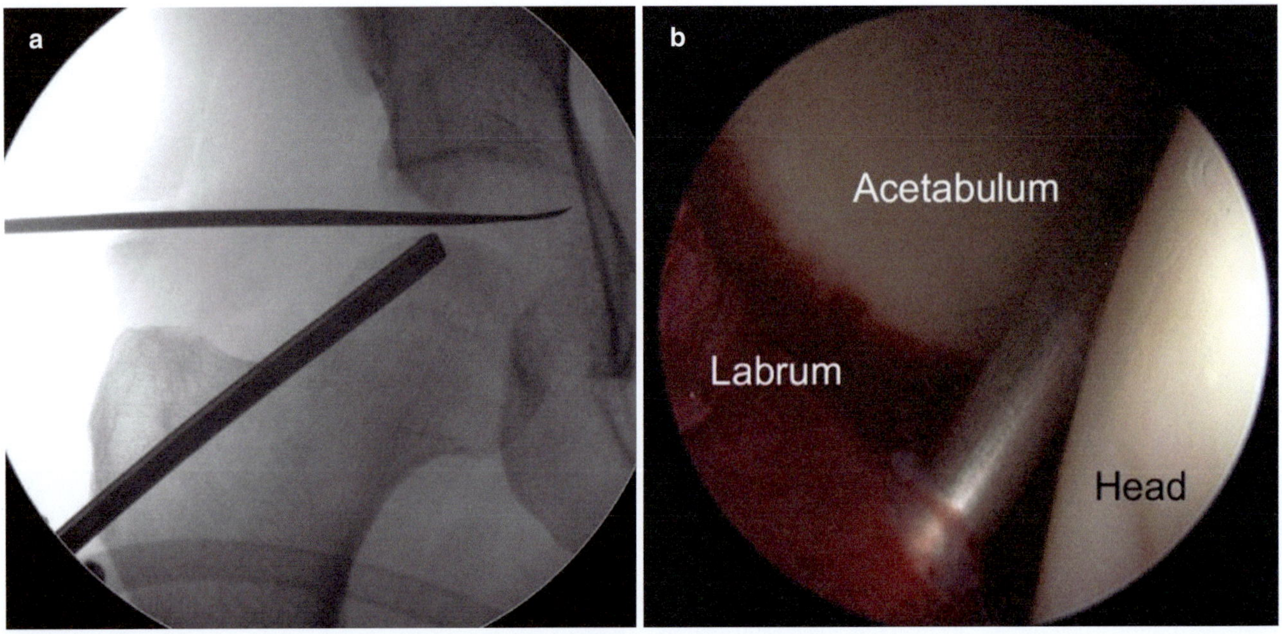

Fig. 7.5 Establishment of anterolateral (AL) access on right hip using "outside-in" technique. (**a**) Fluroscopic picture. (**b**) Arthroscopic viewing from MA mid-anterior (MA) portal

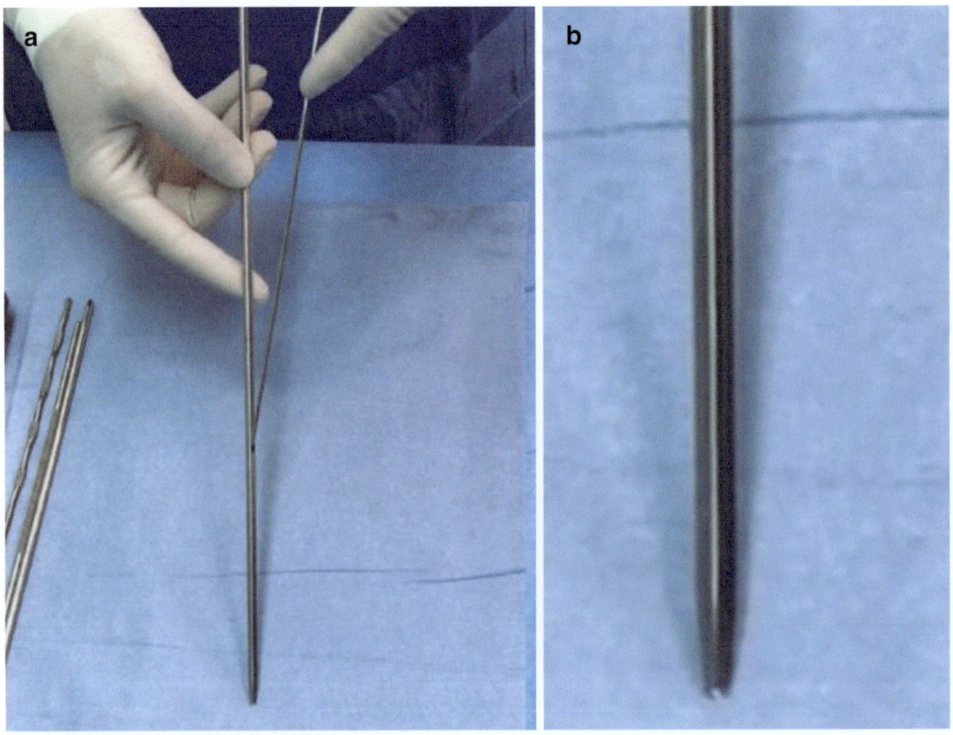

Fig. 7.6 The senior author invents a slotted cannulated guide rod to facilitate the establishment access of MA access. (**a**) The spinal needle into capsule along the chute of the hole guide rod. (**b**) Magnifying picture of the slotted cannulated guide rod

- Under direct arthroscopic vision with occasional fluoroscopic assistance, the MA portal is placed. The spinal needle is entered into the joint through the anterior triangle formed by the labrum, femoral head, and periphery of the arthroscope. To prevent from damaging branches of the lateral femoral cutaneous nerve, a skin incision followed by bluntly dissection using a tonsil clamp.
- Once a cannula is inserted into the joint, let the arthroscopic fluid flow into the joint through AL portal and flow out through MA portal and then the central compartment of the hip can be clearly seen.
- Once a clear view is achieved, inter-portals capsulotomy is performed between the two portals and diagnostic arthroscopy will be performed. To make an exposure of lesions, capsulotomy is suggested to be performed thoroughly, normally 2–3 cm long.
- Acetabuloplasty should be addressed firstly once the diagnostic arthroscopy is done in the hips with pincer deformity. Radiofrequency blade is used to debride partial footprint of acetabular attachment of the capsule to expose the bony pincer deformity. 4 mm Abrader burr is introduced through MA portal to perform the acetabuloplasty (Fig. 7.7). The amount of acetabular rim needed to be resected depends on the preoperative LCE angle of the hip. Prospective data were collected that showed that 1 mm of resection at the 12 o'clock position equaled 2.4° of change, and 5 mm of resection correlated with 5° of change [12]. Chondrolabral junction has to be preserved if it is possible.
- The teared labrum is a major source of the pain in hips with FAI. Once the range of teared labrum is confirmed, resection, refixation, or reconstruction would be performed according to the quality of the labrum. For the labrum that is destroyed too severe, partial or full-thickness resection should be done with a motorized shaver followed by acetabuloplasty. Thermal coagulation on the remaining labral tissue with a radio frequency blade can increase the stability of the labrum.
- If the quality of torn labrum is good enough, refixation of labrum should be selected. Firstly, debride the recess between the labrum and capsule to expose the bony face of the acetabular rim, and then remove the cortical bone to prepare the interface for labral suture refixation. To repair the torn labrum, anchors are introduced through DALA portal and are placed at prepared acetabular rim and 1–2 mm from the articular surface. To prevent from the insertion of anchor into joint, anchors of which diameter less than 3 mm are recommended. The injured labrum will be refixated with looped simple stitch, single-pass or

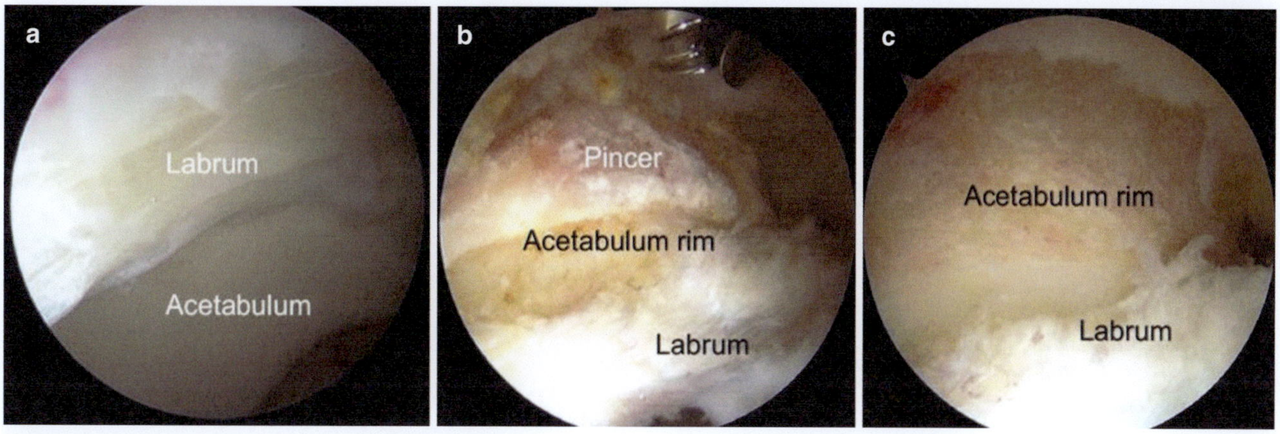

Fig. 7.7 Acetabuloplasty for pincer deformity. (**a**) Torn labrum is confirmed. (**b**) Radiofrequency device is used to debride partial footprint of capsular to expose pincer and 4 mm Abrader burr is introduced through mid-anterior (MA) portal to perform the acetabuloplasty. (**c**) Acetabuloplasty is finished and bony face is prepared for labral repair

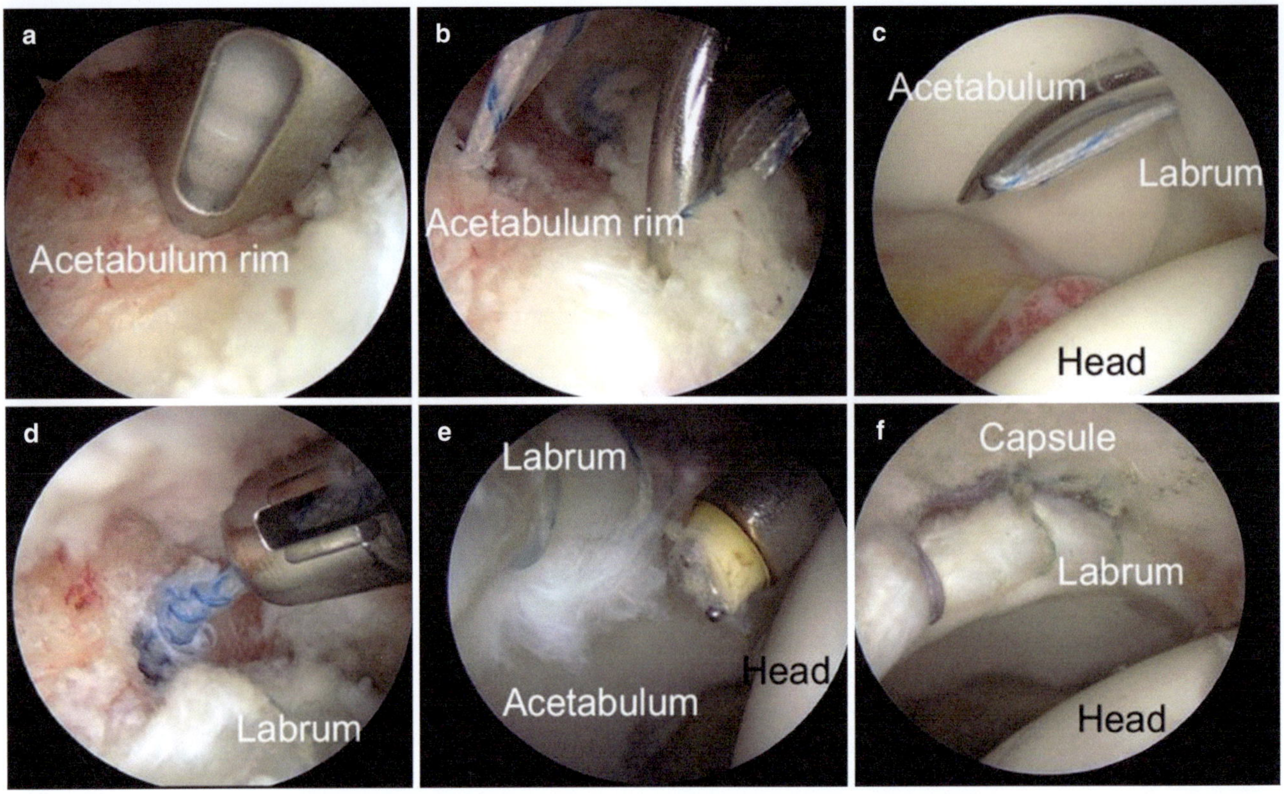

Fig. 7.8 Refixation of labrum of right hip. (**a**) The anchor is placed at prepared acetabular rim and 1–2 mm from the articular surface through distal anterolateral approach (DALA) access. (**b**), (**c**) and (**d**): the injured labrum is refixated with looped simple stitch. (**e**) The injured labralchondral tissue is debrided with radiofrequency device. (**f**) Refixation of labrum is finished

vertical mattress technique according to the thickness of the labrum [13] (Fig. 7.8).

- The distance between two anchors should be 6–8 mm to achieve reliable refixation of the torn labrum. Once the labral repairing work has been completed, any articular cartilage lesions can be addressed using a micro-fracture technique.
- Some labrum of patients in the absence of reparable tissue due to labral calcification or severe full-thickness tear with very poor quality, resection of the damaged labrum and follow by labral reconstruction is necessary to maintain the sealing function of the labrum.
- After central compartment procedure is done, traction on the limbs is slowly released under view of arthroscopy.
- Let the operating hip be flexed to 30°, with neutral rotation, to slight external rotation, the "T" capsulotomy is done, starting approximate at the middle of inter-portals incision of capsule and proceeding down along the femoral neck, which can provide the best exposure of the peripheral compartment (Fig. 7.9).
- The full exposure and checking of cam lesion are critical important. The cam typically located at anterolateral part of the head–neck junction, which could be identified after

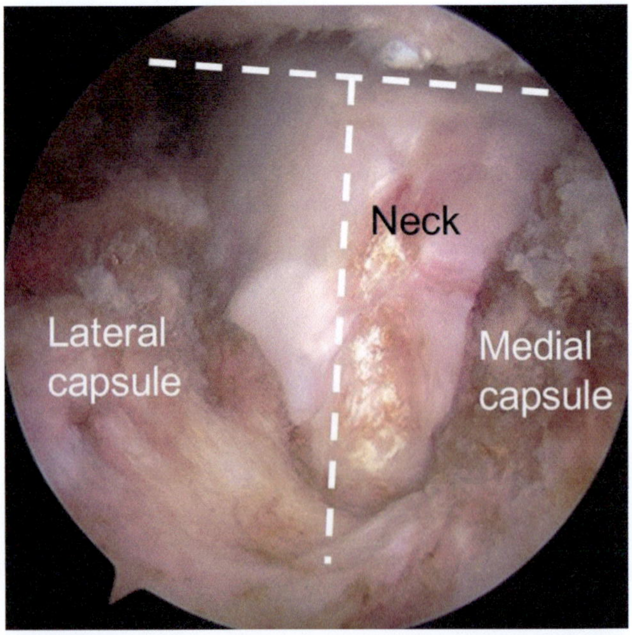

Fig. 7.9 "T" capsulotomy for right hip, starting approximate at the middle of inter-portals incision of capsule and proceeding down along the femoral neck

clearing the fibrocartilage and soft tissue with a radiofrequency device. The proximal border of cam is usually located at the junction from hyaline cartilage to fibrous cartilage of femoral head. The medial and lateral border usually between the medial synovial fold and lateral synovial fold which have the important retinacular vessels go through it.

- The 3D-CT scan and preoperative radiographic parameters including alpha angle and off-set are important references to determine the range and depth of cam decompression. Once the cam is identified, then resect the cam using a 5.5 mm Abrader burr. Maintain the proximal extent of the osteochondroplasty at approximately 5–10 mm distal to the edge of the labrum with the hip flexed to 45°. After the proximal portion of the cam is addressed, the recontouring is tapered distally onto the femoral neck, typically stop at to the junctional zone from spongy bone to cortical bone. During osteochondroplasty, flexion/extension and internal/external rotation of hip are very helpful to aid resection of different portions of the cam lesion. Fluoroscopy at Dunn view of the operating hip flexed at different angles would be applied to check the range and depth of the osteochondroplasty. In addition, we have to visually and dynamically observe whether the hip still has residual impingement when the hip is flexed to more than 90° with internal or external rotation. Addressing any residual impingement is very critical to prevent the patients from postoperative symptoms (Fig. 7.10).
- After cam resection, the anatomic side-to-side stitches with non-absorbable suture on the T-capsulotomy are

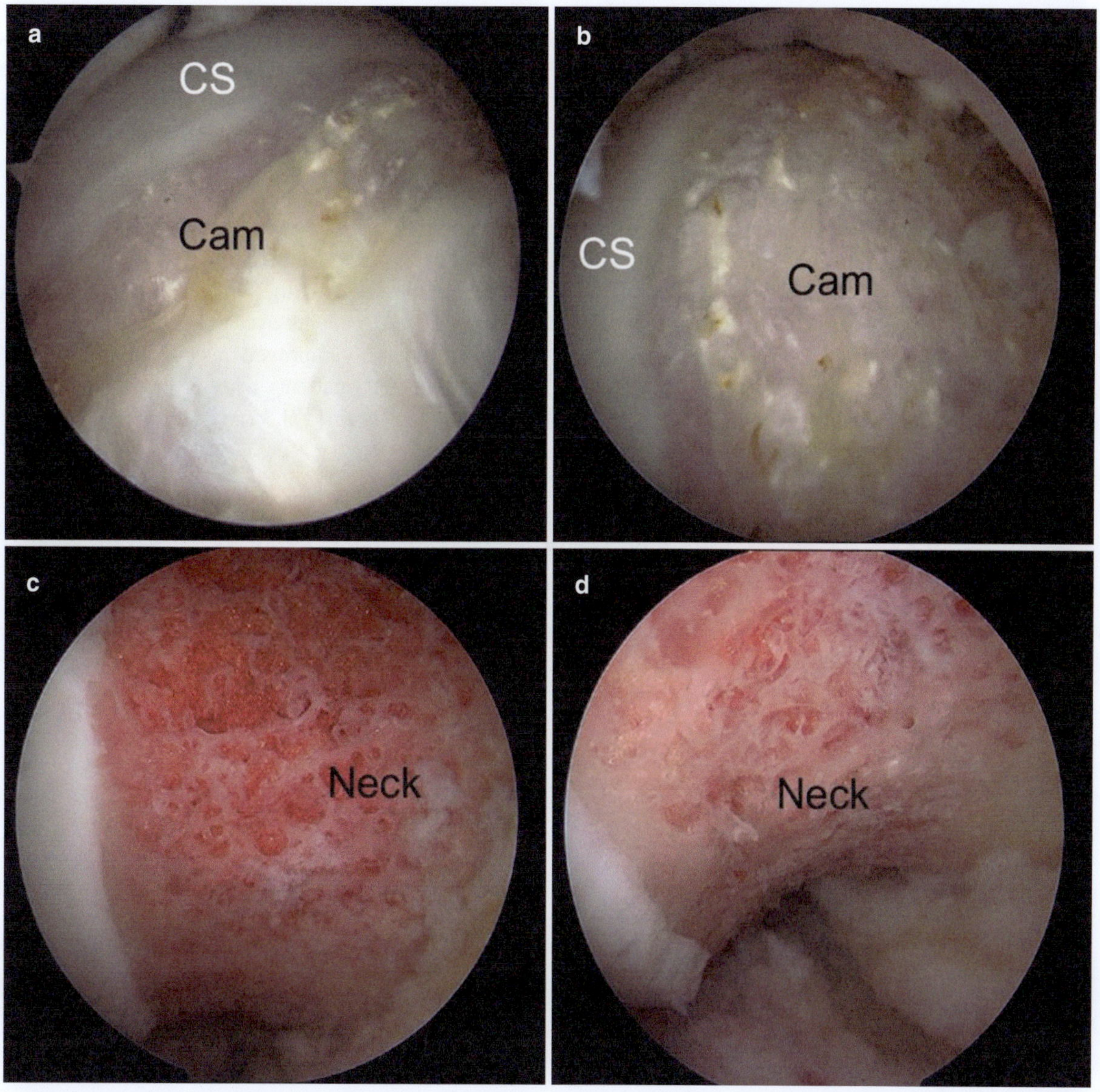

Fig. 7.10 Cam lesion resection and osteochondroplasty on right hip. (**a**, **b**) Fully expose the cam lesion located at anterolateral head–neck junction and remove the fibrous cartilage on the lesion, viewed from anterolateral (AL) portal. (**c**, **d**) Osteochondroplasty is finished. *CS* cartilage surface

performed. Typically, 3 stitches are required at longitudinal incision and 2 for inter-portals incision, respectively.

- 20 ml ropivacaine is injected into the joint to reduce postoperative pain.
- The portals are sutured and the wounds are dressed in the standard fashion with a generous dressing due to the substantial oozing of arthroscopy fluid in the early postoperative period.

7.1.4.5 Complications and Management

- Cartilage and labrum injuries are very common complications during portal establishment. To prevent from the injuries, enough joint space afforded by traction should be checked by fluoroscopy before the establishment of AL access.
- Edema or even cutaneous necrosis at perineum and foot, and nerve injury of the affected leg are the major traction related complications. Controlling the traction time within 2 h and using a big, soft perineum post can prevent these complications effectively.

7.1.4.6 Post-operative Care

- The day after surgery, patients are instructed on partial weight-bearing walking using two crutches. The partial weight-bearing walking on the operated low extremity for 3 weeks, then the patients can try to full weight-bearing walk during the 4th week after surgery. If the patients have no symptom during walking, then they are allowed to walk normally without crutches.
- Motions of the hip are limited after surgery. During the first 4 weeks after surgery, the flexion of the affected hip is limited to 90°. Moderate internal rotation, abduction, and adduction of the hip are allowed whereas the external rotation and hyperextension are forbidden.
- Ankle pump exercises and isometric contraction exercises of the gluteus medius muscle, waist and back muscles, and quadriceps should be exercised postoperatively.
- Patients were prescribed 4 weeks of 200 mg of celecoxib twice daily for pain relief and prevention of heterotopic ossification. Physical therapy began postoperative day one with a protocol specific to the procedure performed.

7.1.4.7 Outcomes

Results of arthroscopic treatment for FAI have been favorable. Multiple studies have shown improvement in symptoms after hip arthroscopy and return to sport in competitive-level athletes with FAI [14, 15]. A retrospective study showed that for the majority of the patients who underwent arthroscopic hip surgery for mild FAI, pain relief was 50% at 6–12 weeks, 75% at 5 months, and 95% at 1 year. A multicenter randomized controlled trial showed that hip arthroscopy and personalized hip therapy both improved hip-related quality of life for patients with FAI syndrome. Hip arthroscopy led to a significantly greater improvement than that did personalized hip therapy [16]. The author investigate a total of 27 FAI patients over the age of 50 years and confirmed considerably improved hip symptoms and function in Chinese elder FAI patients who did not have severe radiographic osteoarthritis [17].

7.2 Endoscopically Assisted Core Decompression of Femoral Head

Qingfeng Yin

7.2.1 Introduction

Osteonecrosis of the femoral head (ONFH) is a clinical condition characterized with the necrosis of trabecular bone and bone marrow caused by multiple factors, which commonly affects young and active patients aged 30s or 40s [18–22]. In the United States, the number of new case of ONFH every year comes up to 20,000 [23]. The clinical presentation of ONFH in early stages could be caused by synovitis and intra-marrow pressure in the femoral head as described by Ficat [24]. Once the collapse of femoral head occurs, the pain and limited range of motion can become severe.

The staging of ONFH is mostly based on the imaging of femoral head. The classification system proposed by Ficat is most commonly used, which basing on plain radiographs of femoral head differentiates early from late-stage ONFH by the presence of collapse of femoral head [24]. The Steinberg classification according to the MRI imaging also uses the "crescent sign" to separate early from late-stage [25]. Another classification developed by Association International research of Circulation Osseous (ARCO) combines plain film radiographs, MRI, and bone scan findings to determine different stages of the disease [26].

According to the presence or not of the collapse, a brief classification of ONFH could be proposed as pre-collapse and post-collapse. In the pre-collapse stage, non-operative modalities include medication of Statins, Stanozolol, and Bisphosphonates [27–29], and the core decompression was the main option of operative modalities. Hungerford and Ficat were among the first to describe the utilization of core decompression for Ficat stages 0, 1, and 2 ONFH [30]. Operative modalities after collapse include vascularized fibula grafts, rotational trans-trochanteric osteotomy, hip resurfacing, joint reconstruction, total hip arthroplasty [31–34].

With the development of technique of hip arthroscopy, the arthroscopic technique was introduced to make a more accurate staging of ONFH. The development of endoscopically assisted core decompression almost brings an evolution of less invasive procedure for ONFH [35, 36].

7.2.2 Indications

- Early stage ONFH (pre-collapse or early-collapsed)
- ONFH concomitant with synovitis or chondrolabral injury

7.2.3 Contra-Indications

- Late stage ONFH (severe collapsed with hip arthritis)

7.2.4 Author Preferred Technique

7.2.4.1 Pre-operative Planning

- The preoperative plan should include the comprehensive radiologic evaluation of hip. The A-P view pelvic radiography, Dunn view of hip joint, CT scan and MRI of hip joint are necessary in our protocol of clinical evaluation for femoral head necrosis.
- Not only the stage of the ONFH should be identified, the size and location of necrotic lesion also should be well evaluated.
- The potential intra-articular pathology including labral lesions, chondral lesions, and synovitis should be diagnosed before surgery.
- Required instruments: C-arm, 4.0 mm, 30-degree arthroscope, lightweight camera, shaver system with 4.0-mm full-radius blades, hip arthroscopic instrument set, such as dilators, probes, baskets, graspers, and curettes, half pipe and an arthroscopic radiofrequency system and its wands.

7.2.4.2 Patient Positioning

The patient is placed supine on the fracture table with a well-padded perineal post, and the feet were fixed in the boots of traction arm to allow for the traction during hip arthroscopy. The operative leg was neutrally placed and the contralateral leg was placed 45-degree abduction.

7.2.4.3 Portal Design

- The anterior lateral portal (ALP, 1 cm anterior and 1 cm distal to the tip of greater trochanter) and middle anterior portal (MAP, 6–8 cm anterior and distal to the ALP) are used to access the hip joint and investigate and address the intra-articular lesion. Another incision is designed distal to the great trochanter for the core decompression of femoral head.

7.2.4.4 Step-by-Step Description of the Technique

- After the routine surgical preparation, traction is applied gently, and satisfactory joint space over 10 mm is confirmed with fluoroscopy.
- An 18-gauge needle is punctured into the hip joint from the ALP under fluoroscopy, and then the dilators are introduced into the hip joint.
- ALP is used as viewing portal, and same procedure is repeated to establish the MAP.

- An inter-portal capsulotomy is conducted to improve the visualization and mobility of instrument in the hip joint.
- The central compartment is comprehensively inspected and the lesions of the labrum, cartilage, and ligamentum teres are addressed (Fig. 7.11a, b).
- Make a 3 cm incision at the distal to the great trochanter, drill one guide pin from the starting point on the lateral cortex of femoral bone aiming to the necrotic area of femoral head. This procedure is conducted under fluoroscopy (Fig. 7.12a).
- 8 or 10 mm diameter bone tunnel is established using a cannulated drill until the tip reaches the subchondral bone of femoral head (Fig. 7.12b, c).
- An expandable reamer (X-REAM™) was introduced through the working cannula, which could make a comprehensive debridement of necrosis (Fig. 7.12d).

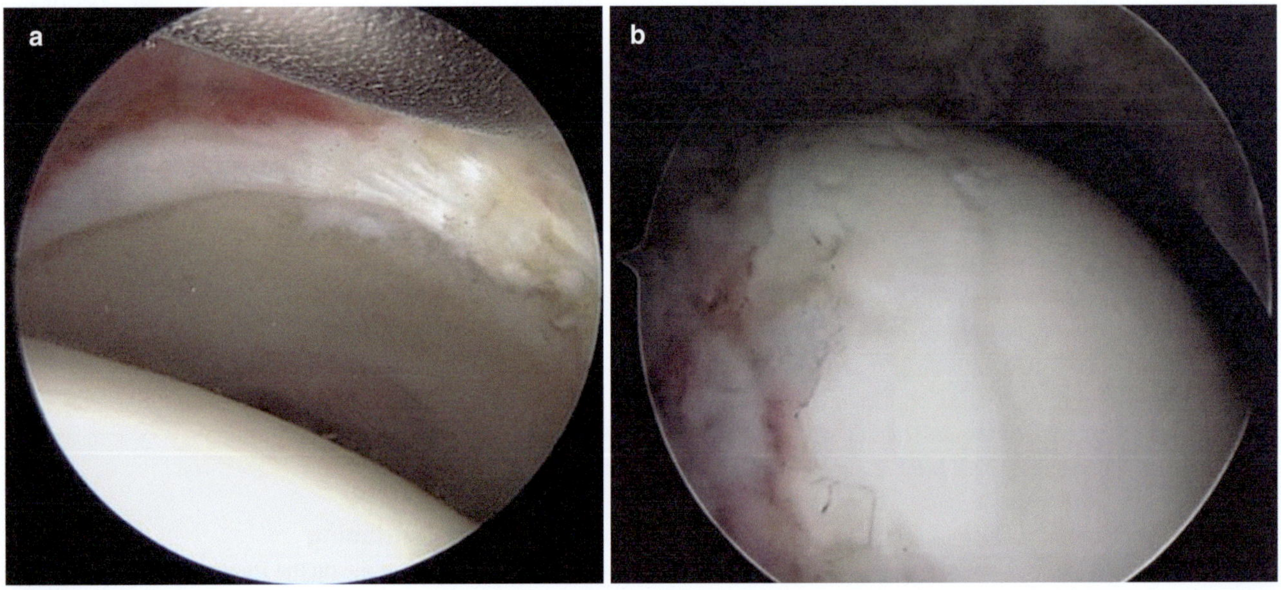

Fig. 7.11 Hip arthroscopy can verify the intra-articular pathology of hip joint. The labral tear and inflammation can be observed (**a**), and the collapsed femoral head and wrinkled cartilage can be found (**b**)

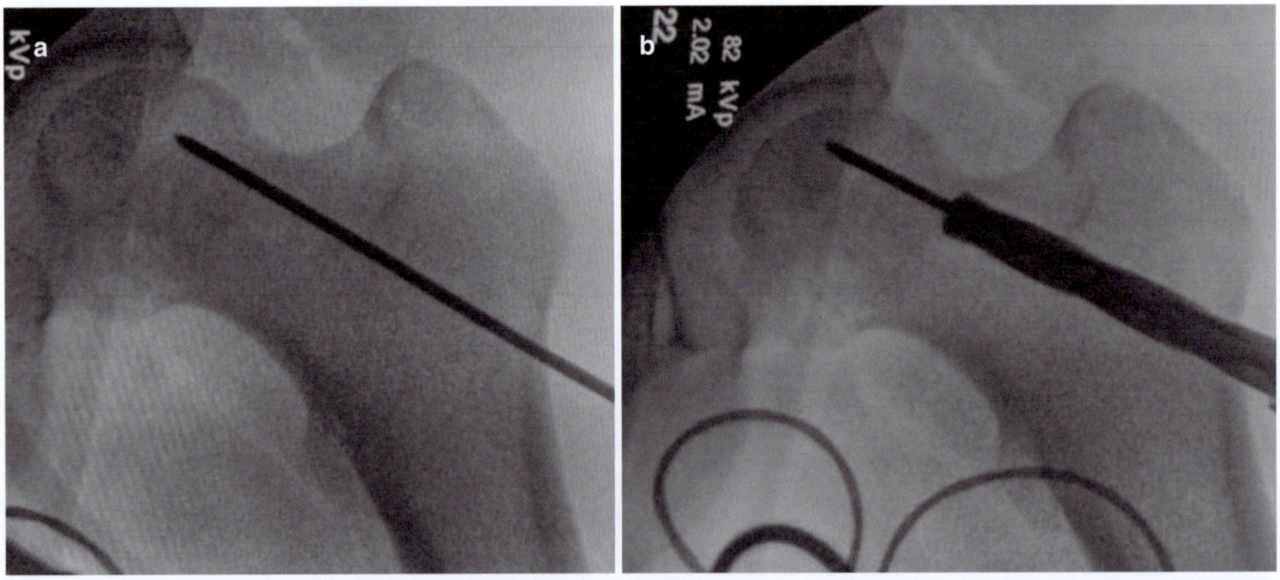

Fig. 7.12 Core decompression under fluoroscopy. Guide pin is drilled into the necrotic lesion (that is identified by preoperative imaging and planning) under fluoroscopy (**a**) and the 8-mm reamer is introduced along the guide pin (**b**), until the reamer penetrates the sclerotic zone and reaches the subchondral plate (**c**). The expandable reamer is then introduced to make a more comprehensive debridement (**d**)

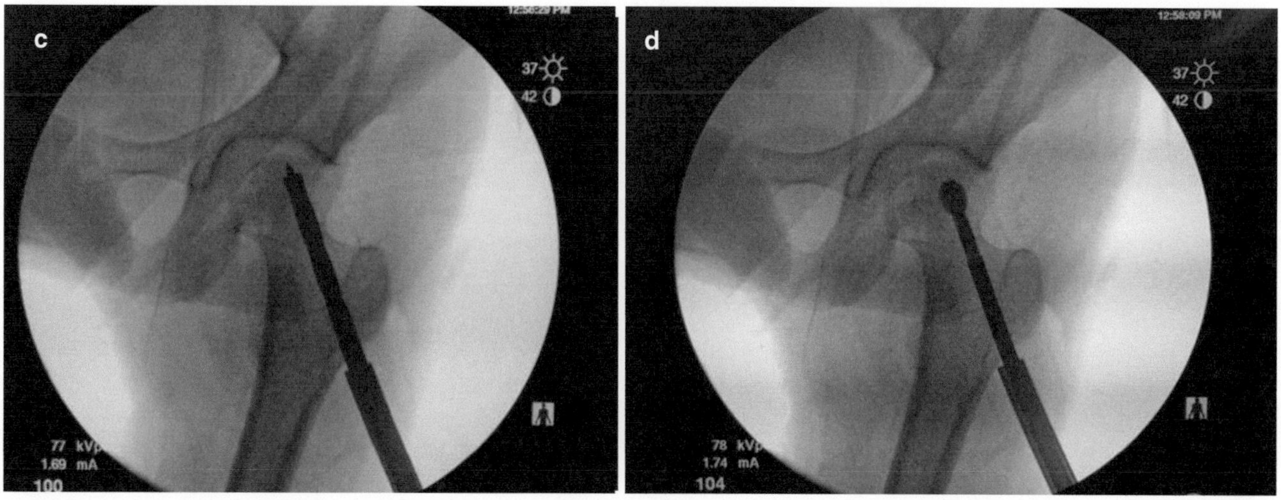

Fig. 7.12 (continued)

- The mild collapsed subchondral bone plate could be elevated through the bone tunnel with impaction of metal rod, which could be continuously inspected under arthroscopy. The arthroscope can also be introduced into the bone tunnel to confirm that the necrotic bone has been completely debrided (Fig. 7.13).
- Bone grafting and backfill of core decompression with artificial materials (PRO-DENSE™) can be done (Fig. 7.14).

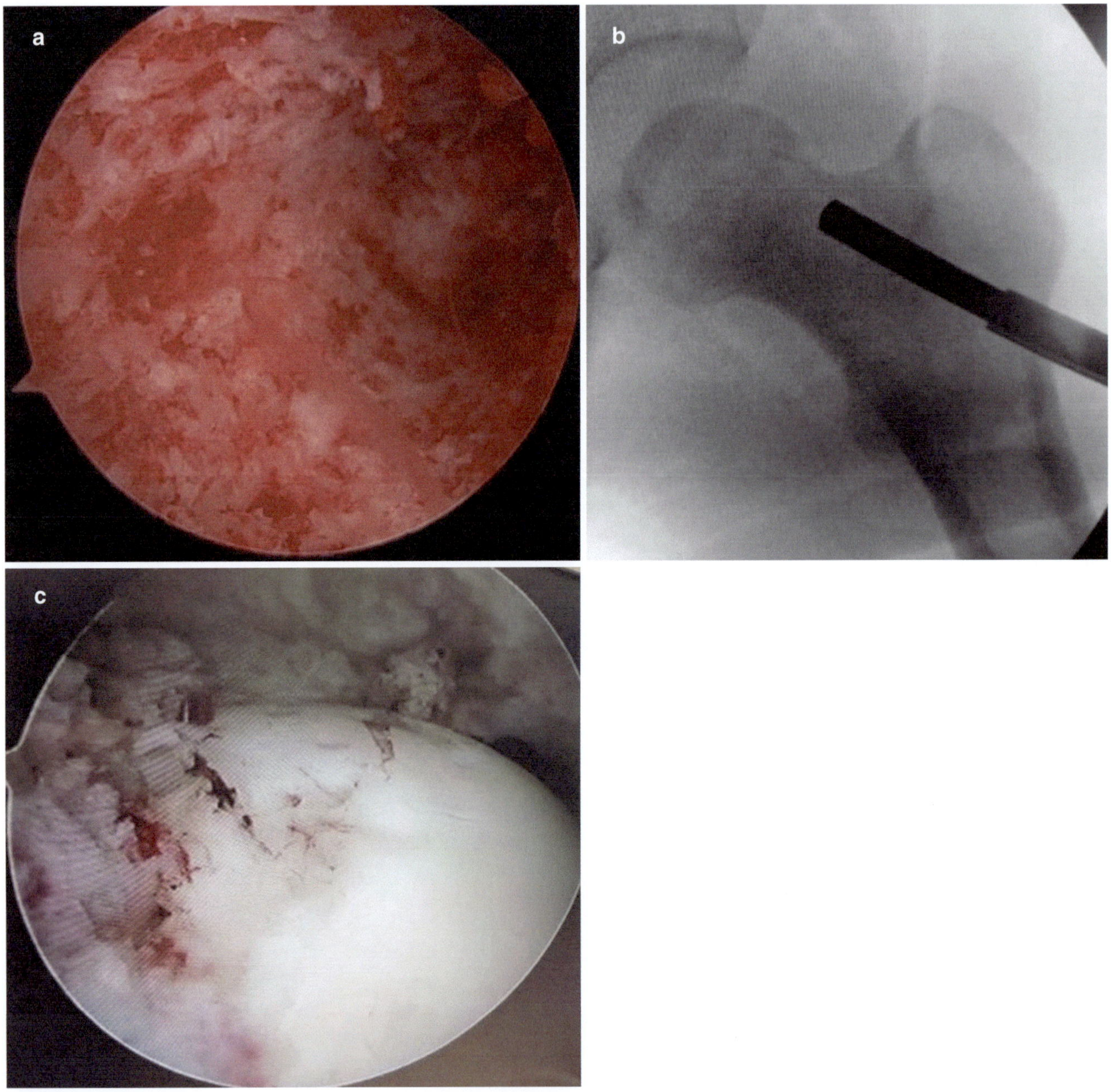

Fig. 7.13 Endoscopically assisted visualization in bone tunnel to verify complete debridement of necrotic bone and only bleeding bone is left (**a**). The collapse is elevated by impaction through the bone tunnel (**b**) and the wrinkled cartilage is confirmed to be smoothened via hip arthroscopy (**c**)

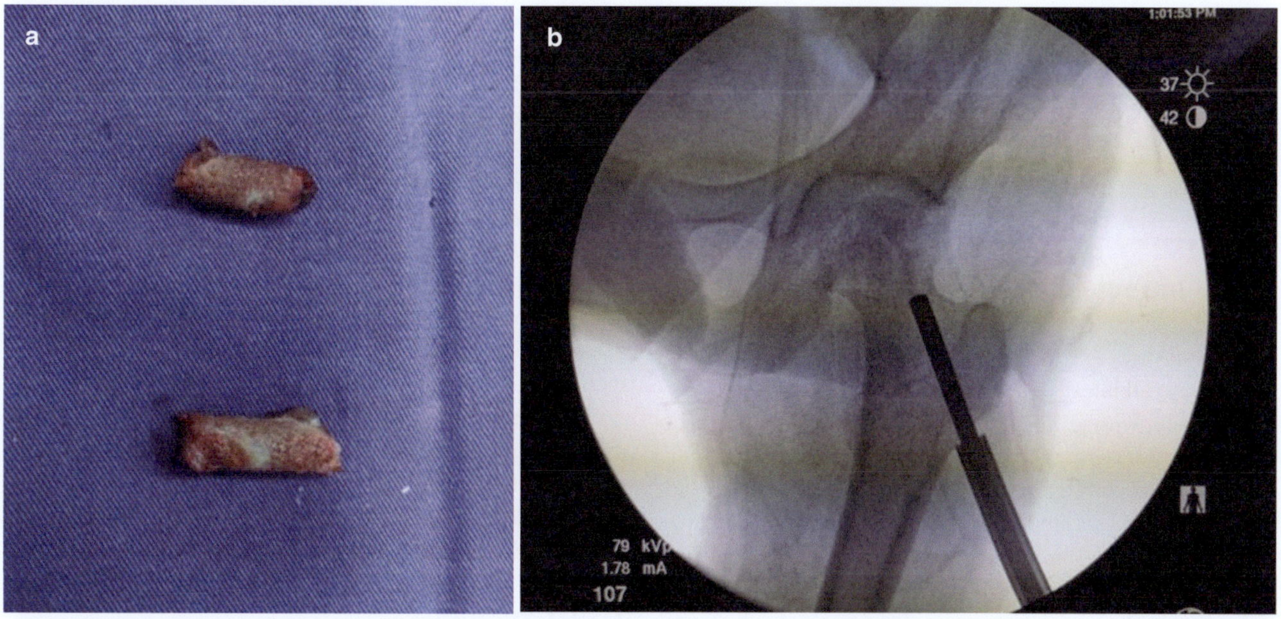

Fig. 7.14 Bone grafting after core decompression. The bone plugs harvest from iliac crest are well prepared (**a**), the bone plugs are introduced into the bone tunnel and impacted (**b**)

7.2.4.5 Complications and Management

- Complication related to the traction including transient pudendal nerve palsy.
- Complication related to the portal establishment including labrum penetration, cartilage injury, and instrument breakage.
- Subcutaneous saline extravasation because of prolonged operation.
- Postoperative femoral head collapse.

7.2.4.6 Post-operative Care

Post-operative cares are various with the treatment proposed, and the 6–12 weeks' partial weight bearing was suggested for most patient with core decompression.

7.2.4.7 Outcome

Several authors have advocated effective results with core decompression for pre-collapse osteonecrosis, including arthroscopic-assisted decompression [37, 38]. Our clinical experience has found that the pain and constrain of range of motion of patient with pre-collapse osteonecrosis could be dramatically relieved through arthroscopic-assisted decompression and debridement of hip joint.

7.2.5 Summary

Hip arthroscopy has been becoming the gold standard for the diagnosis of intra-articular hip pathology. The concomitant soft tissue and/or bony pathology with osteonecrosis of the femoral head are involved in the procession of ONFH. Arthroscopy assisted decompression provides an accurate evaluation to confirm the presence or absence of femoral head subchondral collapse, chondral delamination, and associated labral, capsular, and synovial pathology, which could be addressed simultaneously. Further, arthroscopic inspection could make guidance during drilling and/or reaming to avoid penetration or breakage of cartilage, and confirm totally debridement of necrotic lesion.

7.3 Endoscopic Shelf Acetabuloplasty for the Treatment of Patients in the Setting of Hip Dysplasia

Soshi Uchida
soushi@med.uoeh-u.ac.jp

7.3.1 Introduction

Hip dysplasia is one of the most common causes of hip pain in Japanese athletes [39]. Athletes with hip dysplasia classically present with groin and lateral hip pain, which is associated with intra-articular pathologies, including acetabular labral tear and cartilage damage, predisposing them to osteoarthritis. Numerous studies have reported that anterosuperior and superolateral shallow acetabulum can cause repetitive overload of the hip joint leading to cartilage damage, acetabular labral tear, and sometimes rim stress fracture, which predispose them to osteoarthritis. Additionally, dynamic musculotendinous structures surrounding the hip joint can also contribute as dynamic stabilizers. In the case of patients with intra-articular pathologies, these musculotendinous structures compensate to stabilize the hip joint. In fact, many patients with hip dysplasia also present with groin and lateral hip pain that can result from static overloading of the periarticular musculotendon structures including the gluteus maximus, IT band, and rectus femoris, as well as issues with iliopsoas tendon snapping.

Hip dysplasia is closely linked with sports activities requiring hypermobility such as rhythmic gymnastics, figure skating, and ballet dancing [40]. Another study has shown that 7.9% and 15.9% of throwing athletes (baseball players) have hip dysplasia and borderline hip dysplasia, respectively [41]. Recent studies have shown that cam and hip dysplasia deformities often coexist at rates of 50–80% [42].

Previous studies confirmed that hip arthroscopy is a beneficial treatment for borderline and mild hip dysplasia; however, recent literatures reported a high reoperation rate and progressing osteoarthritis with conversion to total hip arthroplasty. Our study advises against performing hip arthroscopy for hip dysplasia when patients have a broken Shenton line, a femoral neck shaft angle >140°, and lateral center edge angle (LCEA) less than 19°. Recently, some studies have demonstrated that patients with borderline hip dysplasia (BDDH) respond positively to hip arthroscopic labral preservation and capsular plication surgery [43]. Furthermore, our recent study also argues against performing hip arthroscopic labral preservation for BDDH when patients are older than 42 year-old, having a broken Shenton line, a vertical center anterior (VCA) angle <13°, an acetabular inclination >17°, or severe cartilage damage at the time of the surgery [44]. Several studies have shown the effectiveness of various surgical procedures to address hip dysplasia.

Many high-demand athletes, especially hypermobile athletes, do not want to undergo a traditional open approach because it requires longer recovery time and presents cosmetic issues.

Therefore, we devised a new strategy that is less invasive and can concurrently address the capsular, labral, and bony pathologies arthroscopically. The purpose of this book chapter is to describe a new surgical technique of endoscopic shelf acetabuloplasty as treatment of hip dysplasia.

7.3.1.1 Purpose

The purpose of this book chapter is to describe the surgical technique and effectiveness of endoscopic shelf acetabuloplasty for treating patients in the setting of hip dysplasia.

7.3.1.2 Indications

Patient eligibility for endoscopic shelf acetabuloplasty is as follows: (1) patients with symptomatic borderline, mild to moderate DDH (5°<LCEA <25°, 5°< VCA< 25°), (2) patients with Tonnis grade 0 or 1, (3) young and active patients, (4) patients less than 45 years old.

7.3.1.3 Contraindications

This procedure should not be recommended for severe dysplasia (broken Shenton line and LCEA < 5°) and progressive osteoarthritis, including severe chondral damage.

Patients older than 50 years are relatively contraindicated for this procedure.

If femoral anteversion is greater than 40°, femoral derotational osteotomy should be considered at the same time.

7.3.2 Preoperative Radiographic Evaluation

Plain radiographs are readily available and provide good visualization of the overall morphology of the pelvis and the proximal femur. They can also serve as the basis for decision making in joint-preservation surgery, including hip arthroscopy or endoscopic shelf acetabuloplasty.

Anteroposterior radiographs of the pelvis with the patient in supine and standing positions should be checked to assess the Shenton line, lateral center edge angle, femoral neck shaft angle, and Tonnis angle (Fig. 7.15a) [45].

The anterior acetabular coverage or anterosuperior subluxation of the femoral head can be evaluated by the false profile view of Lequesne. This piece of information is particularly important for management of hip [46]. The ventral center anterior (VCA) angle should be measured (Fig. 7.15b). Cam lesion at the femoral head–neck junction is frequently associated with hip dysplasia and can be evaluated by modified Dunn view (Fig. 7.15c).

Preoperative three-dimensional imaging and CT scanning are invaluable for evaluating head/neck junctions, acetabular coverage, morphology of the anterior inferior iliac spine, acetabular and femoral versions (Fig. 7.16). If CT cuts of the distal femoral condyles are also obtained, the femoral neck angle can be evaluated for femoral anteversion [47]. Femoral anteversion is correlated with acetabular version in DDH patients with anterior and global shallow sockets [48]. Increased femoral anteversion is most likely to be associated with osteoarthritis [49]

Magnetic resonance imaging is also invaluable for evaluating labral and cartilage pathologies.

7.3.2.1 Surgical Technique

Hip arthroscopy is performed with the patient under general anesthesia and positioned supine on a traction table.

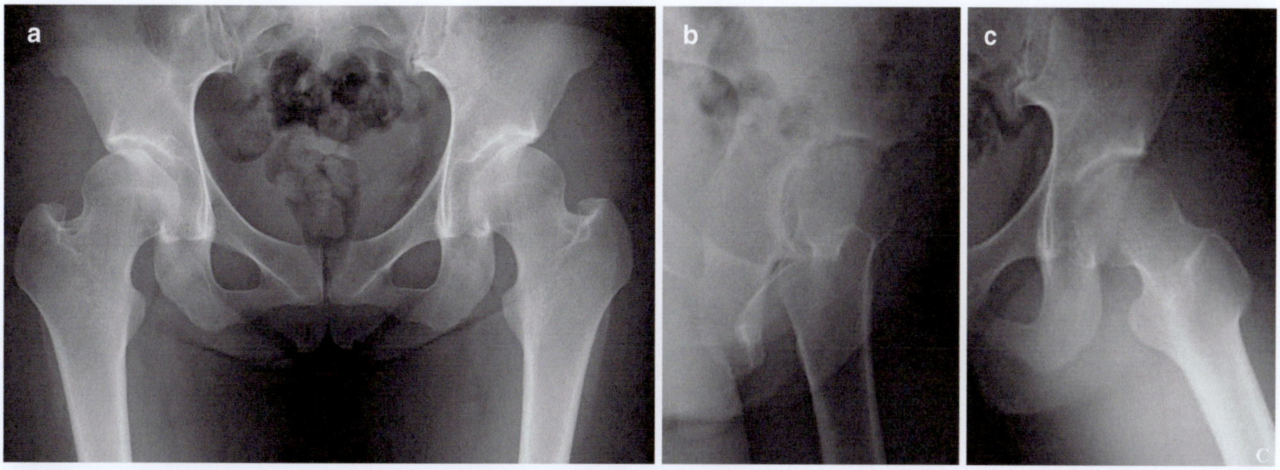

Fig. 7.15 A 29-year-old female ballet dancer with hip dysplasia presented with a 6-month history of right hip pain. (**a**) Preoperative AP radiograph of the pelvis showed hip dysplasia. The center edge angle was 14°, and the Sharp angle was 50°. (**b**) Preoperative false profile view also showed anterior shallowness of the acetabulum. The vertical-center-anterior (VCA) angle was 14°. (**c**) A modified Dunn view showed aspherical shape of the femoral head and alpha angle of 68°, suggesting a cam lesion

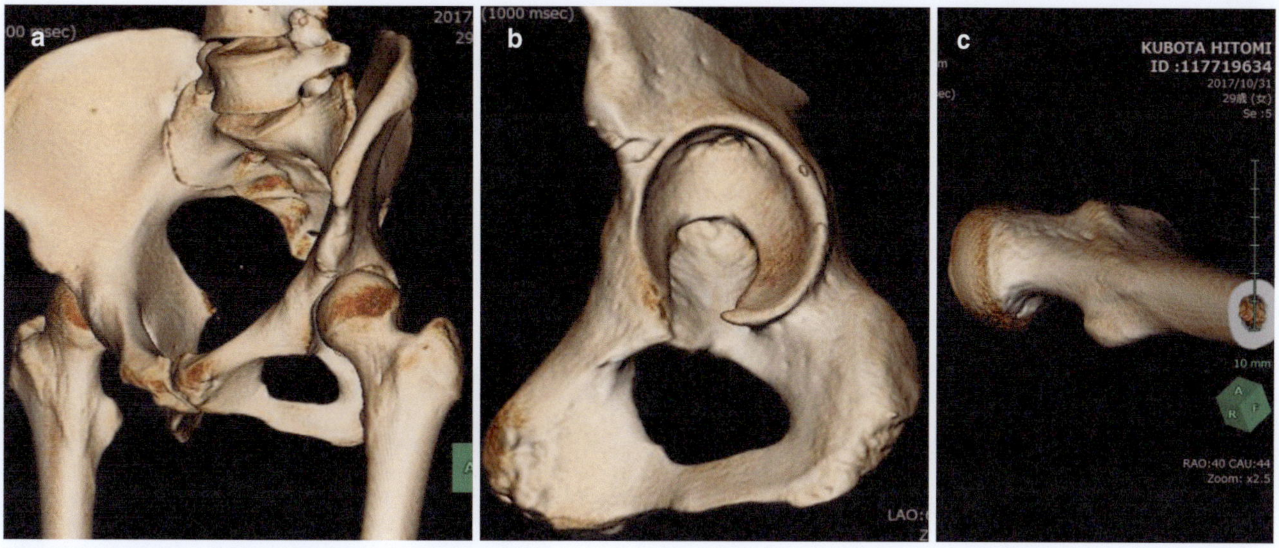

Fig. 7.16 Preoperative three-dimensional computed tomography (**a**) whole pelvic view, (**b**) acetabular view without femur, (**c**) cam at the femoral head–neck junction

Anterolateral portal (ALP), mid-anterior portal (MAP), and proximal mid anterior portal (PMAP) are established and interportal capsulotomy is performed. Arthroscopic assessment of the hip joint is performed and the presence of any intra-articular pathologies, including damage to the acetabular chondrolabral structures and femoral head cartilage are documented (Fig. 7.17a). Microfracture chondroplasty is indicated if there are ICRS grade III or IV cartilage lesions. After that, unstable acetabular labral tears are repaired. The acetabular rim is refreshened to a bleeding bone surface by

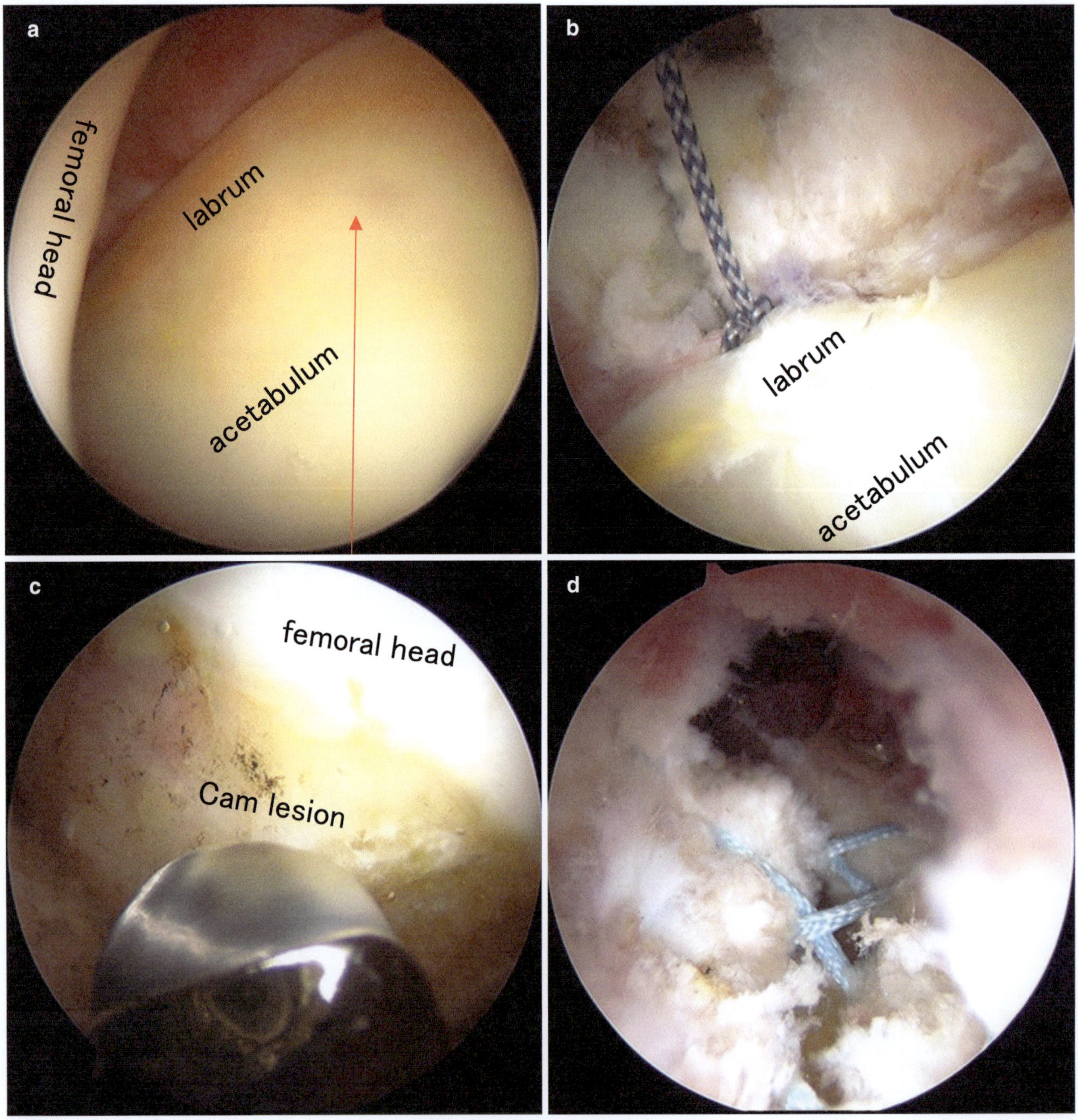

Fig. 7.17 Surgical findings of endoscopic shelf acetabuloplasty. (**a**) Arthroscopic view via the anterolateral portal (ALP) showed an anterosuperior labral tear and suture anchors placed at the acetabulum. (**b**) Labral repair with a suture anchor is visualized via the ALP. (**c**) Arthroscopic view via the mid-anterior portal (MAP) showed the cam osteoplasty. (**d**) Shoelace capsular closure using Ultratape via the mid-anterior portal (MAP) and the proximal mid-anterior portal (PMAP) visualized through the ALP. (**e**) Three 2.4-mm guide wires are inserted via the MAP under fluoroscopy. (**f**) Cannulated drill is utilized via the guide wires to make a shelf slot. (**g**) A tricortical bone graft harvested from the ipsilateral iliac crest with 2 parallel 1.5-mm Kirschner wires. (**h**) The tricortical bone graft is inserted into the slot by means of the guidewires and is secured with press-fit technique

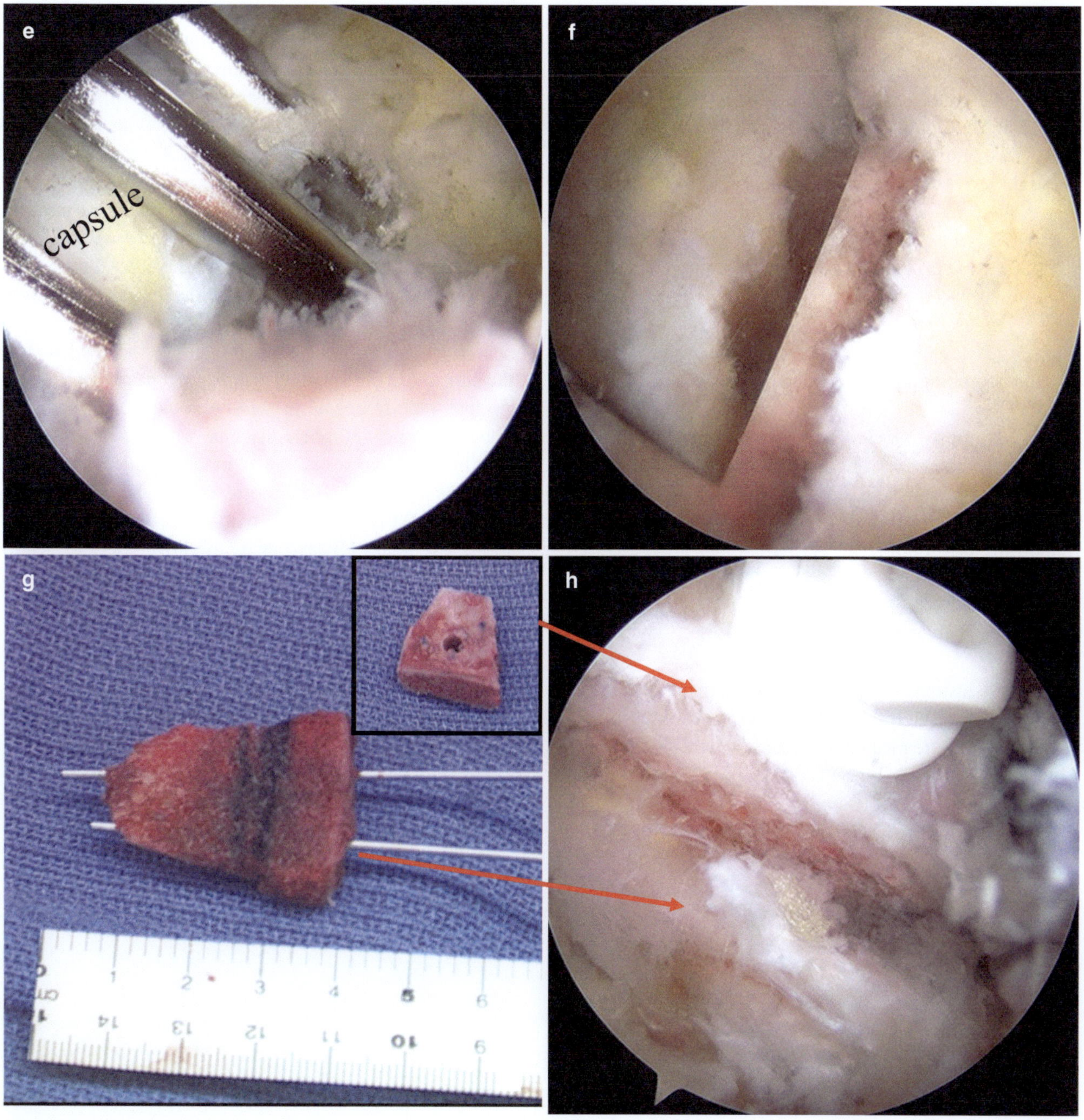

Fig. 7.17 (continued)

means of an arthroscopic burr. The unstable labrum is then repaired with bioabsorbable suture anchors (OsteoRaptor, Smith & Nephew, Andover, MA) and knotting is performed on the capsular side of the labrum (Fig. 7.17b). Cam lesion, if any, is assessed by arthroscopic dynamic examination and cam osteochondroplasty can be performed with a motorized round burr if indicated (Fig. 7.17c). After assessment and treatment of the cam lesion, shoelace repair of the joint capsule with Ultratape (Smith & Nephew, Andover, MA) is performed through the MAP and PMAP with the hip at 40° of flexion (Fig. 7.17d) [50].

After finishing the intra-articular works and capsular repair, endoscopic shelf acetabuloplasty is performed [39, 51]. Under fluoroscopic guidance, a 30° scope is inserted into the extracapsular space. The straight head and reflected head of the rectus femoris are identified and the reflected head is debrided with an arthroscopic shaver and a radiofrequency ablator. After that, two parallel 2.4-mm guidewires are inserted along the anterior acetabular rim close to the capsule by means of drill guide via the MAP to mark the anterolateral periacetabular osteotomy site (Fig. 7.17e). Cannulated drill is utilized via the guide wires to make a shelf slot. The slot is then osteotomized and enlarged with a 10 mm osteotome to a dimension of approximately 5–6 mm in height, 25 mm in width, and at least 20 mm in depth (Fig. 7.17f). Autologous tricortical wedge shaped bone graft is harvested from the ipsilateral iliac crest. Two 1.8 mm drill holes are made in the graft and two 1.5-mm Kirshner wires are inserted into the drill holes to control the graft position during endoscopic insertion into the osteotomy site (Fig. 7.17g). Finally, the wedge-shaped bone graft is secured into the appropriate position (the cortical surface facing the femoral head and in intimate contact with the intervening capsule) by press-fit technique with a cannulated bone tamp (Smith & Nephew, Japan). An additional cortical bone graft is inserted above the new shelf and fixed with a hydroxyapatite PLLA screw and washer under endoscopic guidance to support the shelf graft (Fig. 7.17h).

7.3.3 Postoperative Rehabilitation

Patients are instructed to use flat-foot weight bearing for the first 3 weeks. If microfracture is performed, weight-bearing limitations are extended to 6–8 weeks. Patients are placed in a brace (Philippon hip brace; Bledsoe) for 2–3 weeks to protect the hip and limit flexion (0–120°), abduction (0–45°), and rotation (external rotation 0°). Gentle passive range of motion (ROM) exercise under physiotherapist supervision can be started in the first week. Circumduction with the hip in 70° and neutral flexion is instructed for the first 1 weeks. Then, continuous passive motion (CPM) with hip flexion motion of 0–90° up to 4 h per day for 2 weeks is used to prevent adhesive capsulitis.

During Phase II (weeks 6–12) rehabilitation, patients improved their mobility, stability, and proprioception activity. Endurance strengthening is started only after the range of motion is maximized and good stability in gait and movement is achieved.

Phase III (weeks 12–16) rehabilitation is proceeded only if the patient can demonstrate symmetrical passive ROM and a normal pain-free gait pattern. Aerobic conditioning is advanced using an elliptical machine with a goal of 30 min of continuous exercise at a low to moderate intensity.

Patients are allowed to progress to physical activity only if passive ROM is symmetric, pain-free, with a normal gait pattern. The goal of Phase IV is to allow safe and gentle sports drills and to prepare patients to return to play or work activities. Gentle sport-specific or work agility exercises are initiated [52].

Postoperative radiographs (the AP and the modified Dunn view) showed improvement of LCEA and femoral head–neck offset (Fig. 7.18a, b). X-rays at one year after surgery showed that the shelf graft was inserted into the slot at the anterosuperior border of the hip joint (Fig. 7.18c, d).

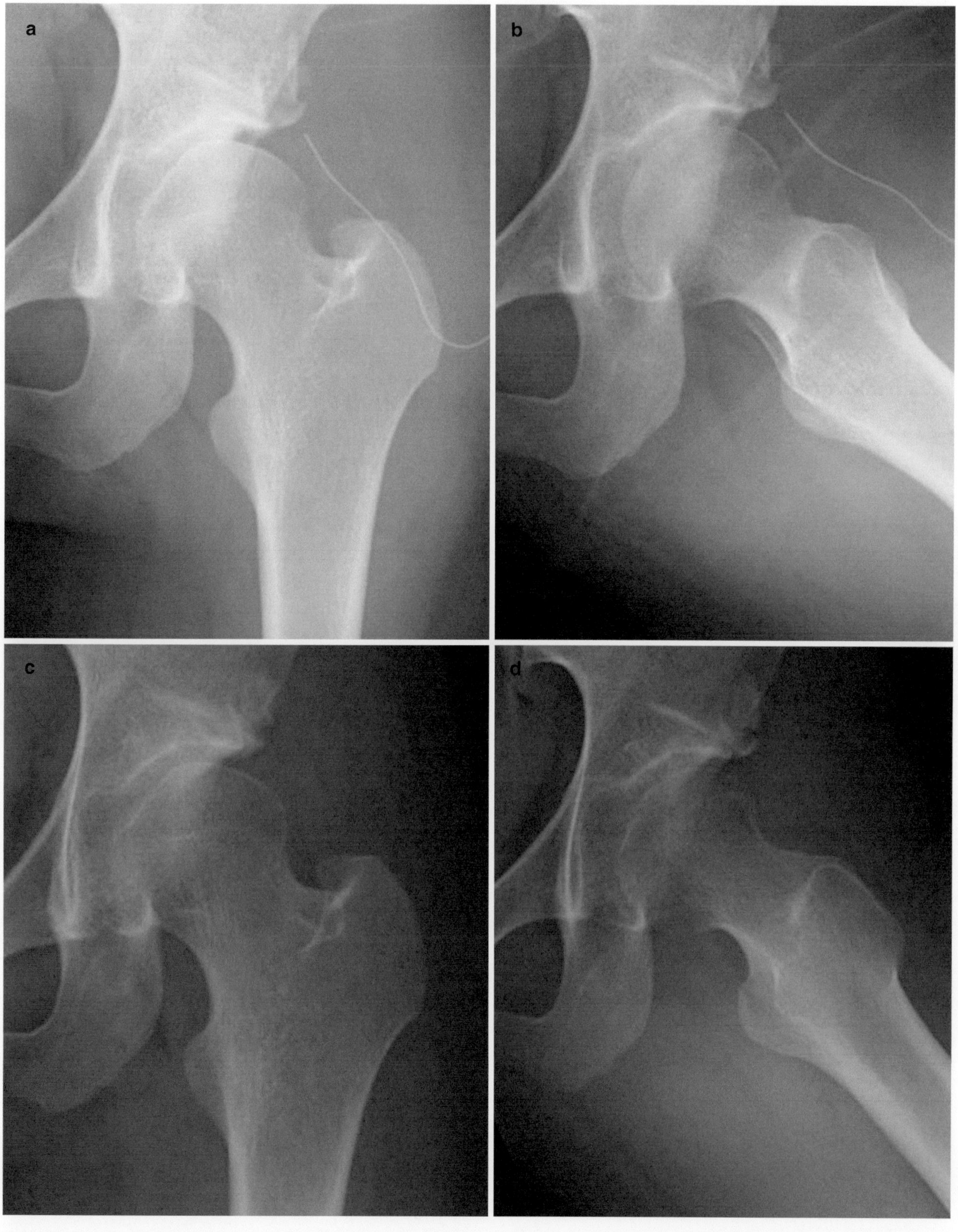

Fig. 7.18 (**a**, **b**) Immediate postoperative pelvic AP and modified Dunn radiograph showed improvement in acetabular coverage with a shelf graft. The LCE angle is 41°. (**c**, **d**) A pelvic AP and modified Dunn views showing proper remodeling of a shelf graft at one year after surgery

7.3.4 Clinical Outcomes of Shelf Acetabuloplasty

In our recent study of a series of 32 active patients undergoing endoscopic shelf acetabuloplasty together with labral repair, the mean PRO scores (modified Harris Hip Score, nonarthritic hip score, and iHot-12) improved significantly after the surgeries, 90% of the patients returned to sport-related activity within an average period of 9 months, and their UCLA activity score also improved significantly [39].

Recent technical reports have demonstrated that endoscopic shelf acetabuloplasty can address hip dysplasia associated with large bone cysts and rim stress fractures [53, 54].

7.3.5 Take-Home Message

Preoperative detailed patient evaluation and surgical planning is the key of success in management of patient with hip dysplasia.

Detailed history taking, clinical examination, and appropriate imaging studies are essential for the surgeon to understand the existing pathology and determine best treatment option.

Patient's point of views and expectations should be respected.

The patients should be educated about their condition, the treatment plan, and the importance of compliance with post-operative rehabilitation.

Acknowledgement The author (Soshi Uchida) is a consultant for Smith & Nephew and Zimmer-Biomet and receives research funds from Smith & Nephew, Pfizer, and Johnson & Johnson. This article is unrelated to that funding. The author reports no other conflicts of interest to disclose that may affect the information and recommendations presented in the manuscript.

The author certifies that he or she has no commercial associations (e.g., consultancies, stock ownership, equity interest, patent/licensing arrangements) that might pose a conflict of interest in connection with the submitted article. Informed consent was obtained from the patient. The patient approved the use of her data for the publication of this manuscript.

References

1. Mont MA, Hungerford DS. Non-traumatic avascular necrosis of the femoral head. J Bone Joint Surg Am. 1995;77(3):459–74.
2. Lieberman JR, Berry DJ, Mont MA, Aaron RK, Callaghan JJ, Rajadhyaksha AD, Urbaniak JR. Osteonecrosis of the hip: management in the 21st century. Instr Course Lect. 2003;52:337–55.
3. Mont MA, et al. Osteonecrosis of the femoral head. Potential treatment with growth and differentiation factors. Clin Orthop Relat Res. 1998;355(Suppl):S314–35.
4. Hungerford DS, Zizic TM. Alcoholism associated ischemic necrosis of the femoral head. Early diagnosis and treatment. Clin Orthop Relat Res. 1978;130:144–53.
5. Cruess RL. Steroid-induced osteonecrosis: a review. Can J Surg (J canadien de chirurgie). 1981;24(6):567–71.
6. Lavernia CJ, Sierra RJ, Grieco FR. Osteonecrosis of the femoral head. J Am Acad Orthop Surg. 1999;7(4):250–61.
7. Ficat RP. Idiopathic bone necrosis of the femoral head. Early diagnosis and treatment. J Bone Joint Surg Br. 1985;67(1):3–9.
8. Steinberg ME, Hayken GD, Steinberg DR. A quantitative system for staging avascular necrosis. J Bone Joint Surg Br. 1995;77(1):34–41.
9. Gardeniers J. A new international classification of osteonecrosis of the ARCO Committee on terminology and classification. J Jpn Orthop Assoc. 1992;66:18–20.
10. Kaneshiro Y, et al. Low hepatic cytochrome P450 3A activity is a risk for corticosteroid-induced osteonecrosis. Clin Pharmacol Ther. 2006;80(4):396–402.
11. Agarwala S, et al. Efficacy of alendronate, a bisphosphonate, in the treatment of AVN of the hip. A prospective open-label study. Rheumatology. 2005;44(3):352–9.
12. Glueck CJ, et al. Idiopathic osteonecrosis, hypofibrinolysis, high plasminogen activator inhibitor, high lipoprotein(a), and therapy with Stanozolol. Am J Hematol. 1995;48(4):213–20.
13. Hungerford DS. Pathogenesis of ischemic necrosis of the femoral head. Instr Course Lect. 1983;32:252–60.
14. Sekiya JK, Ruch DS, Hunter DM, et al. Hip arthroscopy in staging avascular necrosis of the femoral head. J South Orthop Assoc. 2000;9(4):254–61.
15. Gupta AK, Frank RM, Harris JD, McCormick F, Mather RC, Nho SJ. Arthroscopic-assisted core decompression for osteonecrosis of the femoral head. Arthrosc Tech. 2013;3(1):e7–e11.
16. Aldridge JM III, et al. Free vascularized fibular grafting for the treatment of postcollapse osteonecrosis of the femoral head. Surgical technique. J Bone Joint Surg Am. 2004;86-A(Suppl 1):87–101.
17. Sugioka Y. Transtrochanteric rotational osteotomy in the treatment of idiopathic and steroid-induced femoral head necrosis, Perthes' disease, slipped capital femoral epiphysis, and osteoarthritis of the hip. Indications and results. Clin Orthop Relat Res. 1984;184:12–23.
18. Adili A, Trousdale RT. Femoral head resurfacing for the treatment of osteonecrosis in the young patient. Clin Orthop Relat Res. 2003;417:93–101.
19. Garino JP, Steinberg ME. Total hip arthroplasty in patients with avascular necrosis of the femoral head: a 2- to 10-year follow-up. Clin Orthop Relat Res. 1997;334:108–15.
20. Guadilla J, Fiz N, Andia I, Sanchez M. Arthroscopic management and platelet-rich plasma therapy for avascular necrosis of the hip. Knee Surg Sports Traumatol Arthrosc Off J ESSKA. 2012;20(2):393–8.
21. Zhuo N, Wan Y, Lu X, Zhang Z, Tan M, Chen G. Comprehensive management of early stage avascular necrosis of femoral head by arthroscopic minimally invasive surgery. Chin J Repar Reconstr Surg. 2012;26(9):1041–4.
22. Ganz R, Parvizi J, Beck M, Leunig M, Nötzli H, Siebenrock KA. Femoroacetabular impingement: a cause for osteoarthritis of the hip. Clin Orthop Relat Res. 2003;417:112–20.
23. Beck M, Kalhor M, Leunig M, Ganz R. Hip morphology influences the pattern of damage to the acetabular cartilage: femoroacetabular impingement as a cause of early osteoarthritis of the hip. J Bone Joint Surg Br. 2005;87(7):1012–8.
24. Ganz R, Leunig M, Leunig-Ganz K, Harris WH. The etiology of osteoarthritis of the hip: an integrated mechanical concept. Clin Orthop Relat Res. 2008;466(2):264–72.
25. Amanatullah DF, Antkowiak T, Pillay K, Patel J, Refaat M, Toupadakis CA, et al. Femoroacetabular impingement: current concepts in diagnosis and treatment. Orthopedics. 2015;38(3):185–99.
26. McGovern RP, Martin RL, Kivlan BR, Christoforetti JJ. Non-operative management of individuals with non-arthritic hip pain: a literature review. Int J Sports Phys Ther. 2019;14(1):135–47.
27. Griffin DR, Dickenson EJ, O'Donnell J, Agricola R, Awan T, Beck M, et al. The Warwick Agreement on femoroacetabular impingement syndrome (FAI syndrome): an international consensus statement. Br J Sports Med. 2016;50(19):1169–76.
28. Lee YK, Lee GY, Lee JW, Lee E, Kang HS. Intra-articular injections in patients with femoroacetabular impingement: a prospective, randomized, double-blind, cross-over study. J Korean Med Sci. 2016;31(11):1822–7.
29. Maradit Kremers H, Schilz SR, Van Houten HK, Herrin J, Koenig KM, Bozic KJ, et al. Trends in utilization and outcomes of hip arthroscopy in the United States between 2005 and 2013. J Arthroplasty. 2017;32(3):750–5.
30. Kelly BT, Weiland DE, Schenker ML, Philippon MJ. Arthroscopic labral repair in the hip: surgical technique and review of the literature. Arthroscopy. 2005;21(12):1496–504.
31. Philippon MJ, Wolff AB, Briggs KK, Zehms CT, Kuppersmith DA. Acetabular rim reduction for the treatment of femoroacetabular impingement correlates with preoperative and postoperative center-edge angle. Arthroscopy. 2010;26(6):757–61.
32. Fry R, Domb B. Labral base refixation in the hip: rationale and technique for an anatomic approach to labral repair. Arthroscopy. 2010;26(9 Suppl):S81–9.
33. Philippon M, Schenker M, Briggs K, Kuppersmith D. Femoroacetabular impingement in 45 professional athletes: associated pathologies and return to sport following arthroscopic decompression. Knee Surgery, Sports Traumatol Arthrosc. 2007;15(7):908–14.
34. Philippon MJ, Weiss DR, Kuppersmith DA, Briggs KK, Hay CJ. Arthroscopic labral repair and treatment of femoroacetabular impingement in professional hockey players. Am J Sports Med. 2010;38(1):99–104.
35. Sutter R, Pfirrmann CWA. Update on femoroacetabular impingement: what is new, and how should we assess it? Semin Musculoskelet Radiol. 2017;21(5):518–28.
36. Ghaffari A, Davis I, Storey T, Moser M. Current concepts of femoroacetabular impingement. Radiol Clin North Am. 2018;56(6):965–82.
37. Griffin DR, Dickenson EJ, Wall PDH, Achana F, Donovan JL, Griffin J, et al. Hip arthroscopy versus best conservative care for the treatment of femoroacetabular impingement syndrome (UK FASHIoN): a multicentre randomised controlled trial. Lancet (London, England). 2018;391(10136):2225–35.
38. Gao F, Zhang B, Hu B, Lu M, An M, Liu Y, et al. Outcomes of hip arthroscopy for femoroacetabular impingement in Chinese patients aged 50 years or older. Orthop Surg. 2020;12(3):843–51.
39. Uchida S, et al. Endoscopic shelf acetabuloplasty can improve clinical outcomes and achieve return to sports-related activity in active

patients with hip dysplasia. Knee Surg Sports Traumatol Arthrosc. 2018;26(10):3165–77.
40. Charbonnier C, et al. Assessment of congruence and impingement of the hip joint in professional ballet dancers: a motion capture study. Am J Sports Med. 2011;39(3):557–66.
41. Fukushima K, et al. Prevalence of radiological findings related to femoroacetabular impingement in professional baseball players in Japan. J Orthop Sci. 2016;21(6):821–5.
42. Uchida S, et al. Clinical and radiographic predictors for worsened clinical outcomes after hip arthroscopic labral preservation and capsular closure in developmental dysplasia of the hip. Am J Sports Med. 2016;44(1):28–38.
43. Domb BG, et al. Hip arthroscopic surgery with labral preservation and capsular plication in patients with borderline hip dysplasia: minimum 5-year patient-reported outcomes. Am J Sports Med. 2018;46(2):305–13.
44. Hatakeyama A, et al. Predictors of poor clinical outcome following arthroscopic labral preservation, capsular plication and cam osteoplasty in the setting of borderline hip dysplasia. Am J Sports Med. 2017;46(1):135–43.
45. Wiberg G. The anatomy and roentgenographic appearance of a normal hip joint. Acta Chir Scand. 1939;83(Suppl 58):7–38.
46. Chosa E, Tajima N. Anterior acetabular head index of the hip on false-profile views. New index of anterior acetabular cover. J Bone Joint Surg Br. 2003;85(6):826–9.
47. Boster IR, et al. Femoral anteversion in the hip: comparison of measurement by computed tomography, magnetic resonance imaging, and physical examination. Arthroscopy. 2012;28(5):619–27.
48. Akiyama M, et al. Femoral anteversion is correlated with acetabular version and coverage in Asian women with anterior and global deficient subgroups of hip dysplasia: a CT study. Skeletal Radiol. 2012;41(11):1411–8.
49. Tonnis D, Heinecke A. Acetabular and femoral anteversion: relationship with osteoarthritis of the hip. J Bone Joint Surg Am. 1999;81(12):1747–70.
50. Uchida S, et al. Arthroscopic shoelace capsular closure technique in the hip using ultratape. Arthrosc Tech. 2017;6(1):e157–61.
51. Uchida S, et al. Endoscopic shelf acetabuloplasty combined with labral repair, cam osteochondroplasty, and capsular plication for treating developmental hip dysplasia. Arthroscopy Techniques. 2014;3(1):e185–91.
52. Spencer-Gardner L, et al. A comprehensive five-phase rehabilitation programme after hip arthroscopy for femoroacetabular impingement. Knee Surg Sports Traumatol Arthrosc. 2014;22(4):848–59.
53. Uchida S, et al. Arthroscopic management for acetabular rim stress fracture and osteochondritis dissecans in the athlete with hip dysplasia. Arthrosc Tech. 2018;7(5):e533–9.
54. Yamada K, et al. Endoscopic shelf acetabuloplasty for treating acetabular large bone cyst in patient with dysplasia. Arthrosc Tech, 2018.

Hip Endoscopy in Total Hip Arthroplasty: Endoscopic Management of Iliopsoas Tendon Impingement After Hip Arthroplasty

8

Paolo Di Benedetto, Piero Giardini, and Araldo Causero

Abstract

Iliopsoas tendon impingement after hip arthroplasty is a possible cause of painful hip and must always be considered in the differential diagnosis. In these cases, arthroscopic treatment has proven to be safe, guaranteeing superior results compared to open surgery. In this chapter Authors debate the topic of impingement of iliopsoas starting from its etiology up to arthroscopic treatment.

Keywords

Iliopsoas · Hip · Arthroplasty · Arthroscopic · Release

8.1 Introduction: Epidemiology

Total hip arthroplasty (THA) is one of the most successful surgical procedures of the twentieth century and it is often considered the benchmark for clinical outcomes both for orthopedic and non-orthopedic surgical procedures [1]. High satisfaction rate, excellent outcomes, and a very low incidence of complication lead to the well-known "forgotten hip" phenomenon [2, 3].

Despite optimal results in terms of patient related outcomes and implant survival, there is a small percentage of patient complaining of persistent pain about the hip or buttock after their hip replacement in spite of optimal surgery [4–6].

A painful joint replacement requires a careful evaluation and the orthopedic surgeon must follow an algorithm to correctly diagnose and manage the cause of pain [7].

The etiology of a painful THA can be either of articular or extra-articular origin [8]; among the former infection, osteolysis and instability must be primarily ruled out [7].

Within extra-articular causes, lumbar, knee, or neurovascular pathologies, periprosthetic fractures, or heterotopic ossification must be excluded. Inflammation of the soft tissues such as the trochanteric bursa or tendons could be other—often unrecognized—causes of groin pain after THA. Among tendonitis, inflammation of the iliopsoas, greater trochanteric pain syndrome including abductor tendinopathy and snapping hip syndrome are possible conditions of debilitating pain after hip replacement [5].

The etiology of the inflammation of the iliopsoas is strictly related with the course of the muscular-tendon complex and its relation with the native acetabular cavity [9, 10] or with the acetabular cup after hip replacement [3, 4].

The iliopsoas complex is the major flexor of the hip and has a secondary role in the external rotation; its origin takes place by the fusion of the iliacus and the psoas muscles which, respectively, origin by the pelvis and the lumbar

P. Di Benedetto (✉) · A. Causero
Medical Department, University of Udine, Udine, Italy

Clinic of Orthopaedics, Friuli Centrale Healthcare and University Trust (ASUFC), Udine, Italy
e-mail: paolo.dibenedetto@asufc.sanita.fvg.it; paolo.dibenedetto@uniud.it; araldo.causero@asufc.sanita.fvg.it; araldo.causero@uniud.it

P. Giardini
Clinic of Orthopaedics, Friuli Centrale Healthcare and University Trust (ASUFC), Udine, Italy

© The Author(s), under exclusive license to Springer Nature Singapore Pte Ltd. 2021
T. H. Lui (ed.), *Endoscopy of the Hip and Knee*, https://doi.org/10.1007/978-981-16-3488-8_8

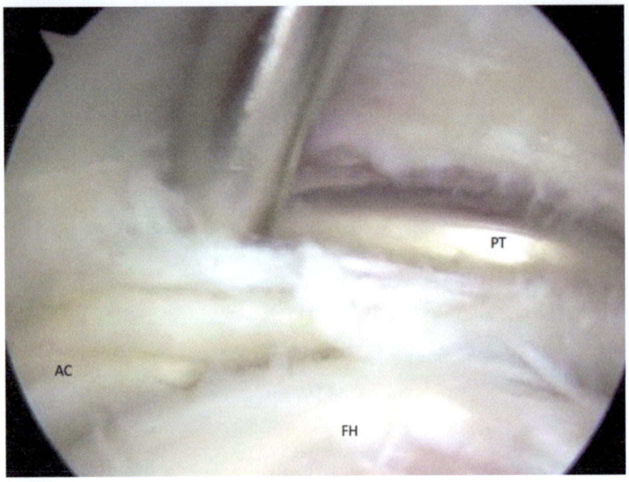

Fig. 8.1 Normal appearance (after medial capsulotomy) of psoas tendon crossing the hip in its anterior-inferior portion. *PT* psoas tendon, *FH* femoral head, *AC* acetabulum

vertebrae and run beneath the inguinal ligament to insert on the lesser trochanter. The iliopsoas muscle crosses the hip in its anterior-inferior portion (Fig. 8.1).

The iliopsoas bursa separates the tendon from the hip capsule and lies between the pubofemoral and iliofemoral ligaments. Although considered extra-articular, the capsulotomy performed during THA implantation makes the tendon intra-articular and therefore intimately associated with the arthroplasty components [3–5].

The tendonitis of the iliopsoas may be related to the mechanical impingement (IPI) of the tendon on the components of the THA or—less commonly—to other reasons such as an increased horizontal offset, an excessive limb-length discrepancy, or as an indirect sign of corrosion of the modular components of the THA [11, 12].

IPI is commonly related with a wrong position of the cup, usually poorly anteverted or wrongly sloped; other causes of impingement have been advocated to the sizing or to the sharp design of the components [3], to the protrusion of an acetabular fixation screws [13], to the overhang of a collared femoral stem [14], to an unstable artificial femoral head [15], or to an anterior osteophytes.

Although traditionally dysplastic hips are potentially at a higher risk of IPI (due to the anatomic disadvantage, the major risk of oversized acetabular component, the frequent implantation of acetabular fixation screws), recent study [15] demonstrated that THA in dysplastic hip patients is not at a higher risk of iliopsoas impingement.

The incidence of the iliopsoas tendonitis is commonly reported around 4% after total hip arthroplasty [6, 12, 16, 17] referring to the bigger case series reported in the literature. Due to its infrequency, most literature on the treatment of iliopsoas impingement after THA is mainly related to small series and retrospective studies [16].

Both conservative and operative treatment (revision of the acetabular component, iliopsoas tenotomy) have been proposed as possible treatment of iliopsoas impingement. Since conservative treatment is related to a high incidence of failures and revision of the acetabular component is associated to a non-negligible percentage of complications [16, 17], arthroscopic release of the iliopsoas is becoming the treatment of choice for IPI. Despite hip arthroscopy in the setting of a THA is a challenging procedure, different studies demonstrated its safeness and its effectiveness [18].

The chapter focuses on the arthroscopic treatment and reports the outcome derived by the personal experience of the main Author (PDB).

8.2 Diagnosis

The diagnosis of iliopsoas impingement is mainly based on clinical findings [4, 5]; nonetheless imaging has a key role in supporting the diagnosis and in ruling out other—more common—causes of painful hip arthroplasty.

Since pain is the principal symptom referred by the patient affected by IPI, a protocol to identify the correct etiology of the painful arthroplasty should be applied. Most important is to rule out a periprosthetic joint infection (PJI) applying the well-known criteria [15]. Secondly, other common causes of hip pain should be excluded such as loosening, osteolysis, or instability [19]. After these major causes are excluded, other less frequent causes of painful THA must be examined.

IPI is responsible of pain in the groin area and it usually presents as an anterior hip pain exacerbated by active hip flexion: resisted straight-leg raise test is positive. Typically, the patient complains of discomfort and pain in activities that require hip flexion, such as walking upstairs and lifting the leg in and out of a car (car sign) [3]. Passive hip flexion is painless while passive hip extension is distressing due to the accentuated impingement of the iliopsoas tendon on the THA components [4, 5, 16, 17].

Rarely, a palpable tenderness in the groin area can be detached during active hip flexion; another—less common—sign is a palpable snapping of the tendon when the patient is asked to move the hip from a flexed to an extended position.

X-Rays are an indispensable tool in the diagnosis of a painful THA; different views permit to assess the position and the integration of the implant. In particular the true lateral view plays an important role in detecting a potential cup-tendon impingement: assessing the version of the acetabular cup permits to suspect—in case of excessive retroversion—or to exclude a potential impingement of the iliopsoas tendon over the anterior-inferior margin of the acetabular cup [20].

A CT scan (MARS technique) is the most accurate method to assess and quantify the prominence of the acetabular component at the anterior-inferior acetabular rim that may determine mechanical irritation to the iliopsoas tendon; recent studies have shown iliopsoas impingement with a prominence of only 2 mm [21]. Nevertheless, normal CT findings do not completely rule out the diagnosis [22].

MRI is a potentially useful imaging method but the presence of the metal cup lead to the presence of artifact that limits its use; Moreta et al. [21] recently described iliopsoas bursitis and iliopsoas tendinopathy as MRI findings related to the IPI between the tendon and the bursa on the anterior rim of the THA. Furthermore, in the same study is postulated that non-contrast sequences have a low sensitivity in detecting iliopsoas tendinopathy.

An US or CT guided-injection of corticosteroid and local anesthetic performed in the sheath of the iliopsoas tendon in a sterile fashion has an important role in confirming the diagnosis; a relief of symptoms after the injection makes the diagnosis of IPI more likely. However, the benefit tested after the injection is transient and only 39–50% [21] of patients are successfully treated conservatively.

8.3 IPI Arthroscopic Treatment

Several treatments for iliopsoas impingement after THA have been proposed; usually a conservative attempt is performed since its failure does not affect a secondary surgical procedure. Conservative treatment usually includes anti-inflammatory medications, physical therapy and local injections of corticosteroid, analgesic or botulinum toxin type A [21].

As previously reported, different studies found a low successful rate of the conservative treatment, with a percentage of failures around 50–61% [21] with a recurrence of symptoms after 3.7 months [17]. A recent study [12] described that only 13.6% of patient affected by IPI and conservatively treated experienced a completely relief from pain and that a same percentage of patient (13.6%) reported that a relatively strong pain remained after conservative treatment.

Surgical procedures of IPI consist on the revision of the component determining impingement on the iliopsoas tendon (usually the cup and the liner) or in the tenotomy of the iliopsoas.

Beside case reports and small case series reporting good results after the revision of a prominent acetabular fixation screws [23], of an overhanging collared stem [14] or other less common causes of IPI [11, 15], the most frequent site of friction of the iliopsoas is at the level of the antero-inferior acetabular rim [21], thus requiring a major revision of the acetabular cup with some concern in regard to the bone stock, in particular in elderly patients.

Both revision of the prominent acetabular component and the tenotomy of the iliopsoas are related with good clinical outcomes [17, 20] but the latter is associated with a lower incidence of complication [17].

Although there is not a clear cut-off, Chalmers et al. developed a treatment algorithm for which IPI associated with a protrusion of the cup greater than 10 mm should be preferably treated with a revision of the acetabular component rather than a tenotomy; conversely, patients affected by IPI with a cup prominence inferior than 10 mm are more successfully treated by tenotomy [16]. Nonetheless, it has recently been published that arthroscopic psoas release provided a high rate of success with no complications even in patients with moderate acetabular component malpositioning [21, 24].

Traditionally, open release of the iliopsoas has been considered the standard of care and it has been performed with different hip surgical approaches (posterior, anterolateral, direct lateral, or medial) [5]. An arthroscopic release is increasingly the favored approach in particular in relation to fewer complication and a higher success rates in relieving groin pain related to IPT compared to open tenotomy (91.8% vs 77.8%) [3, 24].

Moreover, hip arthroscopy has the advantage to be a diagnostic tool as well and permit to confirm the contact between the tendon and the cup rim in a dynamic manner through passive range of motion of the hip. The arthroscopic appearance of the tendon may be either with evidence of inflammation or normal if the site of friction is more proximal or more distal depending at the degree on which the impingement occurs [22].

Hip arthroscopy also allows to assess the integrity of the components and to exclude other causes of pain (osteolysis, synovitis) and consent to collect samples for microbiological or histological evaluation.

While the arthroscopic treatment of the IPI provides a transcapsular release of the tendon, other techniques—commonly referred as endoscopic—provide an extra-capsular release of the tendon; the latter approach has the disadvantage to not assess the intra-articular space but the advantage to make a more reliable tenotomy at the level of the lesser trochanter. However, this endoscopic procedure expose to a potential higher risk of functional impairment do to the higher tendon-muscle ratio [22]. Same consideration can be applied to the US guided-percutaneous tenotomy described by Sampson [25].

Hip arthroscopy requires an unexpectedly long learning curve in a native hip [26] and the complexity and difficulty of the procedures only increase with the presence of the THA: challenges arise mainly due to the decreased ability to traction, the presence of scar tissue and adhesions, and an altered joint contour in the presence of a THA [18].

As recently published [27], the Main Author performs hip arthroscopy by an extra-capsular (OUT-IN) access [28] and tendon release is carried out according to Wettstein technique [29] in the impingement zone on the anterior rim of the acetabular component. Our technique provided in all the patient treated a complete resolution of symptoms without any complication [27]. Our results are similar to those achieved by Moreta and other authors [17, 21] also in terms of any significant hip flexion weakness postoperatively. Our results agree with recent findings among iliopsoas fractional lengthening (IFL) in the context of arthroscopic treatment for femoroacetabular impingement in which the adjunctive procedure (IFL) did not adversely affect clinical outcome compared to the control group [30].

Furthermore, since we perform a careful and targeted tenotomy of the iliopsoas associated with a capsular closure at the end of the procedure [31], we have not experienced any major complications—such as THA dislocation—after arthroscopic debridement of the iliopsoas even if it is a procedure with a potential risk of iatrogenic impairment of important hip stabilizers [32].

8.4 Surgical Technique

Hip arthroscopy was performed in all patients with extracapsular (OUT-IN) access [28].

The surgical procedure is performed under general anesthesia in the supine position using a normal orthopedic table without traction or perineal post. The hip is prepared and draped in the usual fashion. Two standard portals are used for each arthroscopy and established under the use of bony landmarks (ASIS and great trochanter profile). The portals used are the anterior-lateral and the mid-anterior one. The skin is incised following the Langer's lines. After a blunt dissection with scissors, the 30° arthroscope is inserted through the anterior-lateral portal and a radiofrequency probe through the mid-anterior portal. At this point the neo-capsule is visualized and opened from outside with the radiofrequency probe longitudinally to the neck. Scar tissue is dissected until the head and socket are identified. Then a capsulotomy is performed at the iliopsoas notch. After identifying the iliopsoas tendon, the contact between the tendon and the rim of the cup is checked in a dynamic manner through passive range of motion of the hip (Fig. 8.2a, b). The iliopsoas tendon is then released according to the technique described by Wettstein [29] in the impingement zone on the anterior rim of the acetabular component using a radiofrequency probe or a shaver (Fig. 8.3).

After the release of the tendon, the absence of friction between the iliopsoas and the antero-inferior rim of the cup is checked through passive range of motion of the hip. We routinely perform a capsular closure with a side-to-side stitch with high resistance wire at the end of the procedure [31].

In the post-operative period we recommend no weight-bearing walking with crutches and assisted rehabilitation program performing only passive hip mobility for 2 weeks. Active hip flexion with straight-leg raise had to be avoided for 4 weeks as well.

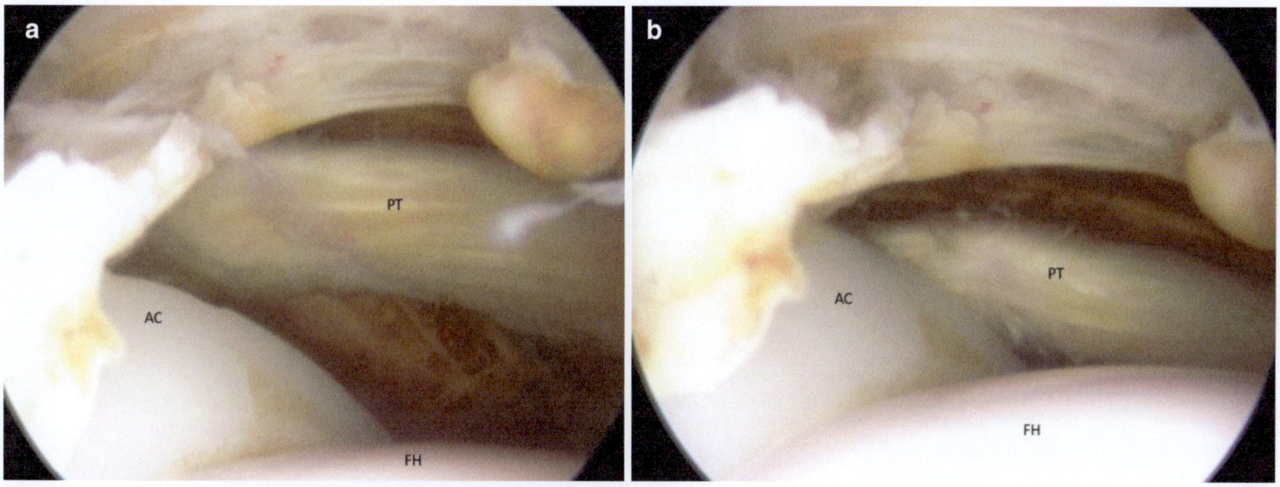

Fig. 8.2 (**a**, **b**) The impingement between the psoas tendon and the acetabular component during flexion/extension movements. *PT* psoas tendon, *FH* femoral head prosthesis, *AC* acetabular cup

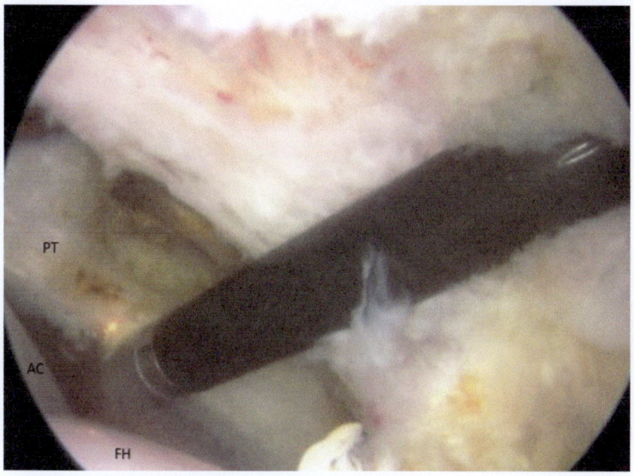

Fig. 8.3 Release of the psoas tendon in the impingement zone on the anterior rim of the acetabular component using a radiofrequency probe. *PT* psoas tendon, *FH* femoral head prosthesis, *AC* acetabular cup

8.5 Conclusion

As previously described for knee arthroscopy performed on total knee replacement, hip arthroscopy in the setting of THA is a recent but safe and effective surgical procedure [18].

Beside a long learning curve, hip arthroscopy is a useful technique with both diagnostic and therapeutic values.

The arthroscopic treatment of the impingement of the iliopsoas after THA should be considered the preferred surgical treatment for different reasons.

First, it is the only procedure that allows to confirm intra operatively and dynamically the exact site of impingement of the tendon on the cup thus to permit an accurate and selective tenotomy in the site of impingement.

Second, arthroscopic treatment of IPI is associated with good results and a low rate of complications compared with other more invasive procedures.

Third, a failure of the arthroscopic treatment does not affect the possibility to perform and the results of a second—more invasive—surgical treatment.

References

1. Schmit PP, et al. No decline in high patient satisfaction after total hip arthroplasty at long-term follow-up, European Journal of Orthopaedic Surgery & Traumatology (2018). Eur J Orthop Surg Traumatol. 2019;29(1):91–5.
2. Swaru I, et al. Implant survival and patient reported outcomes after total hip arthroplasty in young patients. J Arthroplast. 2018;33(9):2893–8. https://doi.org/10.1016/j.arth.2018.04.016.
3. Riemer B, et al. Iliopsoas tendon impingement following total hip replacement surgery. SA Orthop J. 2015;14(4):47.
4. Lachiewic PF, et al. Anterior iliopsoas impingement and tendinitis after total hip arthroplast. J Am Acad Orthop Surg. 2009;17(6):337–44.
5. Capogna BM, et al. Tendon disorders after total hip arthroplasty: evaluation and management. J Arthroplast. 2017;32(10):3249–55. https://doi.org/10.1016/j.arth.2017.04.015.
6. O'Connel RS, et al. A systematic review of arthroscopic vs open tenotomy of iliopsoas tendinitis after total hip replacement. Arthroscopy. 2018;34(4):1332–9. https://doi.org/10.1016/j.arthro.2017.10.051.
7. Monsef JB. Failed total hip arthroplasty. JBJS Rev. 2018;6(11):e3. https://doi.org/10.2106/JBJS.RVW.17.00140.
8. Fink B. Diagnostischer Algorithmus der schmerzhaften Hüfttotalendoprothese. ZOrthop Unfall. 2016;154:527–44.
9. Dom BG, et al. Iliopsoas impingement: a newly identified cause of labral pathology in the hip. HSSJ. 2011;7:145–50.
10. Androni O. Non-arthroplasty iliopsoas impingement in athletes: a narrative literature review. Hip Int. 2019;29(5):460–7. https://doi.org/10.1177/1120700019831945.
11. Ko M, et al. Iliopsoas irritation as presentation of head-neck corrosion after total hip arthroplasty: a case series. Orthop Clin North Am. 2015;46(4):461–8. https://doi.org/10.1016/j.ocl.2015.06.009.
12. Ueno T, et al. Risk factors and cup protrusion thresholds for symptomatic iliopsoas impingement after total hip arthroplasty: a retrospective case-control study. J Arthroplasty. 2018;33(10):3288–3296.e1. https://doi.org/10.1016/j.arth.2018.05.017.
13. Morohashi I, et al. Iliopsoas Impingement After revision total hip arthroplasty treated with iliopsoas muscle transaction. Ann Med Surg (Lond). 2016;7:30–3. https://doi.org/10.1016/j.amsu.2016.03.004.
14. Brew CJ, et al. Iliopsoas tendonitis caused by overhang of a collared femoral prosthesis. J Arthroplasty. 2011;26(3):504.e17–9.
15. Parvizi J, Gehrke T, Mont MA, Callaghan JJ. Introduction: proceedings of international consensus on orthopedic infections. J Arthroplast. 2019;34:S1–2.
16. Chalmers BP. Iliopsoas impingement after primary total hip arthroplasty: operative and nonoperative treatment outcomes. J Bone Joint Surg Am. 2017;99:557–64.
17. Dora C. Iliopsoas impingement after total hip replacement. The Results of non-operative, tenotomy or acetabular revision. J Bone Joint Surg Br. 2007;89-B(8):1031–5.
18. Heaven S, et al. Hip arthroscopy in the setting of hip arthroplasty. Knee Surg Sports Traumatol Arthrosc. 2016;24(1):287–94. https://doi.org/10.1007/s00167-014-3379-5.
19. Kelmer G, et al. Reasons for revision: primary total hip arthroplasty mechanisms of failure. J Am Acad Orthop Surg. 2021;29:78–87. https://doi.org/10.5435/JAAOS-D-19-00860.
20. Schoof B, et al. Anterior iliopsoas impingement due to a malpositioned acetabular component - effective relief by surgical cup reorientation. Hip Int. 2017;27(2):128–33.
21. Moreta J, et al. Outside-in arthroscopic psoas release for anterior iliopsoas impingement after primary total hip arthroplasty. Hip Int. 2020; https://doi.org/10.1117/1120700020909159.
22. May O, et al. Arthroscopic techniques for treating ilio-psoas tendinopathy after hip arthroplasty. Orthop Traumatol Surg Res. 2019;105(1S):S177–85. https://doi.org/10.1016/j.otsr.2018.05.017.
23. Mayne IP, et al. Iliopsoas tendonitis due to the protrusion of an acetabular component fixation screw after total hip arthroplasty. J Arthroplasty. 2010;25(4):659.e5–8.
24. O'Connell RS, et al. A systemic review of arthroscopic versus open tenotomy of iliopsoas tendonitis after total hip replacement. Arthroscopy. 2018;34(4):1332–9.
25. Sampson MJ, et al. Ultrasound-guided percutaneous tenotomy for the treatment of iliopsoas impingement: a description of technique and case study. J Med Imaging Radiat Oncol. 2015;59(2):195–9.
26. Mehta N, et al. Defining the learning curve for hip arthroscopy. A threshold analysis of the volume-outcomes relationship. Am J Sports Med. 2018;46(6):1284–93.
27. Benedetto D, et al. Arthroscopic treatment of iliopsoas impingement syndrome after hip arthroplasty. Acta Biomed. 2019;90(Suppl 1):104–9.
28. Benedetto D, et al. Extracapsular vs standard approach in hip arthroscopy. Acta Bio-Medica Atenei Parm. 2016;87(Suppl 1):41–5.
29. Wettstein M, Jung J, Dienst M. Arthroscopic psoas tenotomy. Arthroscopy. 2006;22:907.e1–4.
30. Maldonado DR, et al. Does iliopsoas lengthening adversely affect clinical outcomes after hip arthroscopy? Am J Sports Med. 2018;46(11):2624–31. https://doi.org/10.1177/036354651878596.
31. Di Benedetto P, et al. Capsular closure after hip arthroscopy: our experience. Acta Biomed. 2020;91(Suppl 4):92–7.
32. Sansone M, et al. Total dislocation of the hip joint after arthroscopy and ilio psoas tenotomy. Knee Surg Sports Traumatol Arthrosc. 2013;21:420–3.

Part III

Knee

Anterior Knee Endoscopy

9

Tsz Lung Choi, Tun Hing Lui, Peter Wai Pan Yau, and Gabriel Ching Ngai Leung

Abstract

Anterior knee endoscopy can access the quadriceps tendon, patellar tendon, Hoffa fat pad, and various bursae. Prepatellar bursa, infrapatellar bursa, and Morel-Lavallée lesion are superficial lesions that are easily approached. However, open resection is associated with poor healing of the surgical wound, decreased sensation over scar area, contracted scar tissue, atrophic skin changes, subcutaneous collection, and scar hypersensitivity. Endoscopic resection is a minimally invasive surgical approach that may reduce the risk of complications associated with open surgery. Acute quadriceps tendon rupture typically occurred in the distal 2 cm of the tendon. While delay in diagnosis was common, it was associated with poor outcome even after open surgical repair. An endoscopic technique of acute quadriceps tendon rupture at the osteotendinous junction and the mid-substance is developed. There is no early post-operation complication and the short-term results are favorable. Patellar tendon pathology typically occurs at the enthesis site; in most cases it occurs at the inferior pole of the patella, but it can occur at the tibial tuberosity. Pathology of the Hoffa pad can be intrinsic, e.g. intracapsular chondroma, localized nodular synovitis, post-surgery or post-traumatic fibrosis, or extrinsic, e.g. pigmented villonodular synovitis, meniscal cyst. Patellar tendoscopy and endoscopy of the Hoffa fat pad are useful minimally invasive approaches to deal with these pathologies with the advantages of better cosmetic result, less post-operative pain, and less surgical trauma. In this chapter, the endoscopic techniques are outlined.

Keywords

Prepatellar bursa · Infrapatellar bursa · Morel-Lavallée lesion · Endoscopy · Resection · Acute · Quadriceps tendon rupture · Endoscopic repair · Tendoscopy Patellar tendon · Hoffa fat pad

The corresponding author of section 9.1 is Tun Hing Lui, Email: luithderek@yahoo.co.uk

The corresponding author of section 9.2 is Peter Wai Pan Yau, Email: peterwpy@hku.hk

The corresponding author of section 9.3 is Tun Hing Lui, Email: luithderek@yahoo.co.uk

T. L. Choi
Department of Orthopaedics and Traumatology, Alice Ho Miu Ling Nethersole Hospital, Hong Kong, China

T. H. Lui (✉)
Department of Orthopaedics and Traumatology, North District Hospital, Hong Kong, China

The Second Affiliated Hospital, Shenzhen University, Shenzhen, China

P. W. P. Yau
Department of Orthopaedics and Traumatology, Li Ka Shing Faculty of Medicine, The University of Hong Kong, Hong Kong, China
e-mail: peterwpy@hku.hk

G. C. N. Leung
Department of Orthopaedics and Traumatology, Queen Mary Hospital, Hong Kong, China
e-mail: LCN126@ha.org.hk

© The Author(s), under exclusive license to Springer Nature Singapore Pte Ltd. 2021
T. H. Lui (ed.), *Endoscopy of the Hip and Knee*, https://doi.org/10.1007/978-981-16-3488-8_9

9.1 Endoscopic Resection of Prepatellar Bursa, Infrapatellar Bursa, and Morel-Lavallée Lesion

Tsz Lung Choi and Tun Hing Lui

9.1.1 Introduction

9.1.1.1 Infrapatellar Bursa Anatomy

Infrapatellar bursa comprises superficial and deep ones. The superficial infrapatellar bursa lies between the subcutaneous tissues and the upper part of the patellar tendon. Superficial infrapatellar bursa may exist as a single bursal sac or, in some patients, as a multisegmented series of loculated sacs. The deep infrapatellar bursa (DIB) is located directly posterior to the distal one third of the patellar tendon, just proximal to its insertion on the tibial tuberosity. It has no communication to the knee joint. Its average width at the most proximal margin of the tibial tuberosity is slightly wider than the average distal width of the patellar tendon [1]. The ventral side of the DIB contains only patellar tendon tissue without synovial covering. The medial and lateral mini recess of DIB consists of a folded synovial membrane based on smooth subsynovial fat tissue, which is responsible for the gliding mechanism of the patellar tendon during knee flexion and extension [1, 2]. The dorsal side of the bursa contains a flat synovial membrane which is based on a loose interstitial connective tissue [2].

9.1.1.2 Disorder of Infrapatellar Bursa

Disorders of infrapatellar bursa can be a source of anterior knee pain. Superficial infrapatellar bursitis, also called clergyman's knee, is due to inflammation and fluid accumulation resulting from chronic stress. Clinically, there is a palpable swelling inferior to the patella [3]. On MRI, it appears as a loculated collection that projects exophytically, anterior to the patellar tendon, forming a swelling [4].

Deep infrapatellar bursa can be site of a number of pathologies, which includes calcification [5], inflammatory bursitis [6], gout, septic bursitis [5], and traumatic hemorrhage [7] and as a possible factor in the infrapatellar contracture syndrome [8]. Inflammatory bursitis of DIB can provoke symptoms like patellofemoral arthralgia [9]. Osgood-Schlatter disease can cause inflammation and pain associated with the DIB [10]. In one study, Rosenberg et al. [11] found distended deep infrapatellar bursa on magnetic resonance imaging in 71% (12 of 17) of cases of Osgood-Schlatter disease. Injection of DIB with lidocaine or a combination of lidocaine and corticosteroids has been reported to result in clinical relief of symptoms [10, 11].

9.1.1.3 Infrapatellar Bursa Endoscopy

Endoscopy is reserved for those who failed conservative treatment. William et al. [2] described a few indications for infrapatellar bursa endoscopy, which include Osgood-Schlatter's disease, infrapatellar bursitis, and patellar tendinopathy. In case of bursitis and soft tissue impingement, the bursa can be removed using a synovial resector. Intratendinous pathology and superficial fraying of the patellar tendon can be cleaned with a shaver [2]. Intratendinous ossicle which can occur in Osgood-Schlatter's disease can produce symptoms. William et al. described a technique by using finger control from outside as counter pressure on the bone piece in the tendon to assist removal [2]. Surgeon must pay special care to patellar tendon and its insertion during removal of the ossicle [2]. Symptomatic osteophytes on the ventral tibial side can be removed with cautions of the patellar tendon insertion in infrapatellar endoscopy as well [2].

9.1.1.4 Prepatellar Bursa Anatomy

A trilaminar arrangement of fibrous soft tissue structures is present anterior to the patella in most knees [12]. From superficial to deep, there are a transversely oriented fascia, an obliquely oriented aponeurosis, and the longitudinally oriented fibers of the rectus femoris tendon [12]. Prepatellar subcutaneous bursa, prepatellar subfascial bursa, and prepatellar subaponeurotic bursa are present between the soft tissue fibrous layers [12]. No potential bursal space exists between the rectus femoris tendon and the anterior patellar bone [12]. The prepatellar bursa usually does not communicate with the knee joint [13].

9.1.1.5 Prepatellar Bursitis and Its Treatment Options

Prepatellar bursitis can be septic or aseptic. Prepatellar aseptic bursitis can occur after repetitive minor trauma. "Housemaid's knee," in those whose occupations require a kneeling posture, such as house cleaners and carpet layers [14]. Acute trauma or low-grade inflammatory conditions, such as gout, syphilis, tuberculosis, rheumatoid arthritis, sarcoid, idiopathic calcification, and calcinosis, Raynaud phenomenon can be other causes of aseptic prepatellar bursitis [13, 15]. In prepatellar septic bursitis, the mechanism of infection is believed to be direct inoculation, not hematogenous seeding, likely because of the poor blood supply to the bursa [13, 14].

Nonoperative treatment is the mainstay of treatment for aseptic prepatellar bursitis. Aspiration, applying compressive dressings, prescribing nonsteroidal anti-inflammatory drugs, and treating underlying causes [13, 15] should be tried before operative treatment.

There are a number of operative treatments for aseptic prepatellar bursitis, which includes aspiration and intrabursal injection of an appropriate drug (corticosteroid, autologous blood, caustic chemical, such as sodium morrhuate) and placement of a short-term indwelling drainage catheter; incision and drainage in cases of acute suppurative bursitis; and excision of chronically inflamed and thickened bursa [13, 15]. Risk of open bursectomy includes poor healing of the surgical wound, decreased sensation over scar area, contracted scar tissue, atrophic skin changes, subcutaneous collection, and scar hypersensitivity [16]. This is related to the poor blood supply to the prepatellar skin and the dense anastomosing network of the vertically descending branches of the anterior divisions of the medial and lateral cutaneous nerves of the thigh, divisions of the intermediate cutaneous nerve, and the infrapatellar branch of the saphenous nerve [13, 15, 17]. Risk of wound complications can be reduced by excising only the posterior half of the prepatellar bursa and leaving the anterior wall intact [18]. Endoscopic bursectomy has been proposed because of the advantages of better cosmetic result and fewer wound complications [16, 19–21].

Septic prepatellar bursitis can usually be treated nonoperatively with resting, compression dressing, aspiration, and antibiotics [22]. Rarely, bursectomy may be required for cases not responding to conservative treatment [22]. Endoscopic bursectomy has the risk of inadequate debridement to prevent recurrence and risk of spreading of the bacteria to the nearby fascia leading to necrotizing fasciitis [23, 24].

9.1.1.6 Morel-Lavallée Lesion

Morel-Lavallée lesion (MLL) is first described by Maurice Morel-Lavallée in 1863. It is a post-traumatic close degloving of soft tissue [25], MLL is caused by shearing blunt trauma which disrupt the perforating blood vessels and separate subcutaneous tissue from underlying fascia. Blood, dead fatty tissue, and lymph fluid then fill the potential space left behind. Pain and persistent swelling can occur if no treatment is given [26]. MLL is usually described around the thigh region in association with pelvic and acetabular fractures. Vanhegan et al. reviewed 204 MLLs and the frequency of occurrence according to site is as follows: pelvis 69.1%, knee 15.7%, Gluteal 6.4%, lumbosacral spine 3.4%, abdominal wall 1.5%, lower leg 1.5%, head 0.5%, and 2% unspecified.

MLL itself is a rare cause of pain and swelling around the knee. It is typically presented as rapid onset, fluctuant collection in anterior knee extending into the suprapatellar area [27]. MRI is considered as the diagnostic imaging modality of choice for MLL. Ultrasonography is a useful adjunct and potential replacement for MRI in diagnosis and monitoring of MLL [27]. MLLs are hypoechoic or anechoic, compressible and located between fascia and underlying deep fat tissue [28, 29].

There is no universally accepted treatment protocol for MLLs [26]. There are studies reported that MLL which is less than 3 weeks old and not encapsulated could be treated conservatively [30]. Conservative treatment includes compression dressing, aspiration of fluid, and injection of sclerosing agent into the MLL [26]. Nickerson et al. showed that aspiration of more than 50 ml of fluid in a MLL is a sign which predicts failure of conservative treatment [31].

As for surgical management of MLL of knee, only a few cases have been reported [26, 32–36]. Mostly are open debridement. Only two cases were reported as endoscopic debridement of MLL [26, 36]. Open debridement can result in wound complication which endoscopic debridement has the advantage of decreasing the chance of wound complication [26, 36]. Baris et al. reported a case of a 33-year-old man with MLL of knee which was treated successfully with endoscopic debridement and fibrin glue injection [26]. While Kim et al. reported a case of successful treatment of a 14-year-old boy with MLL of knee with endoscopic debridement and doxycycline injection.

9.1.2 Indications

For these superficial lesions, endoscopic resection is indicated for symptomatic ones which are recalcitrant to conservative treatment.

9.1.3 Contra-indications

- Skin infection at the planned portal sites
- Recurred lesions after previous endoscopic surgery
- Infected bursitis

9.1.4 Author Preferred Technique

9.1.4.1 Pre-operative Planning

These superficial lesions are obvious clinically. The diagnosis is confirmed by magnetic resonance imaging (Fig. 9.1) or ultrasound study. Any sign of infection or underlying pathologies of the knee joint, quadriceps tendon, and patellar tendon should be examined.

9.1.4.2 Patient Positioning

The patient is in supine position with the legs spread. A thigh tourniquet is used to provide a bloodless operative field. Fluid inflow is driven by gravity and no arthro-pump is used. A 4.0-mm, 30° arthroscope is used for this procedure.

9.1.4.3 Portal Design

Portals can be made at any point of the periphery of the lesion. Usually, two portals, one medial and one lateral to the lesions are sufficient for this procedure. These medial and lateral portals are coaxial portals and interchangeable as the viewing and working portals. The medial and lateral placement of the portals can avoid hindrance of instrument motion. If the lesion has a long longitudinal dimension, one of the portals is placed at the proximal medial corner of the lesion and the other at the distal lateral corner of the lesion or vice versa (Fig. 9.2).

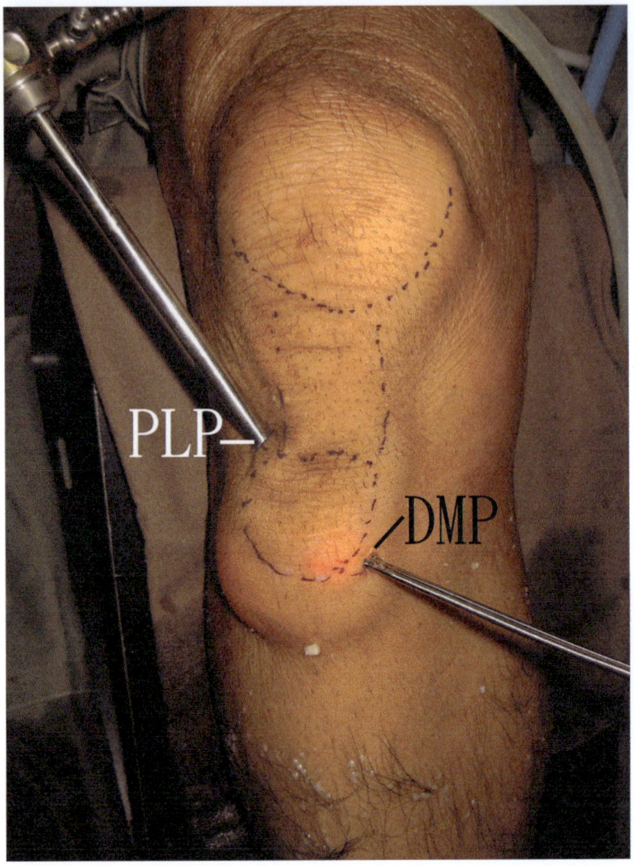

Fig. 9.2 Endoscopic resection is performed via the proximal lateral portal (PLP) and the distal medial portal (DMP)

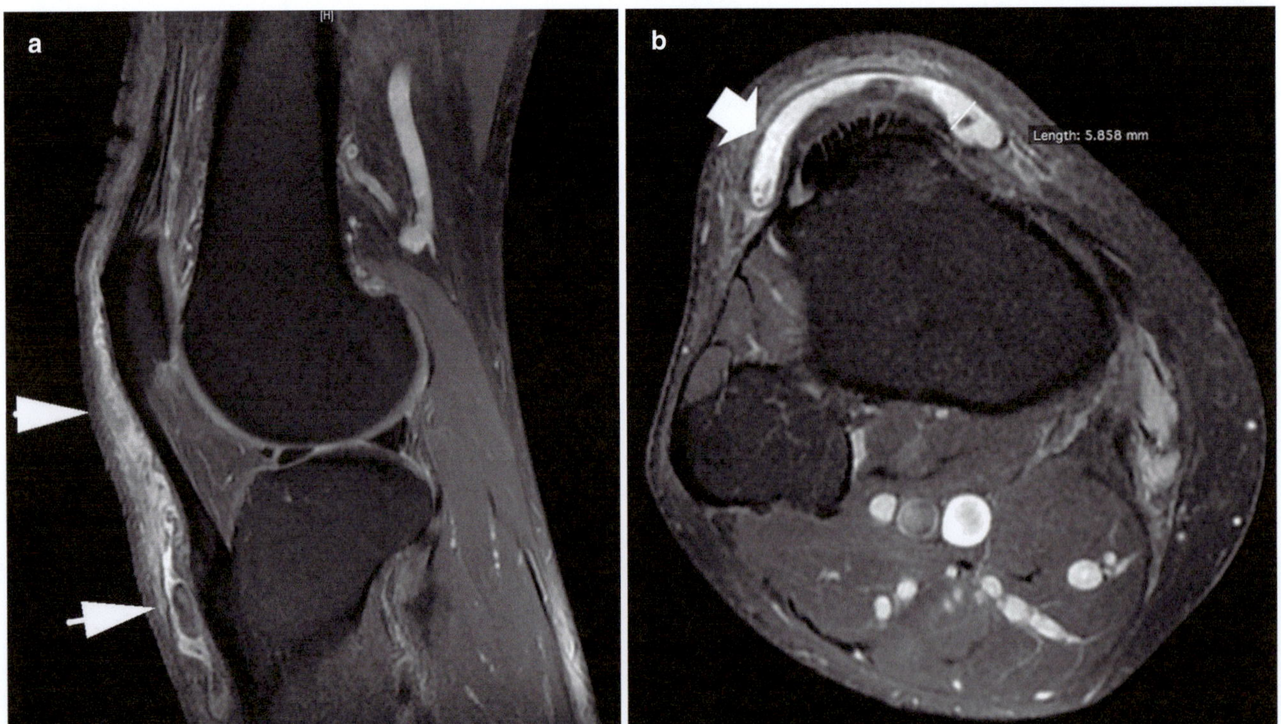

Fig. 9.1 Sagittal (**a**) and transverse (**b**) MRI views of the prepatellar bursa (arrows) of the illustrated case

9.1.4.4 Step-by-Step Description of the Technique

- 5 mm incisions are made at the portal sites.
- Intralesional approach is used for the endoscopic resection procedure. The arthroscope and arthroscopic shaver are inserted into the cavity of the lesion.
- The lesion is resected from inside out with the caution not to injure the underlying structure and the superficial nerve and vascular network (Fig. 9.3).
- The portals can be exchanged as the viewing and working portals by the switching rod technique in order to complete the resection.
- If the working space is collapsed after part of the lesion is resected and may not be distended well with gravity driven fluid inflow, an accessory portal can be used for insertion of small retractor to improve the endoscopic visualization.
- Complete resection of the lesion may not be necessary for subsequent seal off the cavity. The superficial part of the lesion may be preserved in order to avoid injury to the cutaneous nerve and dermal vascular network.
- A drain is inserted into the cavity via the distal medial portal.

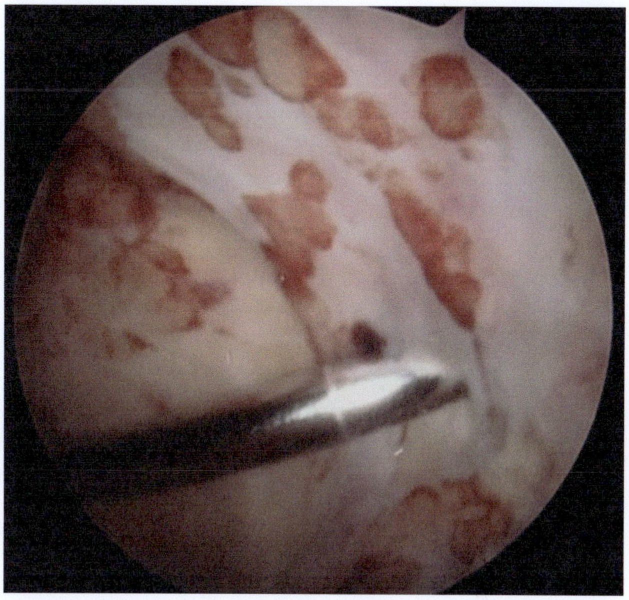

Fig. 9.3 Endoscopic view of the inflamed bursa

9.1.4.5 Complications and Management

- Recurrence of the lesions,
- Cutaneous nerve injury,
- Injury to the cutaneous vascular network leading to patchy skin necrosis,
- Injury to the underlying structures, e.g. quadriceps tendon, patella tendon.

9.1.4.6 Post-operative Care

Compression dressing is applied for 2 weeks to facilitate seal off of the cavity. The patient can start free mobilization of the knee after the compression dressing is taken off. Full weight bearing is allowed immediately after the operation.

9.1.5 Summary

Prepatellar bursa, infrapatellar bursa, and Morel-Lavallée lesion are superficial lesions that are easily approached. However, open resection is associated with poor healing of the surgical wound, decreased sensation over scar area, contracted scar tissue, atrophic skin changes, subcutaneous collection, and scar hypersensitivity. Endoscopic resection is a minimally invasive surgical approach that may reduce the risk of complications associated with open surgery.

9.2 Endoscopic Repair of Acute Rupture of Quadriceps Tendon

Peter Wai Pan Yau and Gabriel Ching Ngai Leung

9.2.1 Introduction

- The prevalence of acute rupture of quadriceps tendon is ranged from 1.3 to 2.8 per 100,000 population [37, 38]. This condition is more commonly seen in patients older than 40 years of age [39], and with propensity for the male sex with a ratio of 9 to 1 [38].
- Histological analysis showed that degenerative changes were present in 64% of the ruptured tendons [40].
- Acute quadriceps tendon rupture typically occurred in the distal 2 cm of the tendon and in the osteotendinous junction of the superior pole of patella [41]. Avulsion fracture of superior pole of patella could be found in a small percentage of cases [39].
- Delay in diagnosis was common. The average time lapse between injury and diagnosis was 7 days (range: 1–40 days) [41]. Late surgical intervention of complete rupture of quadriceps tendon was associated with poor outcome [42]. Persistent extension lag of 5-degree and quadriceps weakness were found in 15–30% of the patients [39, 43, 44].
- Ciriello et al. (2012) published a review article on 319 open surgical repairs of quadriceps tendon rupture [41]. The most common early post-operation complications were infection (superficial wound infection: 1.2%; deep infection: 1.1%) and thromboembolic disease (2.5%). Mid-term complications included re-rupture of repair (average 2%, ranged from 0% to 8.3%) and heterotopic ossification (6.9%).

9.2.2 Indications of Endoscopic Repair of Acute Rupture of Quadriceps Tendon

- Acute or subacute complete rupture of quadriceps tendon, including:
  - Full-thickness, full-width rupture of quadriceps tendon
  - Full-thickness, partial-width rupture in athletes practicing contact sports or high demand individuals [45]

9.2.3 Contra-indications of Endoscopic Repair of Acute Rupture of Quadriceps Tendon

- Chronic full-thickness, full-width tear of more than 4 weeks
- Tear at musculotendinous junction
- Re-rupture of previous quadriceps tendon repair

9.2.4 Author Preferred Technique

9.2.4.1 Pre-operative Planning

- The diagnosis should be confirmed with pre-operative imaging (e.g., MRI or ultrasound). These provide information on the site of tear (at the osteotendinous junction or in the mid-substance) and the extent of retraction of the proximal stump.
- Use of pneumatic tourniquet and arthroscopic fluid management system is advised.
- Leg-holder system for placing the operated knee in full extension, 45-degree flexion, and 90-degree flexion will facilitate the operation.
- Arthroscopes: 30-degree 4-mm diameter arthroscope.
- Instruments: Arthroscopic manual instruments (including probes, basket forceps, graspers, and curettes) and arthroscopic knot-tying instruments (including knot pusher and knot cutter).
- Arthroscopic shaver system and arthroscopic radiofrequency system are required during the operation.
- Arthroscopic video system: the use of two video screens is advised.

9.2.4.2 Patient Positioning

- Surgery can be performed under either general or regional anesthesia with patient lying in supine position.
- Pneumatic tourniquet is inflated after the involved lower limb is exsanguinated.

9.2.4.3 Portal Design

- A total of seven portals are used in the endoscopic assisted acute quadriceps tendon repair described below. They are the anterior-lateral portal, anterior-medial portal, superior-lateral portals (high and low), superior-medial portals (high and low), and superior midline portal (Fig. 9.4).

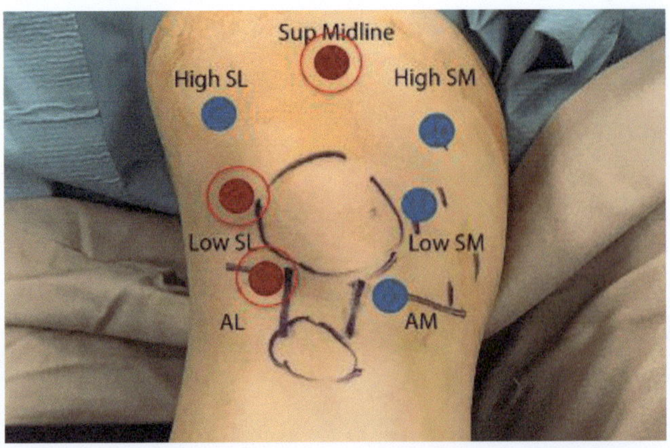

Fig. 9.4 Anterior view of knee, showing the seven portals used in endoscopic assisted quadriceps tendon repair

- The anterior-medial and anterior-lateral portals are the standard portals in conventional knee arthroscopy. They are used for diagnostic arthroscopy of the knee joint.
- The low superior-medial portal and low superior-lateral portal are established at the level of proximal patella, around 1 cm medial and 1 cm lateral to the medial and lateral border of the patella, respectively. They serve as the viewing and working portal within the suprapatellar pouch for surgery on the articular surface of quadriceps tendon.
- The high superior-medial portal and high superior-lateral portal are established at a level 2 cm proximal to the superior pole of patella, around 1 cm medial and 1 cm lateral to the medial and lateral border of the patella. They serve as the viewing and working portal within the prepatellar subfascial bursa [12] for surgery on the bursal surface of quadriceps tendon, repair of the ruptured para-patellar retinaculum, insertion of suture anchors on proximal pole of patella, and preparation of transosseous tunnel for fixation using pulled-out suture technique.
- The superior midline portal is located along the midline, at around 3–4 cm above the superior pole of patella. It is the main viewing portal during preparation of the footprint of quadriceps tendon at the superior pole of patella.

9.2.4.4 Step-by-Step Description of the Techniques

- Anterior-lateral and anterior-medial portals are established using standard arthroscopic technique. Diagnostic knee arthroscopy is performed. Concomitant intra-articular pathology (e.g., meniscus tear, cartilage lesion, etc.) is tackled.
- Knee is then put in full extension. Using the anterior-lateral portal as viewing portal and anterior-medial portal as working portal, the diagnosis of full-thickness quadriceps tendon rupture is confirmed. Debridement of the proximal stump of quadriceps tendon rupture till healthy tendon tissue is carried out (Fig. 9.5).
- Arthroscope was then introduced into the prepatellar subfascial bursa, which is a potential space between the superficial and intermediate layer of prepatellar fibrous tissue in the anterior knee region [12]. This space is easily accessible in full-thickness rupture of quadriceps tendon because the prepatellar subfascial bursa is distended and dissected by the bleeding at the time of injury. The bursal surface of the ruptured quadriceps tendon is dissected up to a level 3–4 cm proximal to the superior pole of patella. The exact level of dissection depends on the site of rupture (Fig. 9.6). The target is to view the whole width of the rectus femoris component of quadriceps tendon up to a level 2–3 cm proximal to the rupture site. After the dissection, the extent of quadriceps tendon tear (full-width versus partial-width) and the involvement of the medial and

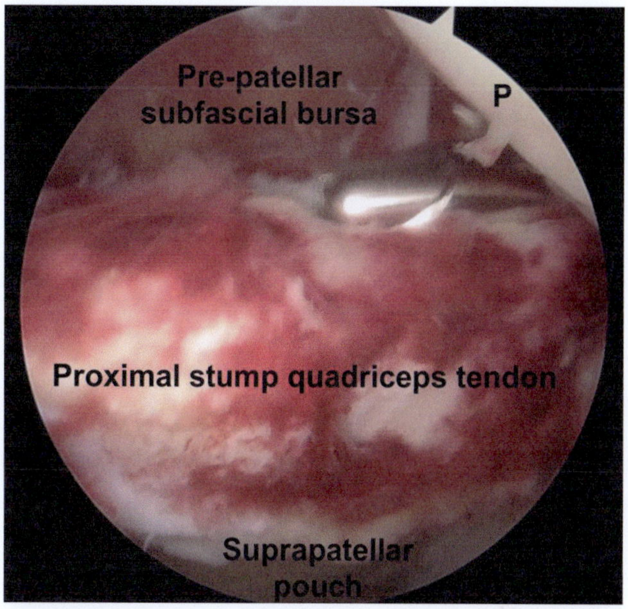

Fig. 9.5 Arthroscopic view of the rupture site of quadriceps tendon (P: Patella)

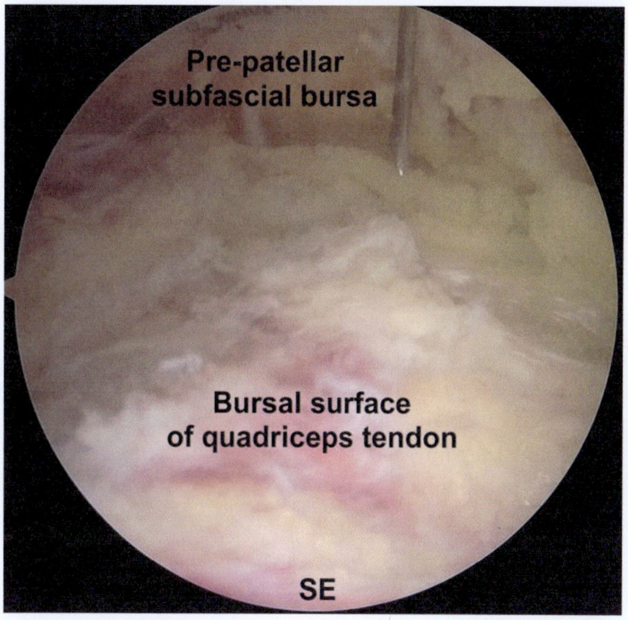

Fig. 9.6 Endoscopic view of bursal surface of quadriceps tendon within the prepatellar subfascial bursa (SE: ruptured end of proximal stump of quadriceps tendon)

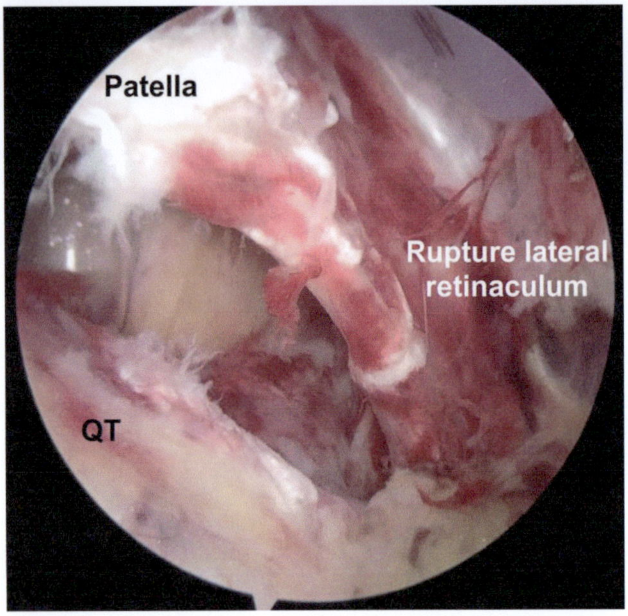

Fig. 9.7 Full-thickness, full-width tear of quadriceps tendon with concomitant full-thickness tear of lateral para-patellar retinaculum (QT: proximal stump of ruptured quadriceps tendon)

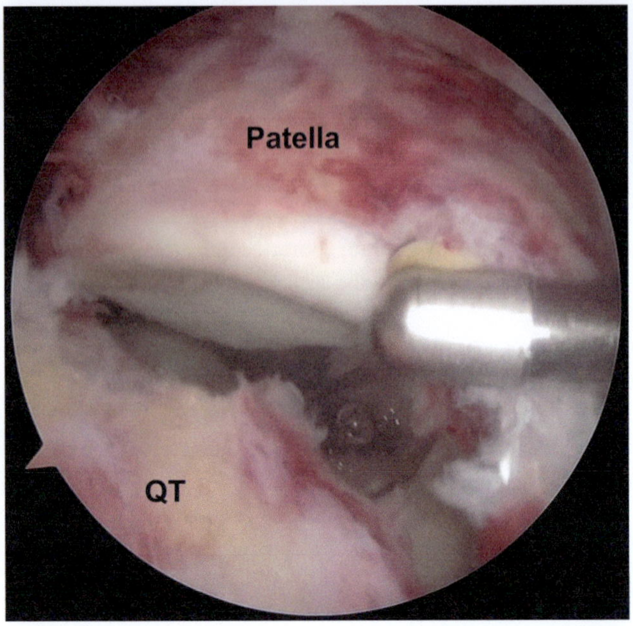

Fig. 9.8 Endoscopic view through the superior midline portal. The quadriceps tendon was found ruptured at the osteotendinous junction of the upper pole of patella (QT: proximal stump of ruptured quadriceps tendon)

lateral para-patellar retinaculum can be assessed accurately (Fig. 9.7).

- The remaining portals (low superior-medial, low superior-lateral, high superior-medial, high superior-lateral, and superior midline portals) are established.
- For majority of acute quadriceps tendon rupture (which occurs within 2 cm from its insertion in superior patella), all the above steps are performed via the anterior-lateral portal and anterior-medial portal.
- But for full-thickness mid-substance quadriceps tendon tear more than 2 cm above the insertion into superior pole of patella; and difficult cases (e.g., subacute tear with significant scarring), early establishment of the low superior-lateral and low superior-medial portals will facilitate the dissection of prepatellar subfascial bursa.
- In case of operating high grade acute partial thickness bursal side tear, one will need to establish an additional low-superior midline portal (which is located along the midline, immediately proximal to the superior pole of patella). This allows direct access into the pre-patella subfascial bursa. The two high superior portals (high superior-medial and high superior-lateral portal) and superior midline portals need to be established at this stage to allow proper dissection of the prepatellar subfascial bursa.
- Arthroscope is then introduced through the superior midline portal and the rupture of the quadriceps tendon at the patellar side is assessed (Fig. 9.8).
- During preparation of the footprint of quadriceps tendon at the superior pole of patella, it will be more convenient for the surgeon to stand in the cranial side of the operated knee. The second video screen should be placed at the end of the operation table to facilitate viewing by the surgeon.

Rupture at the Osteotendinous Junction

- For rupture at the osteotendinous junction or those within 1 cm from the insertion of quadriceps tendon, surgery is best performed by debriding the remaining distal stump and then repairing the proximal stump back to the footprint at the superior pole of patella.
- The footprint of quadriceps tendon insertion is prepared. The superior pole of the patella should be lightly decorticated to expose healthy cancellous bone. However, complete removal of the cortex should be avoided because this will compromise the pull-out strength of suture anchor. The aim is to remove all fibrous tissue on the superior pole of patella and allow the repaired tendon to heal to the bone directly.
- The repair of the tendon can be performed by two methods: (1) suture anchor technique; (2) pulled-out-suture technique.

Repair using suture anchor as distal fixation

- For repair using suture anchor as distal fixation, two to three double-loaded suture anchors should be used. The diameter of the anchors should be around 2–3 mm. Metal anchor is easy to be applied. But anchors made from other materials (e.g., all-suture anchor, bioabsorbable anchor, PEEK anchor) can be used. The author prefers to use 2.8-mm diameter all-suture double-loaded suture anchors.
- The viewing portal is the superior midline portal. The working portal is either the high superior-medial or high superior-lateral portal. The anchors should be inserted at the 11 o'clock and 1 o'clock position of the patella (Figs. 9.9 and 9.10). An optional third suture anchor can be inserted at the 12 o'clock position. During insertion of the suture anchor, the knee should be flexed to around 45-degree flexion. This allows the patella to be engaged in the trochlea and facilitate the drilling of pilot hole and the insertion of the anchors.
- After insertion of suture anchors, the viewing portal is changed to anterior-lateral portal and the knee is put in slight flexion (10–20 degree) for passing of sutures into the proximal stump.

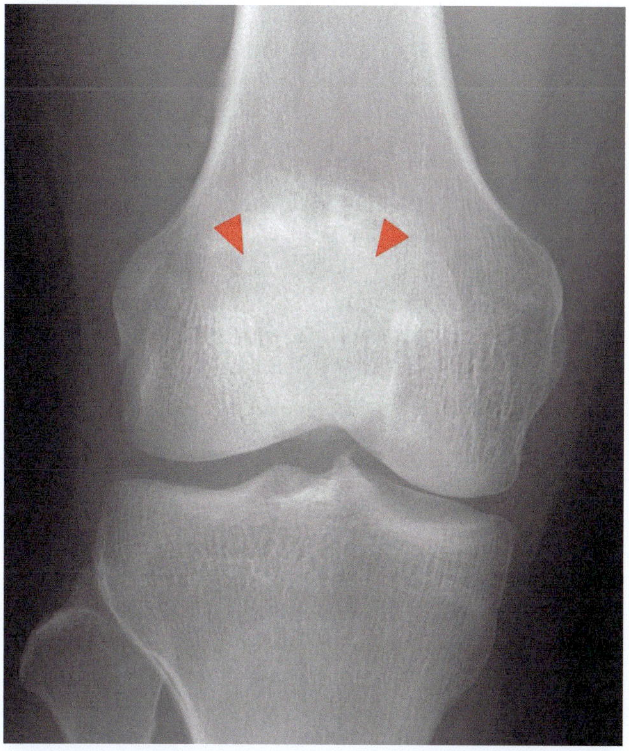

Fig. 9.9 Anterior-posterior view of X-ray of right knee, showing the position of suture anchor at 11 and 1 o'clock position at superior pole of patella

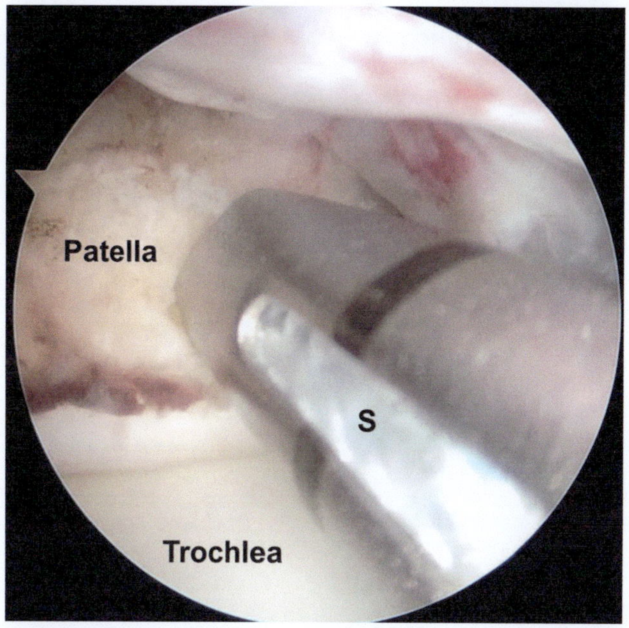

Fig. 9.10 Suture anchor insertion at the superior pole of patella (S: Suture anchor)

- If the quality of the tendon tissue in the proximal stump is satisfactory, the proximal stump can be secured with four horizontal mattress knots with sutures from the two suture anchors (Figs. 9.11 and 9.12). The four mattress knots should be placed at a distance at least 1 cm from the rupture site.

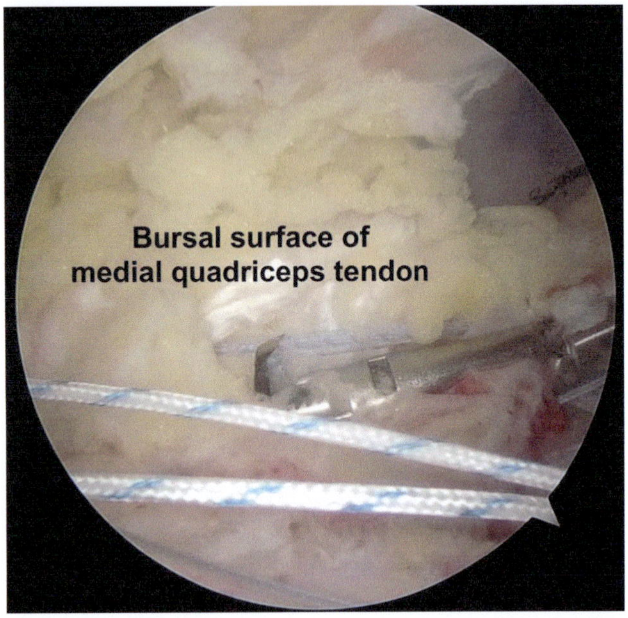

Fig. 9.11 Passing mattress stitches on the medial side of the proximal stump of quadriceps tendon rupture

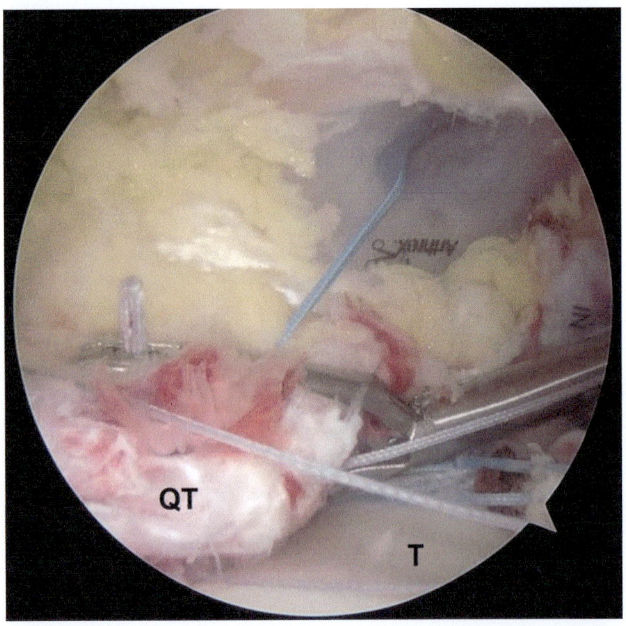

Fig. 9.12 Passing mattress stitches on the lateral side of the proximal stump of quadriceps tendon rupture (QT: Quadriceps tendon; T: Trochlea)

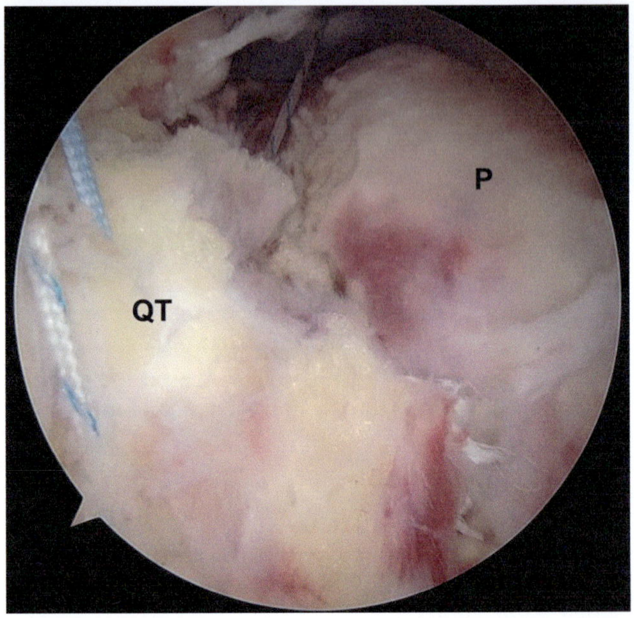

Fig. 9.13 Monitoring of the approximation of tissue at the repair site from the bursal side (QT: Quadriceps tendon; P: Patella)

- If the quality of the tendon in the proximal stump is suboptimal, instead of mattress knots, two grasping stitches (e.g., modified Mason Allen stitch, Bunnell stitch, etc.) should be used. One should be put on the medial side and the other one on the lateral side of the tendon. Use of high-tensile strength tape is recommended to further increase the grasping power of the sutures in the proximal stump.
- During fixation of the repair, the knee should be put in full extension to reduce tension at the repair site. The viewing portal is changed to the superior-lateral portal and the arthroscope is put in the prepatellar subfascial bursa to monitor the approximation of the repair site endoscopically. The target is to ensure good approximation of tissue at the tendon–bone junction (Fig. 9.13).
- After confirming good approximation of the tendon–bone junction on the bursal side, the arthroscope is then introduced into the knee joint through the anterior-lateral portal. The quality of the repair in the articular side is assessed (Fig. 9.14).
- After confirming good approximation of tendon–bone junction in both the bursal and the articular side, the fixation is secured by tying of the knots using standard arthroscopic knot-tying technique.

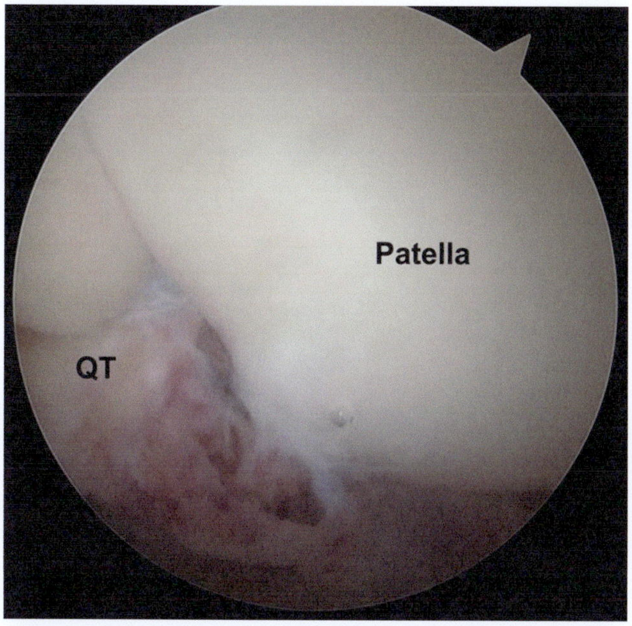

Fig. 9.14 Viewing of the approximation of tissue at the repair site from the articular side (QT: Quadriceps tendon)

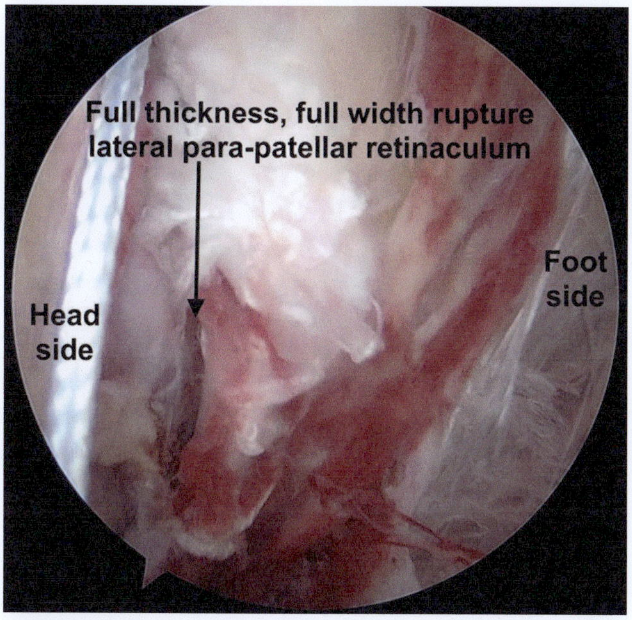

Fig. 9.15 Full-thickness tear of lateral para-patellar retinaculum (view from bursal surface within the prepatellar subfascial bursa)

- If there is concomitant full-thickness para-patellar retinaculum tear (Fig. 9.15), repair of the torn para-patellar retinaculum is done at this stage.
- Over 70% of full-thickness, full-width tear of quadriceps tendon within 2 cm from its insertion in superior pole of patella is associated with full-thickness tear of para-patellar retinaculum.
- Knee is kept in full extension. The arthroscope is put into the prepatellar subfascial bursa again through one of the superior portals. Repair of the para-patellar retinaculum is done using standard side-to-side arthroscopic repair technique with No. 2 high-tensile strength non-absorbable multi-filament suture (Fig. 9.16). If the tissue of para-patellar retinaculum is suboptimal, horizontal mattress stitch should be used (Fig. 9.17).

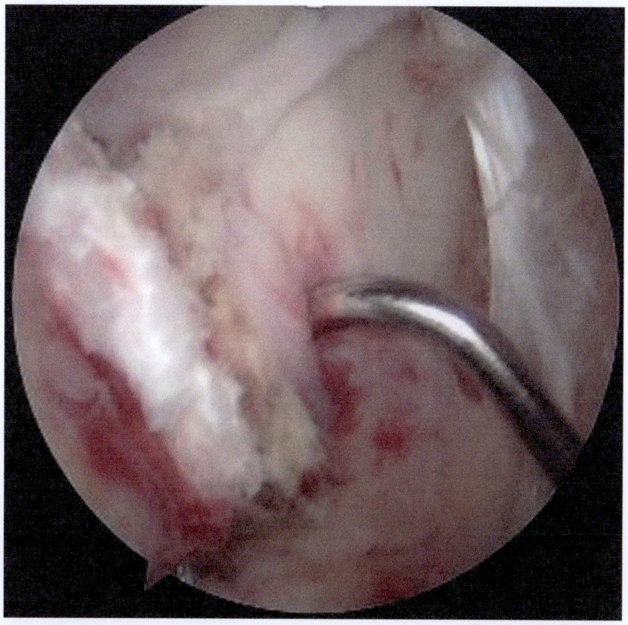

Fig. 9.16 Side-to-side repair of full-thickness tear of lateral para-patellar retinaculum using suture hook

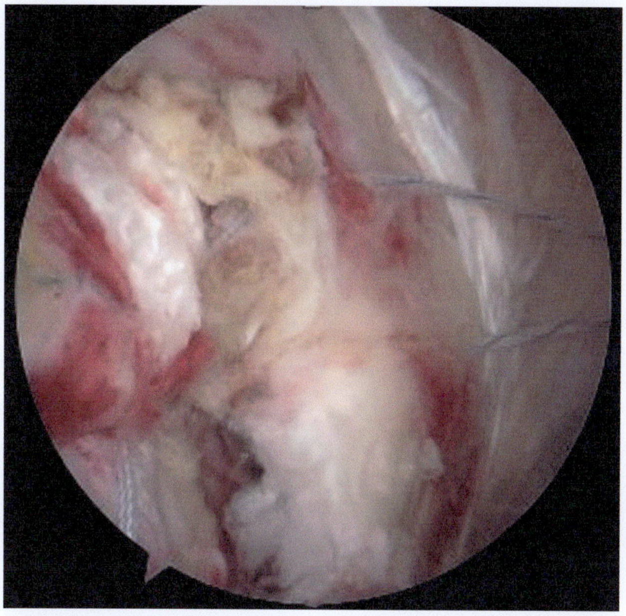

Fig. 9.17 Tying of horizontal mattress stitch for repair of lateral para-patellar retinaculum tear

- After the repair is complete, the integrity of the repair is checked (Figs. 9.18, 9.19, and 9.20).
- Portal wounds are closed in standard manner. Drain is not required as post-operation bleeding is typically minimal.
- The knee is then immobilized in full extension with a long leg back-slab.

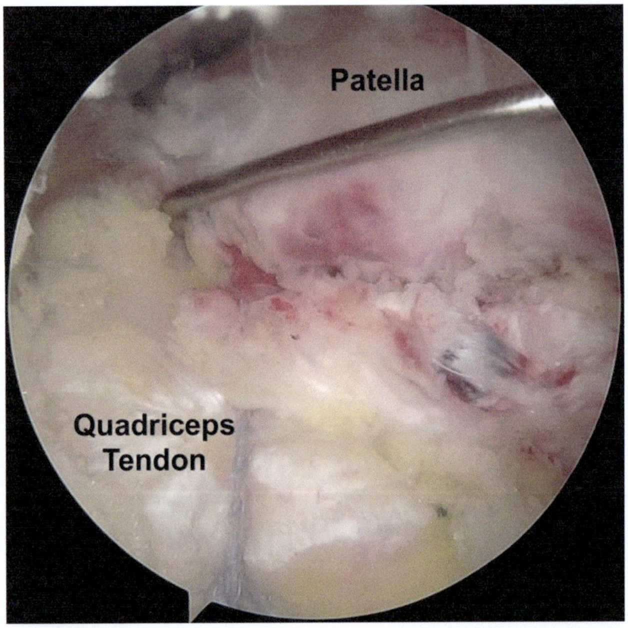

Fig. 9.18 Checking of medial part of repair of quadriceps tendon rupture (view of bursal surface within prepatellar subfascial bursa)

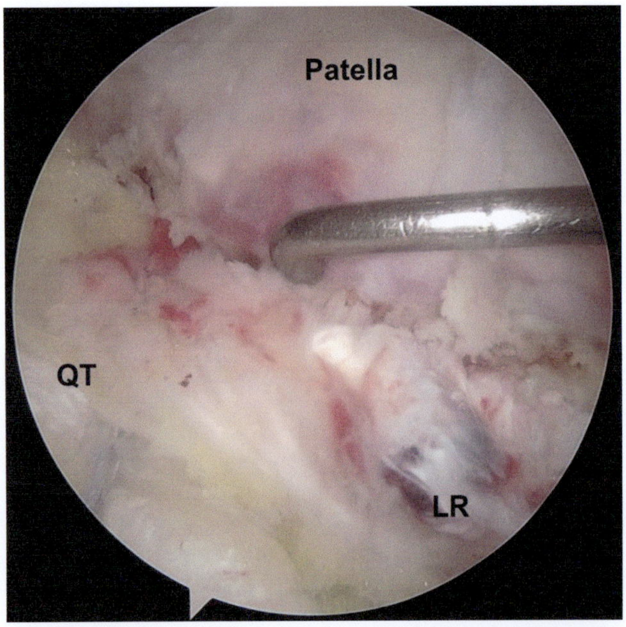

Fig. 9.19 Checking of lateral part of repair of quadriceps tendon rupture (view of bursal surface within prepatellar subfascial bursa) (QT: Quadriceps tendon; LR: Lateral para-patellar retinaculum)

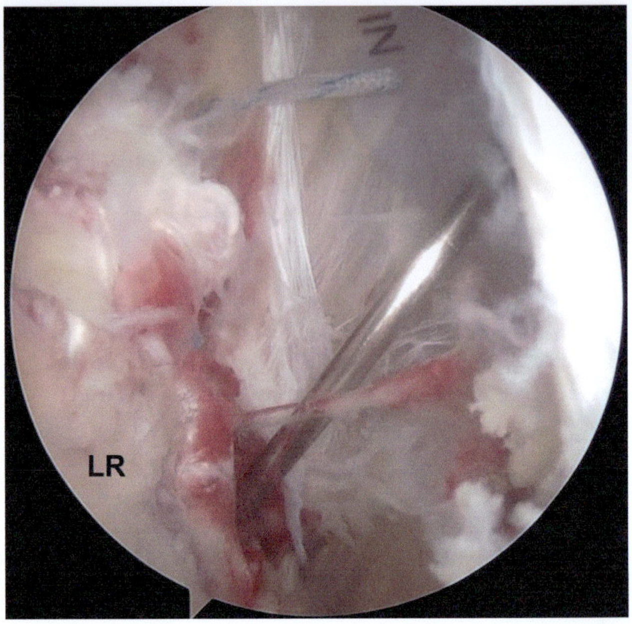

Fig. 9.20 Checking of lateral para-patellar retinaculum repair (view of bursal surface within prepatellar subfascial bursa) (LR: Lateral para-patellar retinaculum)

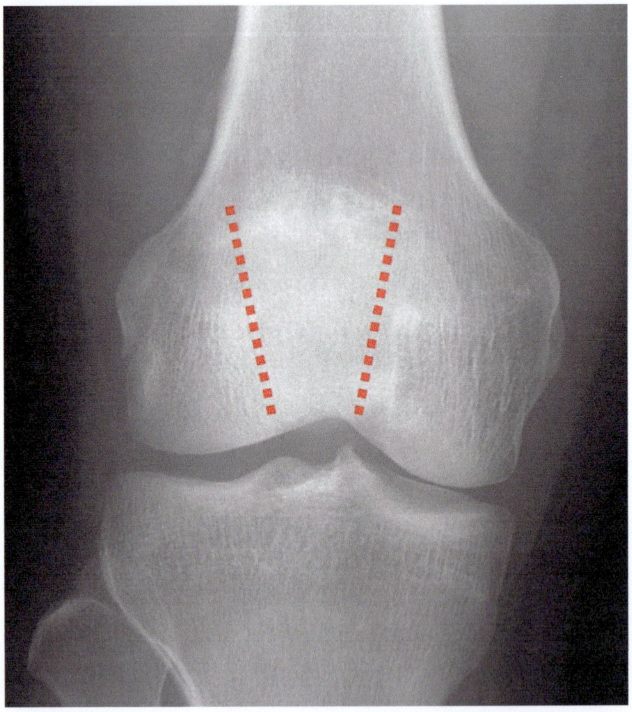

Fig. 9.21 Position of transosseous tunnels for pulled-out-suture

Repair using pulled-out-suture technique as distal fixation

- For repair using pulled-out-suture technique as distal fixation, two longitudinal transosseous tunnels are drilled in the patella with a 2.3-mm diameter guide pin. The entry sites of the guide pin are 11 o'clock and 1 o'clock position of the footprint at superior patella (Figs. 9.21 and 9.22).

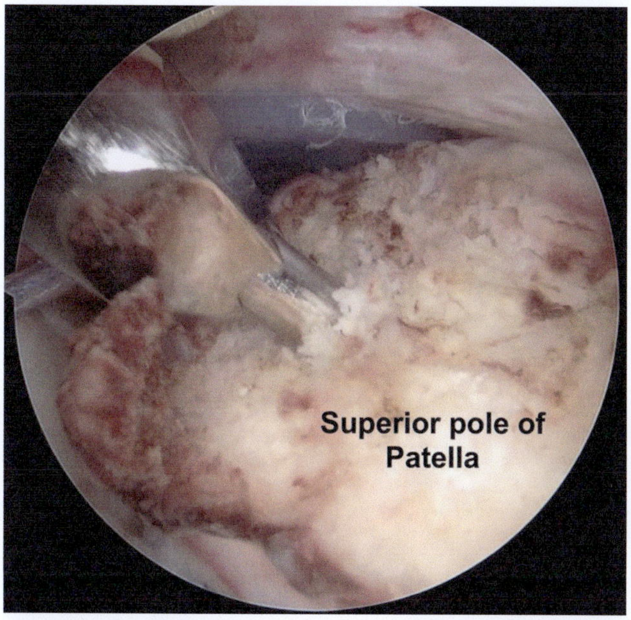

Fig. 9.22 Drilling of transosseous tunnel using 2.3-mm diameter guide pin

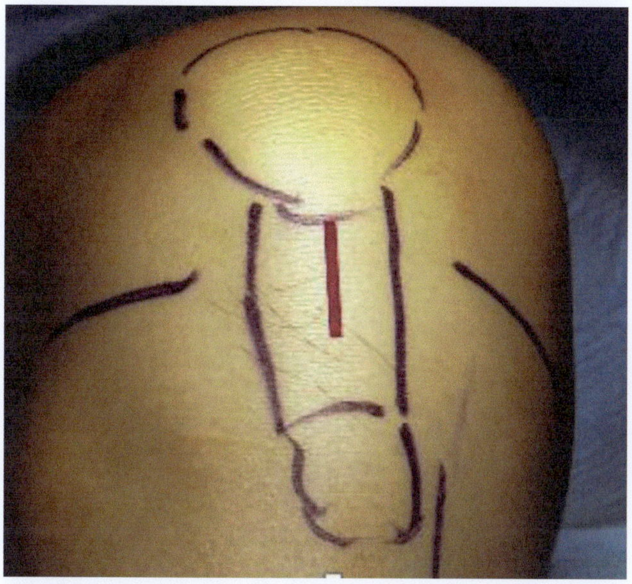

Fig. 9.23 A longitudinal stab wound is made in the skin at the region of patella tendon to facilitate retrieval of the transosseous suture

The exit site is the extra-articular surface at the lower pole of patella. The viewing portal is the superior midline portal. The working portal is either the high superior-medial or high superior-lateral portal. The knee should be flexed to around 45-degree flexion before preparation of the transosseous tunnels. A longitudinal stab wound is made in the skin at the region of patella tendon to facilitate retrieval of the transosseous suture (Fig. 9.23).

- The passage of the transosseous suture can be facilitated using long cannulated arthroscopic needle.
- The guide pin used in preparing the transosseous tunnel is first removed. The cannulated needle is passed into the drill hole in the proximal patella (Fig. 9.24) and the distal end is retrieved from the distal longitudinal wound through a split in the patella tendon (Fig. 9.23).
- A PDS 0 suture is first passed into the cannulated needle and is retrieved from the distal stab wound in the region of patellar tendon.
- After passing the PDS suture, the arthroscopic needle is removed (Fig. 9.25).

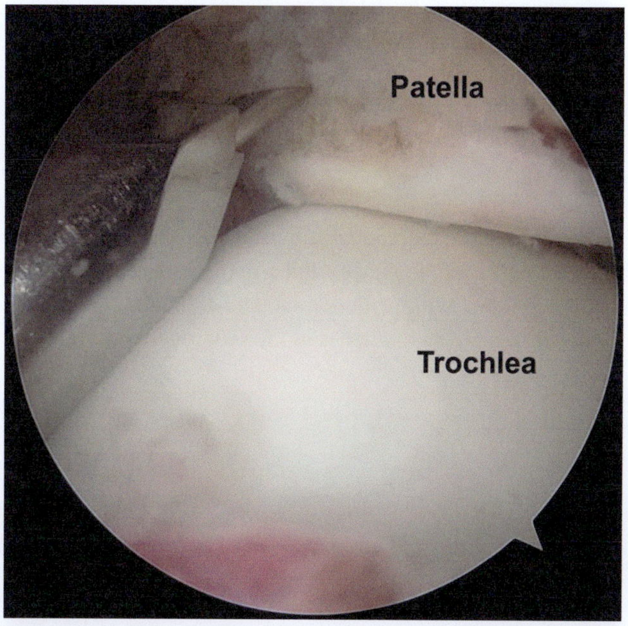

Fig. 9.24 The 2.3-mm diameter guide pin was removed and replaced by a long cannulated arthroscopic needle

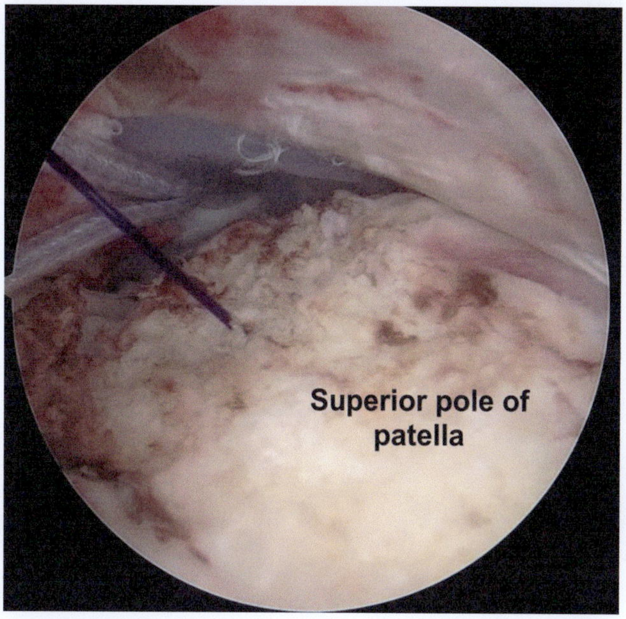

Fig. 9.25 One PDS 0 suture was passed into the cannulated needle and was retrieved from the distal wound. The arthroscopic needle was then removed, leaving the PDS 0 suture passing through the transosseous tunnel

- The PDS suture is used to relay the passage of two No. 2 high-tensile strength non-absorbable multi-filament suture (Fig. 9.26) through the transosseous tunnel. The distal stumps of the transosseous suture are retrieved from the distal wound.
- Afterwards, the surgeon should start to prepare the proximal stump for insertion of two grasping stitches. The knee is put in 10–20-degree of knee flexion. The anterior-lateral portal is used as the viewing portal. The superior-medial and superior-lateral portals are used as the working portals.
- Two grasping stitches are placed in the medial and lateral aspect of the proximal stump of quadriceps tendon using either modified Mason Allen stitch or Bunnell stitch.
- It is important that to ensure good endoscopic view of the bursal surface of the proximal stump of quadriceps tendon within the prepatellar subfascial bursa (Fig. 9.27) and good arthroscopic view of the articular surface of quadriceps tendon within the suprapatellar pouch (Fig. 9.28) during insertion of stitches in the proximal tendon stump.

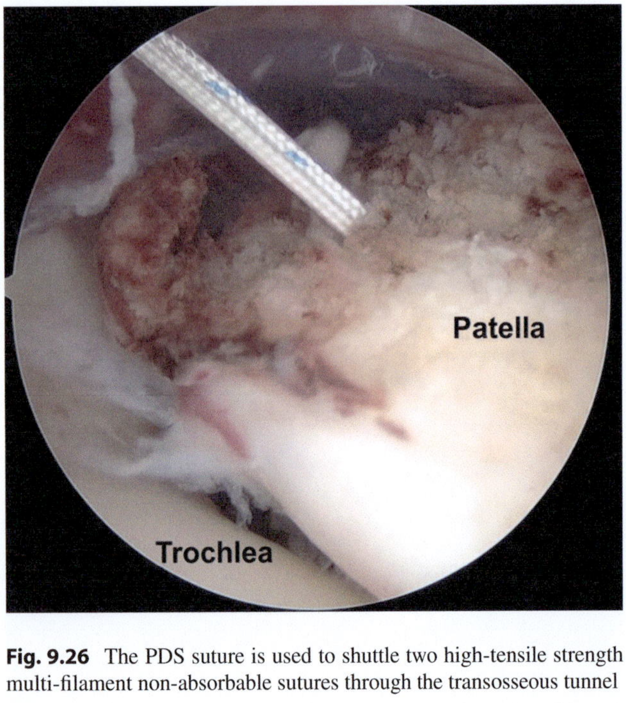

Fig. 9.26 The PDS suture is used to shuttle two high-tensile strength multi-filament non-absorbable sutures through the transosseous tunnel

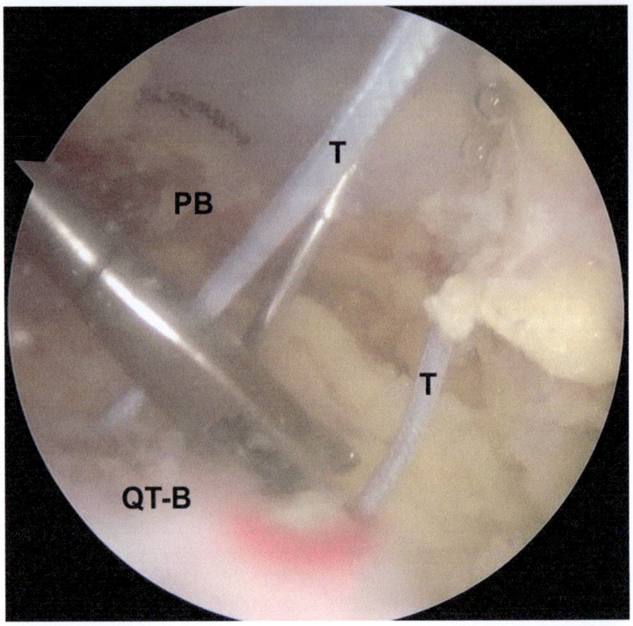

Fig. 9.27 Endoscopic view of bursal surface of proximal stump of quadriceps tendon rupture (QT-B: Bursal surface of quadriceps tendon; T: High-tensile strength multi-filament tape; PB: Prepatellar subfascial bursa)

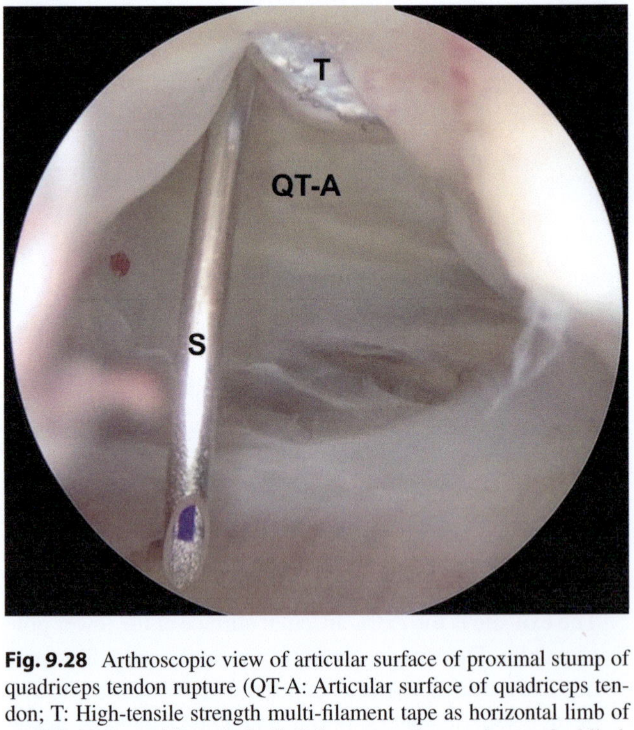

Fig. 9.28 Arthroscopic view of articular surface of proximal stump of quadriceps tendon rupture (QT-A: Articular surface of quadriceps tendon; T: High-tensile strength multi-filament tape as horizontal limb of modified Mason Allen stitch; S: Relay suture for passing vertical limb of modified Mason Allen stitch)

- Two grasping stitches are placed in the medial and lateral aspect of proximal stump of quadriceps tendon rupture (Figs. 9.29 and 9.30). The use of high-tensile strength multi-filament non-absorbable tape increases the mechanical strength of these grasping stitches and reduces the chance of failure of the repair.
- The free ends of the two grasping stitches are then shuttled through the two transosseous tunnel in the patella (Fig. 9.31) and retrieved from the distal stab wound in front of the patella tendon.
- During fixation of the repair, the knee is kept in full extension (Fig. 9.32). The transosseous pulled-out suture is tied at the distal end of patella, anterior to the patellar tendon.

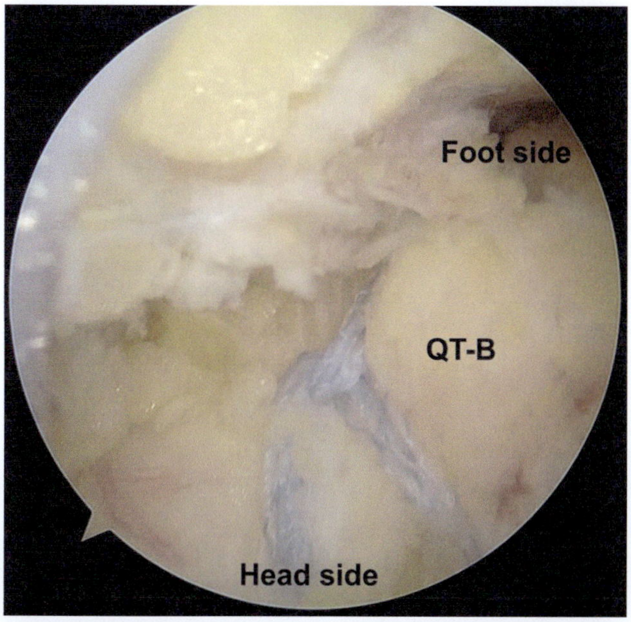

Fig. 9.29 Bursal view of a modified Mason Allen stitch put in the medial side proximal stump of quadriceps tendon with tape (QT-B: Bursal side of quadriceps tendon)

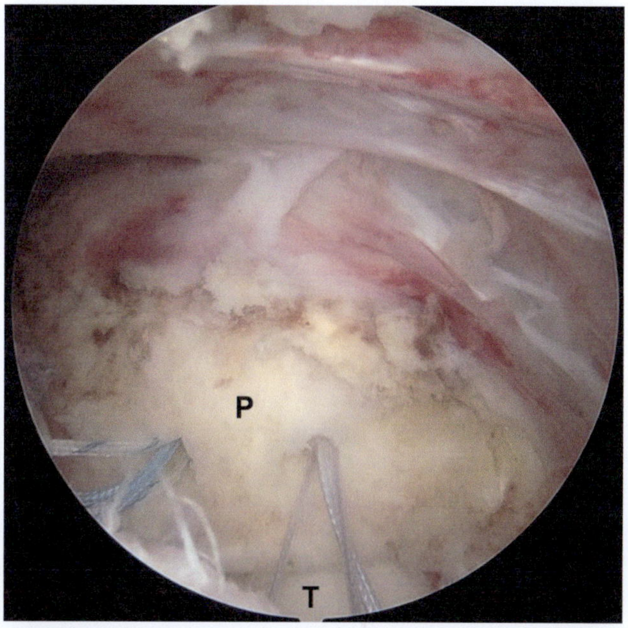

Fig. 9.31 No. 2 high-tensile strength multi-filament non-absorbable suture helps to shuttle the free end of the grasping stitches through the transosseous tunnel (P: Patella; T: Trochlea)

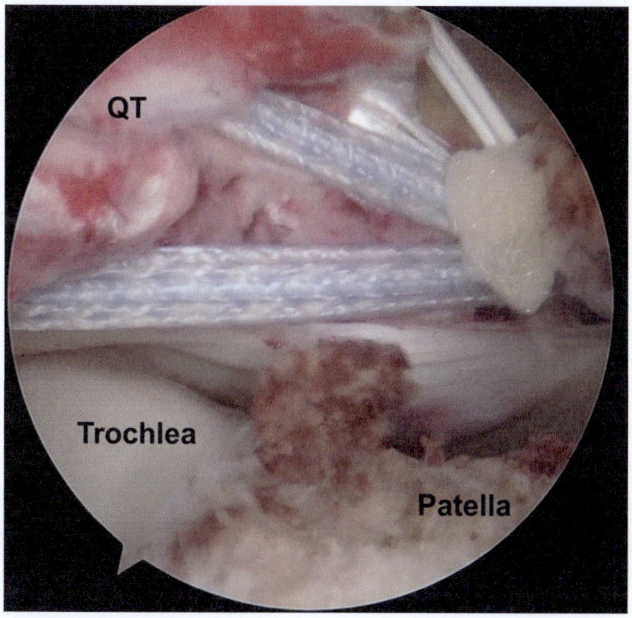

Fig. 9.30 Arthroscopic view of modified Mason Allen stitch with tape at the osteotendinous junction (QT: Rupture end of proximal stump of quadriceps tendon)

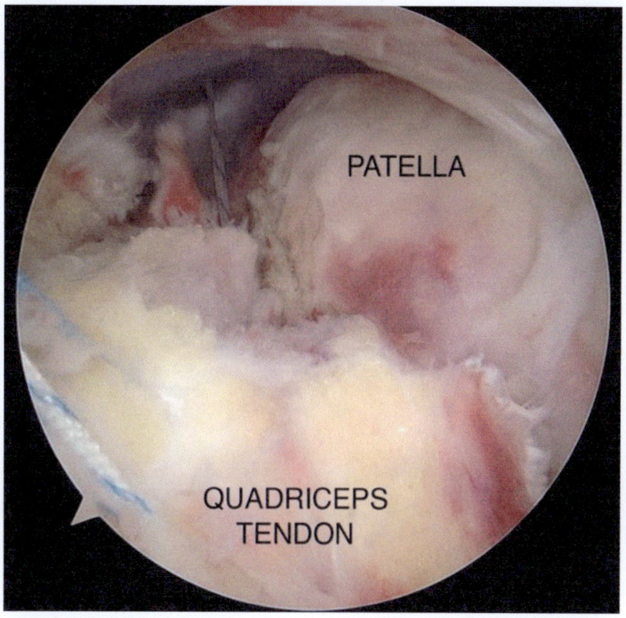

Fig. 9.32 Just before tying of transosseous pulled-out-suture

- The repair of the para-patellar retinaculum is then carried out and the quality of the repair is then checked as described above.

Rupture at the mid-substance

- For rupture at the mid-substance of quadriceps tendon with a distal stump of adequate length, the repair can be done as an end-to-end repair between the two stumps of the quadriceps tendon. The pre-requisite is that the remaining stumps should be healthy enough to allow insertion of grasping stitch to facilitate a strong repair.
- The steps in the placement of the two grasping stitches in the proximal stump are the same as the one described in the section of the pulled-out-suture technique.
- During placement of the grasping stitches in the distal stump, the viewing portal is switched to the superior midline portal. Two grasping stitches are placed in the distal stump of rupture quadriceps tendon.
- The repair is secured by tying the grasping stitches on the proximal stump and that of the distal stump together with knee in full extension. Any full-thickness tear of para-patellar retinaculum is then repaired.

9.2.4.5 Complications and Management

- The author performed a total of seven endoscopic assisted repair of acute quadriceps tendon rupture. There was no early complication (including infection, wound problem, hematoma, neurovascular complication, deep vein thrombosis, and fracture).
- There was one case of re-rupture of quadriceps tendon repair at 3 months after the index operation. The case belonged to a 55-year-old gentleman suffering from simultaneous bilateral quadriceps tendon rupture at the osteotendinous junction. The time lag between injury and surgery was 16-days. One-stage bilateral endoscopic assisted quadriceps tendon repair was performed. The right side healed uneventfully, but the left side re-ruptured at 3-month after the index operation. Revision open repair without augmentation was performed. The proximal stump was repaired to the superior pole of patella using combination of pulled-out suture technique and suture anchor as distal fixation. The revised repair healed uneventfully.

9.2.4.6 Post-operative Care

- Patient's knee is immobilized in long leg cast kept in full extension for 6 weeks. Full weight bearing walking is practiced.
- The cast is taken off from post-operation 7 weeks onwards. This is followed by active and passive mobilization of the operated knee and quadriceps muscle strengthening exercise.
- Squatting is not allowed within the first 3 months.
- Return to pre-injury sport is not advised within the first 6 months.

9.2.5 Summary

- Endoscopic assisted repair of acute quadriceps tendon is a simple operation with good clinical outcomes. Early post-operation complications are rare. Range of motion is usually well preserved.
- A small percentage of patients still suffer from subjective quadriceps weakness and re-rupture of the repair site.
- This operation is indicated in closed, full-thickness rupture of quadriceps tendon at the osteotendinous junction or mid-substance level.

9.3 Tendoscopy of Patellar Tendon and Endoscopy of the Hoffa Fat Pad

Tsz Lung Choi and Tun Hing Lui

9.3.1 Introduction

There are three fat pads found in anterior knee joint compartment, the infrapatellar (Hoffa), quadriceps, and pre-femoral fat pads. The Hoffa fat pad is an intracapsular but extra synovial structure, covered by synovial membrane posteriorly [46]. Gallagher et al. revealed that Hoffa fat pad comprised a central body with medial and lateral extension [46]. Hoffa fat pad is inferior to the inferior pole of patella, posterior to patellar retinacula and patellar tendon (from which the deep infrapatellar bursa separated Hoffa fat pad). The posteroinferior part of the Hoffa fat pad is related to the anterior tibia and anterior horns of the menisci, while the posterior part of the Hoffa fat pad is related to the femoral condyles and intercondylar notch. The Hoffa fat pad is attached to the intercondylar notch by the ligamentum mucosum. The nerve supply of the Hoffa fat pad is mainly from the posterior tibial nerve [47]. The infrapatellar fat pad would be metabolized only in severe malnutrition, implying that it has an essential role in joint function [46, 48].

The Hoffa fad pad acts as a space filler. It may enhance the gliding between the joint capsules and femoral condyles [49]. Inflammation of the Hoffa fat pad can cause bulging on either side of the patella tendon with the synovial membrane compressed against the femoral condyles. It may give rise to pain and effusion [50]. For example, reduced joint space in osteoarthritis may also compress on Hoffa fat pad and result in similar symptoms [51]. Another example is Hoffa's disease, with inflammation and subsequent hypertrophy, compression and trapping of the fat pad. It is characterized by anterior knee pain, functional impairment, and often a bulky effusion. Magnetic resonance imaging would show fibrotic trabeculae and liquid infiltration of fat pads and synovial recesses [52], with an ossifying chondroma being implicated as end-stage Hoffa's disease [53]. Ganglion or meniscal cysts may also increase pressure over Hoffa fat pad and cause symptoms like pain and effusion [46]. Other causes of abnormalities with the Hoffa fat pad include trauma (e.g., post-traumatic or post-surgery fibrosis), synovial diseases (e.g., pigmented villonodular synovitis) and rarely, neoplasm [54].

Injection of hydrocortisone and local anesthetic to the Hoffa fat pad can reduce pain and improve range of motion for the duration of the action of the local anesthetic. Complete or partial resection of Hoffa fat pad can improve symptoms and knee function [55, 56]. It can be done in open surgery or in endoscopy approach. However, Resection of the Hoffa fat pad has been associated with a decrease in patellar blood supply [57].

The patellar tendon extends distally from the infrapatellar pole to the tibial tuberosity. Embryologically there is a single tendon attaching the quadriceps to the tibia in which a mesenchymal condensation develops and becomes the patella, a sesamoid bone. The formation of the patella separates the tendon into two regions, the quadriceps and patellar tendons [58]. The patellar tendon is 25–40 mm wide, 4–6 cm long, and 5–7 mm thick [59, 60]. At the site of bone–tendon junctions of patellar tendons, there is a fibrocartilaginous enthesis with four tissue zones—dense fibrous connective tissue, uncalcified fibrocartilage, calcified cartilage, and bone [61]. The posterior aspect of the patella consisted of an articular zone and a non-articular zone, devoid of patellar tendon attachment and covered by a fold of synovial tissue. The patellar tendon is thin and broad proximally, becoming thick and narrow distally, since the fiber bundles converge as they run towards the tibial tuberosity. In the frontal plane the angle that the bundles formed with the midline axis of patellar tendon is estimated to be 2 degrees in the anterior layers and about 4 degrees in the posterior layers. The patellar tendon becomes narrow toward its tibial attachment. This reflects the shape of the bony attachments of patellar tendon. There is a transition from the flat frontal plane characteristic of the patellar attachment to a medio-laterally convex attachment on the tibial tuberosity [59].

Patellar tendon pathology typically occurs at the enthesis site; in most cases it occurs at the inferior pole of the patella, but it can occur at the tibial tuberosity [62, 63]. Patellar tendinopathy is an overuse injury with the onset typically characterized by no single specific traumatic injury event but gradually increasing tendon pain [58]. There are intrinsic factors and extrinsic risk factors for patella tendinopathy. Intrinsic factors include sex, race, bone structure, bone density, muscle length, muscle strength, joint range of motion, and body composition [58]. Extrinsic factors include training volume, types of conditioning activities, types of sports, surface of training, and environmental conditions [58].

The mainstay of treatment for patella tendinopathy is reduced level of activity or training volume for tendon healing while maintain basic level of exercise to maintain tendon length and strength [58]. Eccentric quadriceps exercise had been discussed in literatures [64–67]. Oral nonsteroidal anti-inflammatory drugs (NSAIDs) and injections of corticosteroids can also reduce inflammation and pain in patellar tendinopathy. Almekinders et al. reported oral NSAIDs may result in some pain relief but the effect on patellar tendon is not known [68]. Fredberg et al. reported injection of corticosteroid in patellar tendon can result in significant reduction in pain and tendon thickness [69].

Operative treatments only reserved for those who do not response to maximal conservative treatments. Principle of operative treatment is excision of diseased tendon tissue, stimulation of active healing response by scarification or drilling on the non-articulating part of distal patellar, and reattachment of tendon to maintain tendon integrity when necessary [70]. It can be achieved by open method or minimal invasive approach such as tendoscopy.

9.3.2 Indications

1. Intrinsic pathology of the Hoffa pad, e.g. intracapsular chondroma, localized nodular synovitis, post-surgery or post-traumatic fibrosis, that is not responsive to conservative treatment [54].
2. Extrinsic pathology of the Hoffa pad, e.g. pigmented villonodular synovitis (PVNS), meniscal cyst [54].
3. Painful bony fragment at the tibial tuberosity as a result of Osgood-Schlatter disease or tophaceous tuberosity [71].
4. Gouty tophus around the patellar tendon [72].
5. Chronic patellar tendinitis and tendinosis [73].
6. Resistant bursitis around the patellar tendon [73].
7. Jumper's knee [73].
8. Synovial lipoma of the patellar tendon [73].

9.3.3 Contra-indications

1. Extensive involvement of the patellar tendon by paratendinous pathology
2. Active infection at the planned portal sites
3. Malignant lesions
4. Vascular lesions

9.3.4 Author Preferred Technique

9.3.4.1 Pre-operative Planning

Magnetic resonance impinging is important to determine location of the pathology and its extent especially the degree of involvement of the patellar tendon.

9.3.4.2 Patient Positioning

The patient is in supine position with a thigh tourniquet to provide a bloodless operative field. The knee can be supported with a triangular frame to keep the knee and hip flexed. The knee can be extended to facilitate approach to the tibial and patellar insertion of the patellar tendon.

9.3.4.3 Portal Design

Portals can be made at any point along the medial and lateral edges of the patellar tendon. The exact locations of the portals depend on the location of pathology. During tendoscopy, different working zones related to the patellar tendon can be accessed:

- Anterior surface of patellar tendon
- Medial and lateral edge of the patellar tendon
- Posterior surface of the patellar tendon
- Hoffa fat pad
- Knee joint

In general, the classic anteromedial and anterolateral portals of knee arthroscopy can be used to approach all working zones related to the patellar tendon. Placement of portals not at the level of the knee joint will affect access to the knee joint proper.

In case of gouty tophus around the patellar tendon, the portals should be placed away from the skin invaded by the tophus in order to prevent unhealed surgical wound with persistent tophaceous discharge.

If the pathology is located at the tibial insertion of the tendon, portal just proximal to the insertion is useful as working portal.

9.3.4.4 Step-by-Step Description of the Technique

- The patella, patellar tendon, and the lesion are outlined with skin marker. Five millimeters incisions are made at the portal site.
- The subcutaneous tissue is bluntly dissected down to the lesion or the respective working zone locating the lesion.
- Whenever possible, extralesional approach is preferred rather than intralesional approach when starting the

endoscopy. A plane superficial to the lesion and the tendon and deep the superficial fascia is developed by a hemostat. This serves as the initial endoscopic working space and allows identification of the lesion and its relationship with the surrounding structure before starting the resection (Fig. 9.33).

- The patellar tendon is the important and consistent endoscopic landmark during patellar tendoscopy.
- The portals are interchangeable as the viewing and working portals.
- The synovial membrane between the Hoffa fat pad and the knee joint proper should be preserved if the knee joint is not involved by the lesion.
- Intra-operative fluoroscopy can be used to identify the osseous lesion, e.g. bony fragment at the tibial tuberosity.
- For lesions surrounding the patellar tendon, circumferential debridement can be performed via the portals (Fig. 9.34).

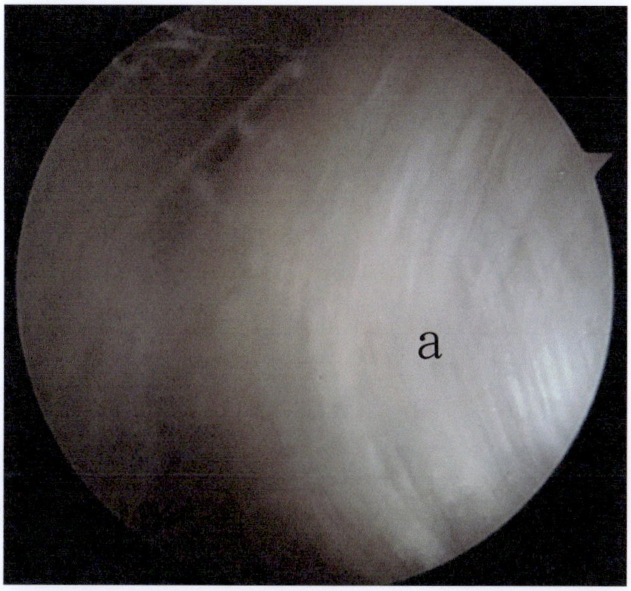

Fig. 9.33 Patellar tendoscopy is performed with the initial working plane superficial to the patellar tendon and its lesion (a)

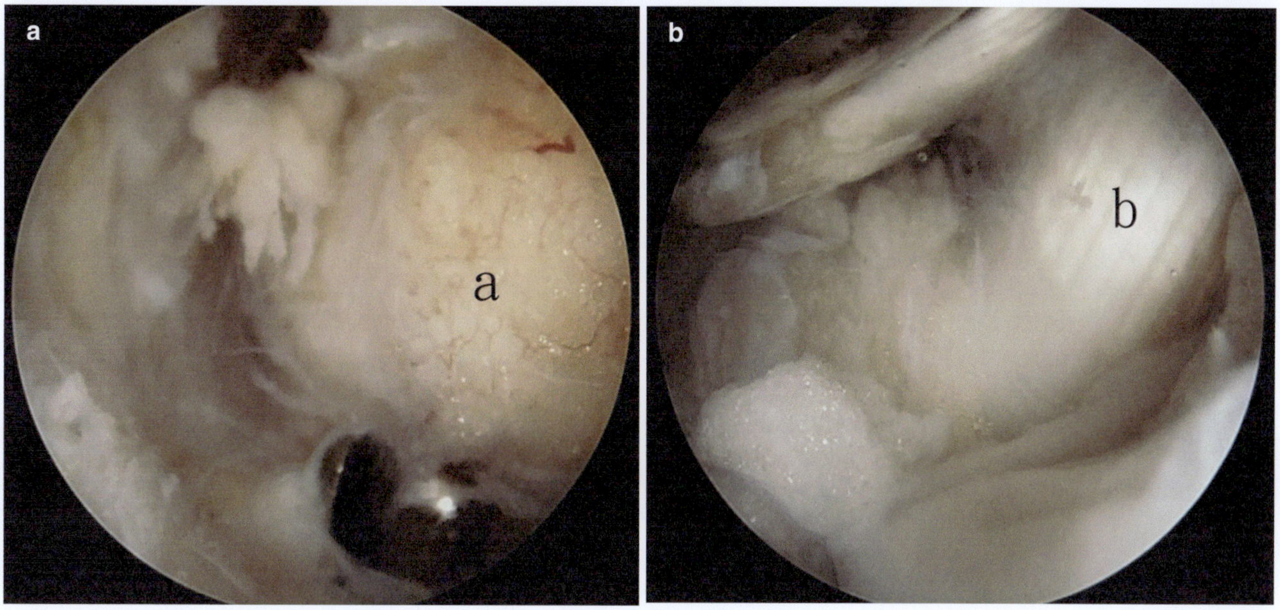

Fig. 9.34 (**a**,**b**) The synovial lipoma (a) surrounding the patellar tendon (b) is resected endoscopically

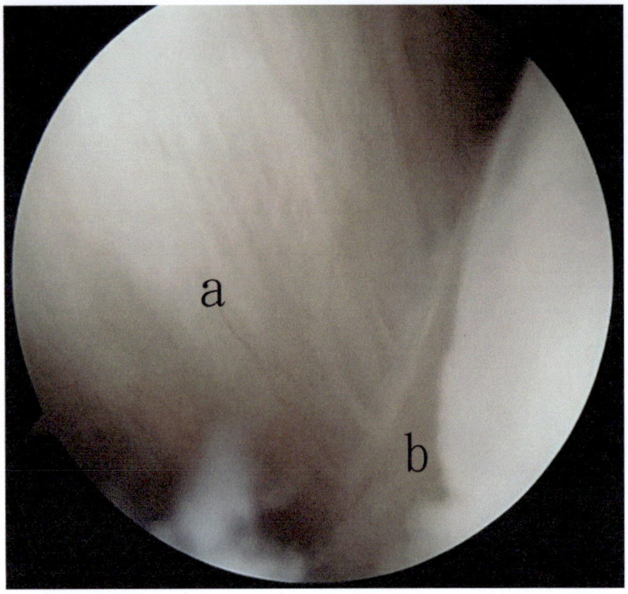

Fig. 9.35 Knee extension can facilitate approach to the tibial insertion of the patellar tendon. a: Patellar tendon; b: tibial tuberosity

- For lesions deep to the patellar tendon and close to its tibial insertion, access can be facilitated by knee extension relaxing the patellar tendon (Fig. 9.35). Access to the tibial insertion of the tendon via proximal portals may be limited as the freedom of motion of the arthroscopic instruments can be hindered by the patella. A distal portal close to the tendon's tibial insertion will be a useful working portal.
- The Hoffa fat pad is pyramidal in shape with the anterior synovial membrane of the knee joint very close to the patellar insertion of the patellar tendon. Caution should be paid not to breach the thin anterior synovial membrane of the knee joint during endoscopic resection of lesion at this area, in order to avoid spreading of the lesion (e.g., PVNS) into the knee joint.
- For lesion at the Hoffa fat pad, the space is obscured by fatty tissue and identification of lesion in this zone can be difficult. The appropriate endoscopic approach can be determined by careful study of the MRI about the location of the lesion related to the patellar tendon and the anterior synovial membrane of the knee joint. If the lesion is close to the deep surface of the patellar tendon, the initial endoscopic working space is developed at the deep surface of the tendon by hemostat via the portals and the fatty tissue is resected from anterior to posterior till the lesion is seen (Fig. 9.36). If the lesion is abutting to the anterior synovial membrane of the knee joint, knee arthroscopy can be performed and the anterior synovial membrane is resected to expose the lesion. However, this is chance of spreading of the disease into the knee joint. This approach is more appropriate if the knee joint is already involved by the disease.

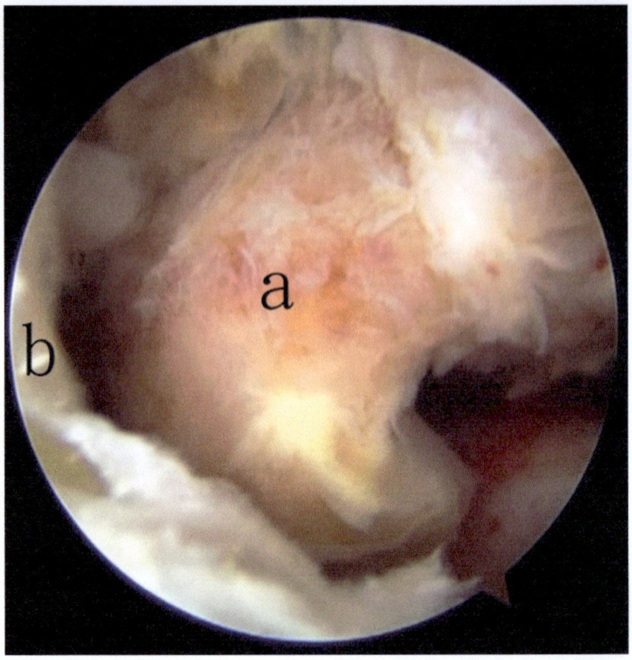

Fig. 9.36 Endoscopy of the Hoffa fat pad. a: Nodular PVNS of the Hoffa fat pad; b: patellar tendon

9.3.4.5 Complications

- Injury to the infrapatellar branch of saphenous nerve
- Spreading of pathology, e.g. PVNS
- Injury to the patellar tendon and its patellar or tibial insertion

9.3.4.6 Post-operative Care

Free mobilization of the knee is allowed immediately after the procedure. Physiotherapy can be offered to control local soft tissue edema and strengthening exercise.

9.3.5 Summary

Patellar tendoscopy and endoscopy of the Hoffa fat pad are useful minimally invasive approaches to deal with different pathologies of the patellar tendon and the Hoffa fat pad with the advantages of better cosmetic result, less post-operative pain, and less surgical trauma.

References

1. Robert F. LaPrade: the anatomy of the deep infrapatellar bursa of the knee. Am J Med. 1998;26(1).
2. Wilhelm Klein MD. Endoscopy of the deep infrapatellar bursa. Arthroscopy. 1996;12(1):127–31.
3. De Miguel ME, Cobo Ibáñez T, Usón Jaeger J, Bonilla Hernán G, Martín ME. Clinical and ultrasonographic findings related to knee pain in osteoarthritis. Osteoarthritis Cartilage. 2006;14:540–4.
4. Chatra PS. Bursae around the knee joints. Indian J Radiol Imaging. 2012;22(1):27–30. https://doi.org/10.4103/0971-3026.95400.
5. Norley T, Bickel WH. Calcification of the bursae of the knee. J Bone Joint Surg. 1949;31A:417–20.
6. Albert J, Lagier R. Enthesopathic erosive lesions of patella and tibial tuberosity in juvenile ankylosing spondylitis. Anatomico-radiological study of a case with tibial bursitis. ROFO Fortschr Geb Rontgenstr Nuklearmed. 1983;139:544–8.
7. Reicher MA, Hartzman S, Bassett LW, et al. MR imaging of the knee. Part I. Traumatic disorders. Radiology. 1987;162:547–51.
8. Paulos LE, Wnorowski DC, Greenwald AE. Infrapatellar contraction syndrome. Diagnosis, treatment, and long-term followup. Am J Sports Med. 1994;22:440–9.
9. Fulkerson RP, Hungerford DS. Evaluation and rehabilitation of nonarthritic anterior knee pain. In: Disorders of the Patellofemoral Joint. Baltimore: Williams & Wilkins; 1990. p. 94–5.
10. Reichmister J. Injection of the deep infrapatellar bursa for Osgood-Schlatter's disease. Clin Proc Child Hosp DC. 1969;25:21–4.
11. Rosenberg ZS, Kawelblum M, Cheung YY, et al. Osgood-Schlatter lesion: fracture or tendinitis? Scintigraphic, CT, and MR imaging features. Radiology. 1992;185:853–8.
12. Dye SF, Campagna-Pinta D, Dye CC, Shifflett S, Eiman T. Soft tissue anatomy anterior to the human patella. J Bone Joint Surg Am. 2003;85A:1012–7.
13. Aaron DL, Patel A, Kayiaros S, Calfee R. Four common types of bursitis: diagnosis and management. J Am Acad Orthop Surg. 2011;19:359–67.
14. Thompson TL, Simpson BM, Burgess D, Wilson RH. Massive prepatellar bursa. J Natl Med Assoc. 2006;98:90–2.
15. Huang YC, Yeh WL. Endoscopic treatment of prepatellar bursitis. Int Orthop. 2011;35:355–8.
16. Luk WCB, Lui TH. Endoscopic Resection of Prepatellar Bursa. Arthrosc Tech. 2020:E1057–60.
17. Ger R. The skin incision in the excision of the prepatellar bursa. J Dermatol Surg Oncol. 1978;4:166–7.
18. Quayle JB, Robinson MP. An operation for chronic prepatellar bursitis. J Bone Joint Surg Br. 1976;58:504–6.
19. Ogilvie-Harris DJ, Gilbart M. Endoscopic bursal resection: the olecranon bursa and prepatellar bursa. Arthroscopy. 2000;16:249–53.
20. Kaalund S, Breddam M, Kristensen G. Endoscopic resection of the septic prepatellar bursa. Arthroscopy. 1998;14:757–8.
21. Steinacker T, Verdonck AJ. Endoscopic therapy of prepatellar bursitis. Sportverletz Sportschaden. 1998;12:162–4.
22. Gendernalik JD, Sechriest VF II. Prepatellar septic bursitis: a case report of skin necrosis associated with open bursectomy. Mil Med. 2009;174:666–9.
23. Meade TC, Briones MS, Fosnaugh AW, Daily JM. Surgical outcomes in endoscopic versus open bursectomy of the septic prepatellar or olecranon bursa. Orthopedics. 2019;42:e381–4.
24. Schlesinger NH, Friis-Moller A, Hvolris J. Necrotizing fasciitis after arthroscopic synovectomy of an infected prepatellar bursa. Ugeskr Laeger. 2007;169:1693–5.
25. Morel-Lavallee M. Decollements traumatiques de la peau et des couches sousjacentes. Arch Gen Med. 1863;1:20–38.
26. Koc BB, Somorjai N, Kiesouw E, et al. Endoscopic debridement and fibrin glue injection of a chronic Morel-Lavallée lesion of the knee in a professional soccer player: a case report and literature review. Knee. 2017;24(1):144–8.
27. Greenhill D, Haydel C, Rehman S. Management of the Morel-Lavallée lesion. Orthop Clin North Am. 2016;47(1):115–25.
28. Goodman BS, Smith MT, Mallempati S, Nuthakki P. A comparison of ultrasound and magnetic resonance imaging findings of a Morel-Lavallée lesion of the knee. PM R. 2013;5(1):70–3.
29. Neal C, Jacobson JA, Brandon C, Kalume-Brigido M, Morag Y, Girish G. Sonography of Morel-Lavallee lesions. J Ultrasound Med. 2008;27(7):1077–81.
30. Bansal A, Bhatia N, Singh A, Singh AK. Doxycycline sclerodesis as a treatment option for persistent Morel-Lavallée lesions. Injury. 2013;44(1):66–9.
31. Nickerson TP, Zielinski MD, Jenkins DH, Schiller HJ. The Mayo Clinic experience with Morel-Lavallée lesions: establishment of a practice management guideline. J Trauma Acute Care Surg. 2014;76(2):493–7.
32. van Gennip S, van Bokhoven SC, van den Eede E. Pain at the knee: the Morel-Lavallée lesion, a case series. Clin J Sport Med. 2012;22(2):163–6.
33. Jones RM, Hart AM. Surgical treatment of a Morel-Lavallée lesion of the distal thigh with the use of lymphatic mapping and fibrin sealant. J Plast Reconstr Aesthet Surg. 2012;65(11):1589–91.
34. Kumar S, Kumar S. Morel-Lavallee lesion in distal thigh: a case report. J Clin Orthopaed Trauma. 2014;5:161–6.
35. Weiss NA, Johnson JJ, Anderson SB. Morel-LAvallee lesion initially diagnosed as quadriceps contusion: ultrasound, MRI, and importance of early intervention. West J Emerg Med. 2015;16(3):438–41.
36. Kim S. Endoscopic treatment of Morel-Lavallee lesion. Injury. 2016;47(5):1064–6.
37. Clayton RA, Court-Brown CM. The epidemiology of musculoskeletal tendinous and ligamentous injuries. Injury. 2008;39(12):1338–44. https://doi.org/10.1016/j.injury.2008.06.021.
38. Reito A, Paloneva J, Mattila VM, Launonen AP. The increasing incidence of surgically treated quadriceps tendon ruptures. Knee Surg Sports Traumatol Arthrosc. 2019;27:3644–9. https://doi.org/10.1007/s00167-019-05453-y.
39. Rougraff BT, Reeck CC, Essenmacher J. Complete quadriceps tendon rupture. Orthopaedics. 1996;19(6):509–14.
40. Trobisch PD, Bauman M, Weise K, Stuby F, Hak DJ. Histologic analysis of ruptured quadriceps tendon. Knee Surg Sports Traumatol Arthrosc. 2010;18(1):85–8. https://doi.org/10.1007/s00167-009-0884-z.
41. Ciriello V, Gudipati S, Tosounidis T, Soucacos PN, Giannoudis PV. Clinical outcomes after repair of quadriceps tendon rupture: a systematic review. Injury. 2012;43(11):1931–8. https://doi.org/10.1016/j.injury.2012.08.044.
42. Wenzl ME, Kirchner R, Seide K, Strametz S, Jurgens C. Quadriceps tendon ruptures – is there a complete functional restitution. Injury. 2004;35:922–6. https://doi.org/10.1016/S0020-1383(03)00261-4.
43. Konrath GA, Chen D, Lock T, Goltz HT, Watson JT, Mode BR, D'Ambrosio G. Outcomes following repair of quadriceps tendon ruptures. J Orthopaed Trauma. 1998;12(4):273–9.
44. O'Shea K, Kenny P, Donovan J, Condon F, McElwain JP. Outcomes following quadriceps tendon ruptures. Injury. 2002;33:257–60.
45. Boublik M, Schlegel TF, Koonce RC, Genuario JW, Kinkartz D. Quadriceps tendon injuries in National Football League Players. Am J Sports Med. 2013;41:1841–6. https://doi.org/10.1177/0363546513490655.
46. Gallagher J, Tierney P, Murray P, O'Brien M. The infrapatellar fat pad: anatomy and clinical correlations. Knee Surg Sports Traumatol Arthrosc. 2005;13(4):268–72. https://doi.org/10.1007/s00167-004-0592-7. Epub 2005 Jan 28. PMID: 15678298.
47. Kennedy JC, Alexander IJ, Hayes KC. Nerve supply of the knee joint and its functional importance. Am J Sports Med. 1982;10(6):329–35.

48. Apostolaki E, Cassar-Pullicino VN, Tyrrell PN, McCall IW. MRI appearances of the infrapatellar fat pad in occult traumatic patellar dislocation. Clin Radiol. 1999;54(11):743–7.
49. Smillie IS. Diseases of the knee joint. London: Churchill Livingstone; 1974. 152 pp.
50. Schweitzer ME, Falk A, Berthoty D, Mitchell M, Resnick D. Knee effusion: normal distribution of Fluid. AJR Am J Roentgenol. 1992;159:361–3.
51. Creamer P, Hochberg MC. Osteoarthritis. Lancet. 1997;350(9076):503–8.
52. Morini G, Chiodi E, Centanni F, Gattazzo D. Hoffas disease of the adipose pad: magnetic resonance versus surgical findings. Radiol Med (Torino). 1998;95(4):278–85.
53. Krebs VE, Parker RD. Arthroscopic resection of an extrasynovial ossifying chondroma of the infrapatellar fat pad: end-stage Hoffas disease? Arthroscopy. 1994;10(3):301–4.
54. Fan AKH, Lui TH. Endoscopic resection of localized pigmented villonodular synovitis in the Hoffa fat pad. Arthrosc Tech. 2019;8(11):e1309–12.
55. Ogilive-Harris DJ, Giddens J. Hoffas disease: arthroscopic resection of the infrapatellar fat pad. Arthroscopy. 1994;10(2):184–7.
56. Wu H, Xu Q, Zhou W. Hoffa disease: diagnosis and arthroscopic treatment. Zhonghua Wai Ke Za Zhi. 1995;33(10):581–3.
57. Hughes SS, Cammarata A, Steinmann SP, Pellegrini VD. Effect of standard total knee arthroplasty surgical dissection on human patellar blood flow in vivo. J South Orthop Assoc. 1998;7(3):198–204.
58. Reinking MF. CURRENT CONCEPTS IN THE TREATMENT OF PATELLAR TENDINOPATHY. Int J Sports Phys Ther. 2016;11(6):854–66.
59. Basso O, Johnson D, Amis A. The anatomy of the patellar tendon. Knee Surg Sports Traumatol Art. 2001;9:2–5.
60. Panni AS, Tartarone M, Maffulli N. Patellar tendinopathy in athletes. Outcome of nonoperative and operative management. Am J Sports Med. 2000;28(3):392–7.
61. Benjamin M, Kumai T, Milz S, Boszczyk BM, Boszczyk AA, Ralphs JR. The skeletal attachment of tendons–tendon "entheses". Comp Biochem Physiol A Mol Integr Physiol. 2002;133(4):931–45.
62. Ferretti A. Epidemiology of jumper's knee. Sports Med. 1986;3(4):289–95.
63. Ashford RL, Cassella JP, McNamara S, Stevens RM, Turner P. A retrospective magnetic resonance image study of patellar tendinosis. Phys Ther Sport. 2002;3(3):134–42.
64. Fincher AL. Managing patellar tendinosis. Athl Ther Today. 2001;6(2):34–5.
65. Milne AD, Evans NA, Stanish WD. Detecting and managing jumper's knee: early intervention and adequate rest can prevent chronicity. J Musculoskelet Med. 2001;18(5):261–7.
66. Warden SJ, Brukner P. Patellar tendinopathy. Clin Sports Med. 2003;22(4):743–59.
67. Fredberg U, Bolvig L. Jumper's knee. Review of the literature. Scand J Med Sci Sports. 1999;9(2):66–73.
68. Almekinders LC, Temple JD. Etiology, diagnosis, and treatment of tendonitis: an analysis of the literature. Med Sci Sports Exerc. 1998;30(8):1183–90.
69. Fredberg U, Bolvig L, Pfeiffer-Jensen M, Clemmensen D, Jakobsen BW, Stengaard-Pedersen K. Ultrasonography as a tool for diagnosis, guidance of local steroid injection and, together with pressure algometry, monitoring of the treatment of athletes with chronic jumper's knee and Achilles tendinitis: a randomized, double-blind, placebo-controlled study. Scand J Rheumatol. 2004;33(2):94–101.
70. Griffiths GP, Selesnick FH. Operative treatment and arthroscopic findings in chronic patellar tendinitis. Arthroscopy. 1998;14(8): 836–9. https://doi.org/10.1016/s0749-8063(98)70020-9. PMID: 9848595.
71. Lui TH. Endoscopic resection of avulsed fragment of tibial tuberosity and endoscopic-assisted repair of patellar tendon. Arthrosc Tech. 2015;4(6):e851–4.
72. Lui TH. Endoscopic resection of gouty tophus of the patellar tendon. Arthrosc Tech. 2015;4(4):e379–82.
73. Lui TH. Endoscopic resection of lipoma of the patellar tendon. Arthrosc Tech. 2015;4(1):e19–22.

Medial Knee Endoscopy

10

Keith Hay-Man Wan, Tun Hing Lui, and Tianlong Huang

Abstract

Medial knee endoscopy can be utilized for management of cysts of the medial knee and repair and reconstruction of the medial patellofemoral ligament. Cysts of the medial knee vary in size. Surgery is indicated for symptomatic ones and surgical options include open resection, arthroscopic internal drainage, and endoscopic resection. Regardless the treatment choice of the cyst, the underlying intra-articular lesions should be addressed. Preoperative magnetic imaging is essential for preoperative planning not only to study the architecture of the cyst but also to detect any associated intra-articular pathology. This chapter describes the technique of endoscopic resection, which is indicated for large and multi-loculated cyst. Patellar lateral dislocation is a prevalent musculoskeletal disorder affecting young and middle-aged population. Medial patellofemoral ligament (MPFL) has been recognized the dominating soft tissue restraint for patella lateral displacement. MPFL repair and reconstruction is an effective and classical procedure for treatment of patellar lateral dislocation, with/without other corrective bony procedures. With the advancement of knee arthroscopy, endoscopically MPFL repair and reconstruction has been demonstrated to be a more accurate and effective procedure compared with the traditional method.

Keywords

Medial · Knee · Cyst · Parameniscal · Endoscopy Patellar lateral dislocation · Medial patellofemoral ligament · Repair · Reconstruction · Endoscopically assisted

10.1 Endoscopic Resection of Cysts of the Medial Knee

Keith Hay-Man Wan and Tun Hing Lui

10.1.1 Introduction

10.1.1.1 Anatomy and Pathology

First described by Nicaise in 1883 [1], meniscal cyst is not an uncommon condition around the knee, with a prevalence ranging from 1.5% to 4% [2, 3]. It can be classified into parameniscal, intrameniscal, or both [4], with parameniscal cysts being far more common than intrameniscal cysts [5]. Medial meniscal cysts are more common than the lateral ones [3, 6]. In parameniscal cysts, the fluid is extruded outside the meniscus, giving rise to cystic lesions along the periphery of the meniscus. Whereas in intrameniscal cysts, the fluid is collected within the substance of the meniscus.

There are several accepted theories explaining the etiologies, including *trauma* which results in accumulation of joint fluid at the substance of broken meniscus, with subsequent extravasation of the fluid towards the adjacent soft tissue and mucoid degeneration. The most common mechanism of trauma occurs after a twisting/rotational injury to the knee while weight bearing [7]; *degeneration with age*, which

The corresponding author of Section 10.1 is Tun Hing Lui, Email: luithderek@yahoo.co.uk
The corresponding author of Section 10.2 is Tianlong Huang, Email: tianlong.huang@csu.edu.cn

K. H.-M. Wan
Department of Orthopaedics and Traumatology, Kwong Wah Hospital, Hong Kong, SAR, China

T. H. Lui (✉)
Department of Orthopaedics and Traumatology, North District Hospital, Hong Kong, SAR, China

The Second Affiliated Hospital, Shenzhen University, Shenzhen, China

T. Huang
The Second Xiangya Hospital of Central South University, Changsha, China
e-mail: tianlong.huang@csu.edu.cn

© The Author(s), under exclusive license to Springer Nature Singapore Pte Ltd. 2021
T. H. Lui (ed.), *Endoscopy of the Hip and Knee*, https://doi.org/10.1007/978-981-16-3488-8_10

results in local necrosis and mucoid degeneration into a cyst; more recently, formation of meniscal cysts has been suggested to be resulted from the influx of synovial fluid through the microscopic and macroscopic tears within the substance of the meniscus. On MRI meniscal cysts demonstrate direct contact with an adjacent meniscal tear in 98% of cases [3], supporting the theory that paramensical cysts arise as the result of extravasation of fluid through a meniscal tear.

Meniscal cysts are almost always associated with meniscal pathologies, in particular horizontal meniscal tears, with extrusion of synovial fluid through the adjacent meniscal tear via a one-way valve mechanism [1, 8]. Barrie observed that nearly all meniscal cysts were associated with meniscal tear and that the meniscal tears were either primarily horizontal or had a horizontal component [9].

10.1.1.2 Symptomatology

Meniscal cysts are often asymptomatic and incidentally picked up during MRI of the knee. However, as their size increases and expands outside the joint, patients would often complain of varying symptoms of palpable masses with pain, swelling, and snapping.

Patients are more likely to pick up cysts located in the lateral compartment owing to the fact that the soft tissue around the lateral aspect of the knee is thinner than that in the medial compartment. Because the medial knee capsule is covered by a thick soft tissue envelope including muscle and fat, cysts arising from the medial knee are often not recognized until they become larger in size. Because of that, meniscal cysts from the medial compartment tend to grow larger than those from the lateral compartment. Medial meniscal cysts are more likely to extend away from their site of origin owing to the fact that the medial collateral ligament limits their direction of expansion [10].

When the cystic lesion is clinically visible and palpable, the diagnosis of meniscal cyst can easily be made. However, ganglion cyst, inflamed bursa, synovial inflammation, baker cyst, hematoma, loose bodies, and tumors should be considered as the differential diagnoses.

Piscani reported that meniscal cysts are characteristically more prominent with knee extension and less so with knee flexion [11]. Pain is usually the main presenting complaint and is exacerbated by activity. The size of the cyst may vary according to the degree of activity. If the cyst is associated with meniscal tear, classical signs of meniscal tear such as clicking, snatching, and popping would also be present.

10.1.1.3 Investigations

Magnetic resonance imaging (MRI) is the investigation of choice to confirm the cystic nature of the lesions. It is a useful investigation to differentiate meniscal cysts from the other aforementioned differential diagnoses, and to pick up other associated intra-articular pathologies like meniscal tears.

Meniscal cysts have high water content and on MRI they exhibit the signal features of fluid, hypointense on T1-weighted images, intermediate signal on proton density images, and hyperintense on T2-weighted images [12].

On MRI, meniscal cyst would appear as a cystic mass on T2 weighted images. By looking at the axial, coronal and sagittal views one can identify the location of the cyst, whether it is non-loculated or multi-loculated and its anatomical relationship to the joint and surrounding structures.

Intrameniscal cyst appears as lesion of fluid signal change within the meniscus. Sometimes it appears as focal enlargement of the meniscus with an adjacent cleavage tear. Parameniscal cysts appear as well-defined, frequently septated lesions at the periphery of the meniscus.

With the recent improvement in sonographic technology, ultrasound has emerged as a sensitive modality for the detection of meniscal cysts, with sensitivity and specificity of 94% and 100%, respectively [13]. The dynamic real-time nature of ultrasound enables us to observe the size and its relationship with surrounding muscles during the range of motion of the knee. It is particularly useful to look for the cause of snapping.

10.1.1.4 Treatment

Conservative treatments, including non-steroidal anti-inflammatory medication and injection of steroid [14, 15], are rarely useful and result in no more than temporary relief of symptoms. The current recommended treatment of choice is surgery. Options include open excision of meniscal cyst, arthroscopic partial meniscectomy and meniscal cyst decompression, and endoscopic resection.

Open excision of the meniscal cysts can be considered if the symptoms are of relatively short duration, with relatively normal appearance of the meniscus and capsular attachment. Another indication for open excision is for large multi-loculated cysts. A small incision can be made directly over the cyst and its pedicle traced into the periphery of the meniscus to expose the area to a vascular access channel. The junction between the meniscus and the cyst can then be sutured with multiple interrupted sutures.

Because of the fact that meniscal cysts are almost always associated with horizontal meniscal tear with subsequent extrusion of synovial fluid through the tear, intra-articular decompression of cyst by resection or closure of the one-way valvular system between the cyst and the knee joint has been proposed [16, 17]. Standard knee arthroscopy portals are established and diagnostic arthroscopy of the knee joint is performed. The menisci should be probed to identify the extent of the tear. Depending on the tear configuration, the torn meniscus is trimmed and partially resected. The communication between the cyst and the knee joint is identified either by applying external pressure onto the cyst, and if not successful, a spinal needle can be placed percutaneously through the cystic mass to help locating the track. This is followed by placing a punch forceps or low-suction shaver to widen the track to convert the one-way valve into a bi-directional communication. If necessary, a shaver can be placed into the cyst to break up the loculations. Arthroscopic excision of cysts has been reported with [16, 18, 19] or without [20] a trans-cystic portal. In cases when there is no communication between the cysts and the joints, the cysts can either be excised or decompressed internally by resecting a portion of the cyst wall and adjacent knee capsule that is away from the meniscus. This can create a communication between the cyst and the knee joint, which is described as an "arthroscopic marsupialization" [21].

The drawback of arthroscopic approaches is limited freedom of motion of the arthroscope through the knee joint that limits the visualization field during the excision. Arthroscopic cyst decompression through partial meniscectomy to the menisco-capsular junction to expose the communication between the cyst and the knee joint may sacrificed some of the healthy parts of meniscus especially when meniscal tear is peripheral [22]. Moreover, internal drainage may not be an adequate treatment for cyst larger than 5 cm in size or multi-loculated cyst [7].

Endoscopic excision of the cysts has been proposed with the advantage of good visualization of the cyst and the adjacent extra-articular structures that is unrestricted by the boundary of the knee joint [22]. These can ensure complete resection of the cyst.

10.1.2 Indication of Endoscopic Resection of Cysts of the Medial Knee

- Symptomatic extra-articular cysts at the medial side of the knee with peripheral or no tear of the medial meniscus, especially for large and multi-loculated cysts.

10.1.3 Contra-indications

- Severe symptomatic knee osteoarthrosis that is indicated for total knee arthroplasty.
- Malignant tumor with cystic change.
- Cysts extending posteriorly to the popliteal neurovascular bundle.

10.1.4 Author Preferred Technique

10.1.4.1 Preoperative Planning

Magnetic resonance imaging is important for preoperative planning because the diagnosis can be confirmed and the extent of the lesion and involvement of adjacent structures can be determined (Fig. 10.1). Any intra-articular pathology especially associated meniscal tear can also be detected.

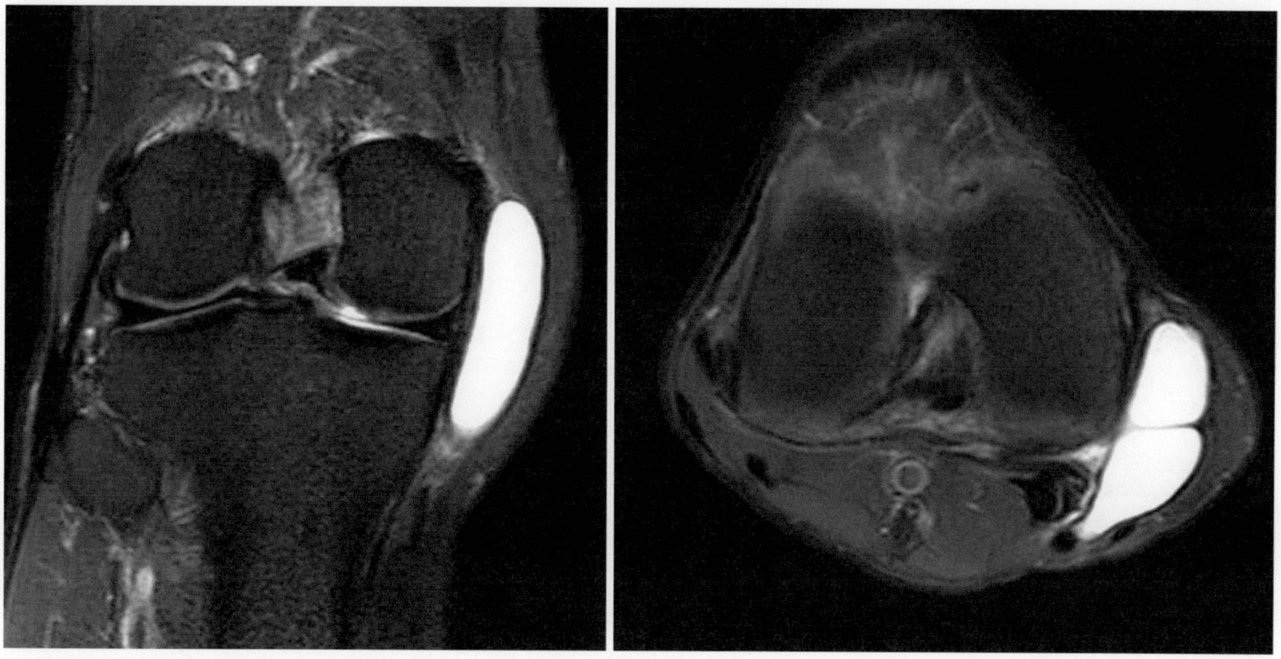

Fig. 10.1 Magnetic imaging shows a large cyst at the medial knee

10.1.4.2 Patient Positioning

The patient is in supine position with the legs spread. A thigh tourniquet is applied to provide a bloodless operative field. Fluid inflow is driven by gravity and no arthro-pump is used. A 4.0 mm 30° arthroscope is used for this procedure.

10.1.4.3 Portal Design

The cyst, the medial haemstring tendons, the medial head of gastrocnemius, and the proximal edge of the medial femoral condyle are outlined by skin marker. The posterior distal and anterior proximal portals are used for this procedure. The posterior distal portal is located between the medial hamstring tendons and the medial head of gastrocnemius and just distal to the medial knee joint line. The anterior proximal portal is located at the anterior corner of upper edge of the medial femoral condyle and is established by inside-out technique (Fig. 10.2).

10.1.4.4 Step-by-Step Description of the Technique

- A 5 mm longitudinal incision is made at the posterior distal portal. The subcutaneous tissue is bluntly dissected down to the cyst with a haemostat using nick and spread technique.
- The arthroscopic tocar-cannula is inserted between the medial gastrocnemius and hamstring tendons and perforates the cyst. The trocar is replaced by the arthroscope and the correct intra-cystic placement of the scope can be confirmed by arthroscopic view. Then, the scope is replaced by the trocar and the trocar-cannula is advanced pointing to the anterior corner of the upper border of medial femoral condyle. A 5 mm longitudinal incision is made at the trocar tip to create the anterior proximal portal.
- These two portals are interchangeable as the viewing and working portals (Fig. 10.3). Exchange of portals should be performed with Wissinger rod technique.
- This is an intra-lesional endoscopic approach as the resection is performed with the arthroscope and arthroscopic shaver inside the cyst (Fig. 10.4).
- In order to achieve complete resection of multi-loculated cyst, all the septa and cyst wall are resected to expose the surrounding normal structures including the medial collateral ligament of the knee, medial hamstring muscle and tendon, medial gastrocnemius, and fatty tissue of the pos-

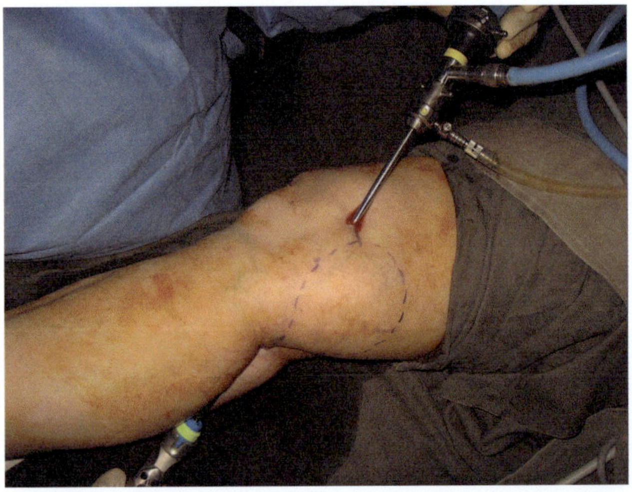

Fig. 10.3 Endoscopic cyst resection is performed via the posterior distal and anterior proximal portals

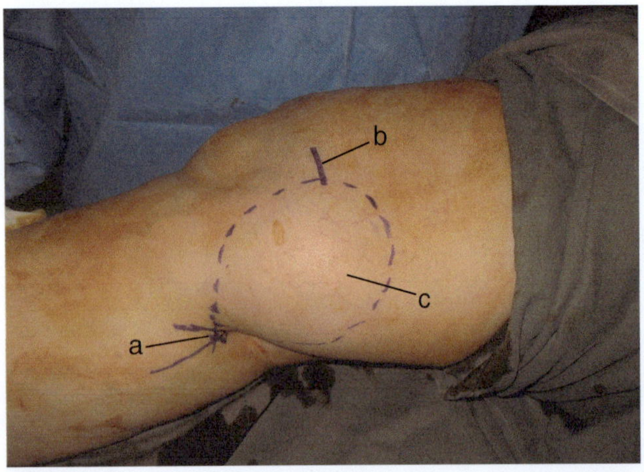

Fig. 10.2 Endoscopic cyst resection is performed via the posterior distal and anterior proximal portals. The posterior distal portal is located between the medial hamstring tendons and the medial head of gastrocnemius and just distal to the medial knee joint line. The anterior proximal portal is located at the anterior corner of upper edge of the medial femoral condyle. a: Posterior distal portal; b: anterior proximal portal; c: cyst of the medial knee

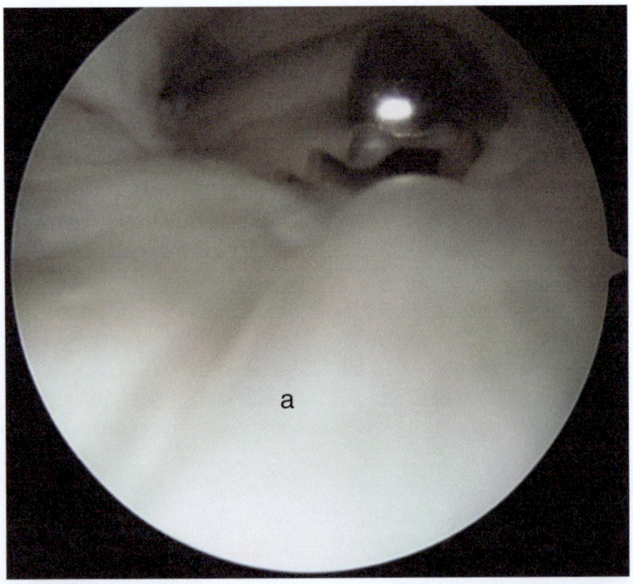

Fig. 10.4 Endoscopic cyst resection with the arthroscope and arthroscopic shaver inside the cyst. a: Cyst wall

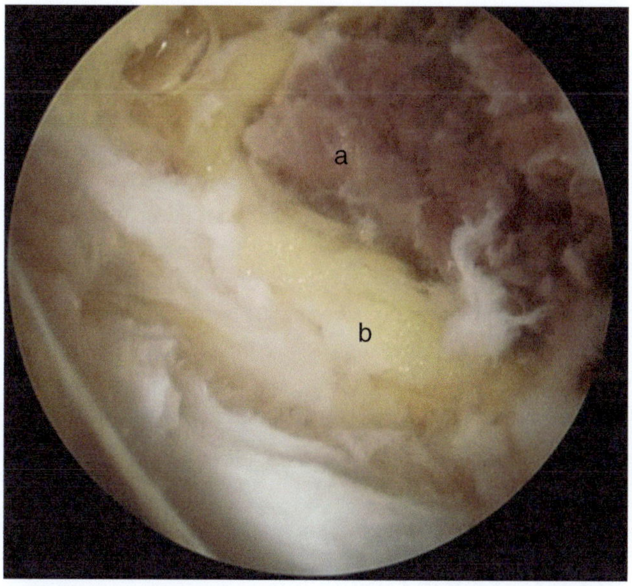

Fig. 10.5 After endoscopic cyst resection, a: the medial hamstring muscle and b: posterior knee fatty tissue are exposed

terior knee are seen (Fig. 10.5). The normal structures should be preserved.

- Any capsular hiatus or peripheral tears of the medial meniscus, if present, can be repaired endoscopically.
- Knee arthroscopy can be performed to deal with concomitant intra-articular pathology.

10.1.4.5 Complications and Management

- The potential risks of this technique include injury to the popliteal vessels and nerve, saphenous nerve and its infra-patellar branch, medial collateral ligament of the knee, and semimembrosus and semitendinosus tendons.
- The medial head of gastrocnemius protect the popliteal vessels and nerve and the medial hamstrings protect saphenous nerve during instrumentation via the posterior distal portal.
- The proximal placement of the anterior portal can avoid injury to the infra-patellar branch of saphenous nerve.
- Dissection into the posterior knee fatty tissue should be avoided in order to present injury to the popliteal neurovascular bundle.

10.1.4.6 Post-operative Care

The wounds are closed by simple suture. Crepe bandage is applied to the knee for 2–4 weeks.

10.1.5 Summary

Regardless the treatment choice of the cyst, the underlying intra-articular lesions should be addressed. Preoperative magnetic imaging is essential for preoperative planning not only to study the architecture of the cyst but also to detect any associated intra-articular pathology. Endoscopic resection of cyst of the medial knee is an effective minimally invasive approach especially for large and multi-loculated cyst.

10.2 Endoscopically Assisted Medial Patellofemoral Ligament Repair and Reconstruction

Tianlong Huang

10.2.1 Introduction

Primary patellar lateral dislocation occurs in 23–42 per 100,000 people per year, with further dislocations reported in 17–66% of those who undergo nonsurgical management [23, 24].

The medial patellofemoral ligament (MPFL) is an extra-capsular fascial band that lies within the second of three layers of soft tissue envelope on the medial side of the knee, and it has been recognized as the primary and most important stabilizer against lateral patellar dislocation or subluxation [24–26]. A multitude of repair and reconstruction procedures of the MPFL are recommended in literature and show promising outcomes. The author prefers using semitendinosus, gracilis or allograft for MPFL reconstruction.

10.2.2 Indications

Recurrent patellar lateral dislocation

10.2.3 Contra-indications

- Patellofemoral pain without instability
- Patellofemoral osteoarthritis

10.2.4 Author Preferred Technique

10.2.4.1 Preoperative Planning

- Comprehensive physical examination especially the following entries, some of them may need be done under anesthesia.
  - Varus or valgus knee
  - Medial sided patellar tenderness,
  - Beighton scores
  - Grade the medial and lateral translation of patella by quadrants,
  - Whether we can evert the patella to neutral, if it will be tilted laterally, try to correct this to neutral. If we cannot correct, it means the lateral side is tight
  - Any instability or patellar apprehension tests through full range of motion,
  - J sign,
- Knee AP and lateral X-rays, 30°, 60°, 90° patellar axial X-rays, full-length lower extremities X ray and CT scan, knee MRI.
- Based on these radiographs, we can measure the patellar height, the alignment of lower extremities, patellar tilt angle, tibial tubercle-trochlear groove distance (TTTG), femoral anteversion, angle and tibial torsion angle.
- Check the area and extension of bone edema, especially exclude the loose body and concomitant injury.
- Required instruments: C arm, 4.0 mm, 30-degree arthroscope, lightweight camera, shaver system with 4.0-mm full-radius blades, knee arthroscopic instrument set, such as dilators, probes, baskets, graspers, and curettes, half pipe and an arthroscopic radiofrequency system and its wands. Two 2.0 Kirschner wire and one 1.2 Kirschner wire.

10.2.4.2 Patient Positioning

The patient is placed supine on the operative table with a well-padded thigh tourniquet. The feet should be at the end of operative table.

10.2.4.3 Portal Design

- Anterolateral portal: place knee in approximately 60–90 degrees of flexion, 1 cm lateral to the patella tendon and just parallel to the distal pole of the patella.
- Anteromedial portal: place knee in approximately 60–90 degrees of flexion, 1 cm medial to the patella tendon and just parallel to the distal pole of the patella. We can use an 18-gauge spinal needle to assess appropriate direction visualizing the entrance from the lateral viewing portal.
- Superolateral portal: place knee in 0 degrees of extension but no hyperextension. 1 cm lateral to the patella and 1 cm proximal to the proximal pole of the patella. We can use a 18 gauge spinal needle to assess appropriate direction visualizing the entrance from the lateral viewing portal.
- Medial parapatellar portal: place knee in approximately 0 degrees of extension but no hyperextension. The portal is at the middle between the medial margin of the patella and the femoral medial epicondyle, located at the level of midpoint of longitudinal axis of the patella.

10.2.4.4 Step-by-Step Description of the Technique

- Anterolateral portal is the viewing portal for complete arthroscopic examination of knee joint. With the anteromedial portal as the working portal, all ligaments and meniscus, especially for the cartilage or avulsion fractures of medial patella is examined with arthroscopic probe. The medial and lateral sulcus should be examined for any loose osteochondral body. The concomitant injuries if present should be managed.

- Assess the patellofemoral joint again from the superolateral portal. Find the accurate angle when the patella begin to dislocate from 0° to 60° flexion, this will be the right position of the knee that we fix our graft.
- Get and prepare the autograft or allograft for reconstruction. Notably, remember to modify the two thin distal sections of graft, it could be hard to pull into bone tunnel if the end is too fat.
- According to anatomic position of the adductor tubercle and medial femoral epicondyle, mark the position of MPFL femoral insertion with a 2.0 Kirschner wire. Use C arm to check the anatomic insertion [27] via true lateral view of the knee (superimposition of the medial and lateral condyles of the distal femur). The Kirschner wire is inserted percutaneously heading from medial to lateral, slightly from distal to proximal, and slightly from posterior to anterior. The Kirschner wire is left in situ for subsequent step.
- At the medial parapatellar portal, the interval between the extensor retinaculum and knee joint capsule is carefully dissected from the superior pole of the patella distally to 2/5 of the length of the patella and from the medial half of the anterior surface of the patella to the MPFL femoral insertion as marked by the Kirschner wire. The joint capsule must be carefully protected.
- Expose the medial aspect of patella. A Kirschner wire is inserted at the level of 2/5 of the length of the patella (not distal than 1/2, not proximal than 1/3) (Fig. 10.6) and 2–3 mm from the articular surface of the patella. The direction of Kirschner wire insertion should be adjusted to make sure that it exits the patella surface where should be at the 1/2 width of the patella, not less than 1/3 but not over 2/3 (Fig. 10.7). Use 4.5 mm reamer to build the patellar bone tunnel and Ethicon MB66 for patellar tunnel (suture1).

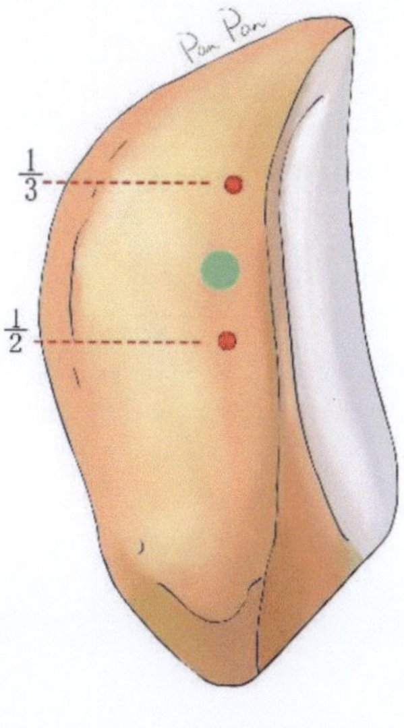

Fig. 10.6 The position of bone tunnel should be at 2/5 of the length of the patella (not distal than 1/2, not proximal than 1/3)

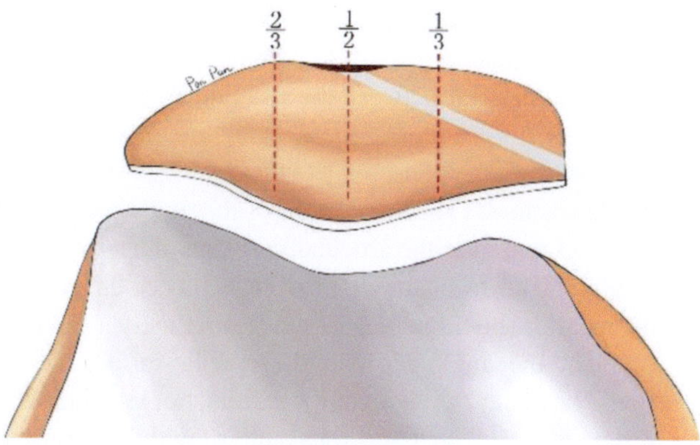

Fig. 10.7 The bone tunnel should just over the articular cartilage in height of the patella, make sure it exit the patella surface where should be at the 1/2 width of the patella, not less than1/3 but not over 2/3

- Pass the MB66 suture around the Kirschner wire in the MPFL femoral insertion, move the knee from 0 to 90 degree flexion to test the isometry of the suture, less than 5 mm changes in 0 to 90 degree flexion means good isometry.
- To establish the femoral tunnel, use 4.5 mm reamer to drill to lateral femoral cortex and then 6 mm reamer to get a 30 mm 6 mm tunnel along the Kirschner wire. Use another Ethicon MB66 for femoral tunnel (suture2). The traction end of the suture 2 is outside of the lateral thigh skin, and the loop of the suture 2 should be moved to the medial parapatellar portal from the interval using grab clamp or curved clamp.
- Use suture 1 to pull the graft to the patellar bone tunnel and use suture 2 to pull the two graft ends into femoral bone tunnel after aligning the graft end.
- Observe the PF joint from superolateral portal, flex the knee to about 20°, and toggle the patella back and forth to make sure it is engaged and the patella tracks centrally. If there exist contracture of lateral retinaculum, radiofrequency ablation can be used for delicate individualized release, never over release the lateral retinaculum.
- Use 1.2 mm Kirschner wire as the guide pin for femoral tunnel, find the right tension of graft for the good congruence of PF joint and then get the 6 × 25 mm screw in femoral bone tunnel, the depth should be at least 30 mm. The assistant needs to be holding the patella still so it does not over reduce it as the screw is advanced
- Check patellar mobility and make sure full knee ROM, explore the knee by arthroscopy again. And then exclude all joint fluids and cut the traction suture closed to skin. Inject the cocktail into joint and portal for analgesia.

10.2.4.5 Complications and Management

- Capsule damage: It is easy to damage the capsule when isolate the interval between the second and third soft tissue layers (retinaculum and capsule). Be careful but no matter when it happens.
- Patella fracture: (1) The position of the guide pin should be at 2–3 mm over the articular cartilage in height of the patella, too far from articular cartilage may be dangerous, the operator should adjust the guide pin timely. (2) Make sure that the guide pin exit the patella surface where should be at the 1/2 width of the patella, not less than 1/3. If not, it could be dangerous and should be adjusted timely.
- Excessive lateral retinaculum release: some surgeons prefer to do lateral retinaculum release for all cases, which may lead to the medial patellofemoral instability, the author seldom do lateral release when the patella can be medially moved 1/3 quadrant and everted. Only do delicate individualized release of the contracture of lateral retinaculum under arthroscopic view.

10.2.4.6 Post-operative Care

Post-operative cares include pain management, rehabilitation, and early complication prevention.

- Pain management: regular oral NSAIDs drug, opioid with/without hypnotics if necessary. Adductor canal nerve block can be done if the patient is hyperalgesia.
- Rehabilitation: isometric quadriceps and hamstring contractions, straight leg raise when pain is relieved. Closed chain (foot planted) exercises is better than open chain exercises.
- Early complication: regular wound check and prophylactic antibiotics.

10.2.4.7 Outcome

Medial patellofemoral ligament repair and reconstruction is a feasible solution for isolated MPFL reconstruction in patients with recurrent patellofemoral instability. Several authors [25, 26, 28–32] have reported the positive outcomes and low re-dislocation rate for bone tunnel techniques. Although anterior knee pain after bone tunnel techniques has been proposed in some articles, it is tolerable and will vanish in 1 year.

10.2.5 Summary

Medial patellofemoral ligament (MPFL) reconstructions have promising perspective with few complications notwithstanding varied techniques used. The techniques recommended in this chapter can be done in total endoscopic surgery with six portals, some patients will prefer this less invasive operation.

References

1. Nicaise A. Ganglion articulaire du genou. Rev Chir. 1883;3:463–5.
2. Beaman FD, Peterson JJ. MR imaging of cysts, ganglia, and bursae about the knee. Radiol Clin North Am. 2007;45:969–82.
3. Campbell SE, Sanders TG, Morrison WB. MR imaging of meniscal cysts: incidence, location, and clinical significance. Am J Roentgenol. 2001;177(2):409–13.
4. Anderson JJ, Connor GF, Helms CA. New observations on meniscal cysts. Skeletal Radiol. 2010;39:1187–91.
5. Lektrakul N, Skaf A, Yeh LR, et al. Pericruciate meniscal cysts arising from tears of the posterior horn of the medial meniscus: MR imaging features that simulate posterior cruciate ganglion cysts. AJR Am J Roentgenol. 1999;172:1575–9.
6. Tasker AD, Ostlere SJ. Relative incidence and morphology of lateral and medial meniscal cysts detected by magnetic resonance imaging. Clin Radiol. 1995;50(11):778–81.
7. Kose O, Erol B, Ozyurek S, Ege T. A giant medial parameniscal cyst of the knee joint. BMJ Case Rep. 2013;2013. https://doi.org/10.1136/bcr-2013-009440.
8. Choi EH, Huang J, Bryk D, Bryk E. Giant medial parameniscal cyst in an osteoarthritic knee. Orthopedics. 2009;32. https://doi.org/10.3928/01477447-20090818-26.
9. Barrie HJ. Pathogenesis and significance of meniscal cysts. J Bone Joint Surg Br. 1979;61(2):184–9.
10. Spina M, Sabbioni G, Tigani D. Medial meniscal cyst: a case report. La Chirurgia Degli Organi di Movimento. 2008;92(3):175–8.
11. Pisani AJ. Pathognomonic sign for cyst of knee cartilage. Arch Surg. 1947;54:188–90.
12. McCarthy C, McNally E. The MRI appearance of cystic lesions around the knee. Skeletal Radiol. 2004;33:187–209.
13. Sorrentino F, Iovane A, Nicosia A, et al. High-resolution ultrasonography (HRUS) of the meniscal cyst of the knee: our experience. Radiologia Medica. 2007;112(5):732–9.
14. Muddu BN, Barrie JL, Morris MA. Aspiration and injection for meniscal cysts. J Bone Joint Surg Br. 1992;74(4):627–8.
15. MacMahon PJ, Brennan DD, Duke D, Forde S, Eustace SJ. Ultrasound-guided percutaneous drainage of meniscal cysts: preliminary clinical experience. Clin Radiol. 2007;62(7):683–7.
16. Ohishi T, Suzuki D, Yamamoto K, et al. Snapping knee caused by medial meniscal cyst. Case Rep Orthop. 2014;2014:151580.
17. Asopa V, Douglas RJ, Heysen J, Martin D. Diagnosing snapping sartorius tendon secondary to a meniscal cyst using dynamic ultrasound avoids incorrect surgical procedure. Case Rep Radiol. 2013;2013:813232.
18. Ahn JH, Yoo JC, Lee SH, Lee YS. Arthroscopic cystectomy for popliteal cysts through the posteromedial cystic portal. Arthroscopy. 2007;23:559.e1–4.
19. Shetty GM, Wang JH, Ahn JH, Lee YS, Kim BH, Kim JG. Giant synovial cyst of knee treated arthroscopically through a cystic portal. Knee Surg Sports Traumatol Arthrosc. 2008;16:175–8.
20. Franceschi F, Rizzello G, Maffei MV, Papalia R, Denaro V. Arthroscopic ganglion cyst excision in the anterolateral aspect of the knee. Arthroscopy. 2003;19:E32.
21. Howe TS, Koh JS. Arthroscopic internal marsupialization of meniscal cysts. Knee. 2007;14:408–10.
22. Lui TH. Endoscopic resection of medial extra-articular cysts of the knee. Arthrosc Tech. 2017;6:e461–6.
23. Gravesen KS, Kallemose T, Blønd L, Troelsen A, Barfod KW. High incidence of acute and recurrent patellar dislocations: a retrospective nationwide epidemiological study involving 24.154 primary dislocations. Knee Surg Sports Traumatol Arthrosc. 2018;26(4):1204–9.
24. Sanders TL, Pareek A, Hewett TE, Stuart MJ, Dahm DL, Krych AJ. Incidence of first-time lateral patellar dislocation: a 21-year population-based study. Sports Health. 2018;10(2):146–51.
25. Neri T, Philippot R, Carnesecchi O, Boyer B, Farizon F. Medial patellofemoral ligament reconstruction: clinical and radiographic results in a series of 90 cases. Orthop Traumatol Surg Res. 2015;101(1):65–9.
26. Niu J, Qi Q, Fu K, Duan G, Liu C, Wang F. Medial patellofemoral ligament reconstruction with semi-patellar tunnel fixation: surgical technique and mid-term follow-up. Med Sci Monit. 2017;23:5870–5.
27. Redfern J, Kamath G, Burks R. Anatomical confirmation of the use of radiographic landmarks in medial patellofemoral ligament reconstruction. Am J Sports Med. 2010;38(2):293–7.
28. Panni AS, Alam M, Cerciello S, Vasso M, Maffulli N. Medial patellofemoral ligament reconstruction with a divergent patellar transverse 2-tunnel technique. Am J Sports Med. 2011;39(12):2647–55.
29. Raghuveer RK, Mishra CB. Reconstruction of medial patellofemoral ligament for chronic patellar instability. Indian J Orthop. 2012;46(4):447–54.
30. Smith TO, Mann CJ, Donell ST. Does knee joint proprioception alter following medial patellofemoral ligament reconstruction? Knee. 2014;21(1):21–7.
31. Song SY, Kim IS, Chang HG, Shin JH, Kim HJ, Seo YJ. Anatomic medial patellofemoral ligament reconstruction using patellar suture anchor fixation for recurrent patellar instability. Knee Surg Sports Traumatol Arthrosc. 2014;22(10):2431–7.
32. Toritsuka Y, Amano H, Mae T, Uchida R, Hamada M, Ohzono K, et al. Dual tunnel medial patellofemoral ligament reconstruction for patients with patellar dislocation using a semitendinosus tendon autograft. Knee. 2011;18(4):214–9.

Lateral Knee Endoscopy and Proximal Tibiofibular Endoscopy

11

Lok Yiu Cheng, Tun Hing Lui, Tze Wang Chan, Iciar M. Dávila Castrodad, Matthew J. Kraeutler, and Anthony J. Scillia

Abstract

Lateral knee endoscopy can approach the cysts of the lateral knee, distal part of the iliotibial band, the proximal tibiofibular joint, and the fibular head and it can be used for creation of the posterior portals for posterior knee arthroscopy. Endoscopic resection of cyst of the knee is a feasible minimally invasive approach for symptomatic cystic lesion of the lateral knee. It is particularly useful for multi-loculated cysts. Pre-operative magnetic resonance imaging is important to confirm the diagnosis and study the multi-loculation of the cyst and its relationship to surrounding important structures. The proximal tibiofibular joint can be considered as the fourth compartment of the knee to explain subtle knee problems. Endoscopic approach to proximal tibiofibular joint can reach adjacent capsulo-ligamentous structures including biceps femoris tendon, lateral collateral ligament, popliteofibular ligament, fibular head, and posterolateral corner of the knee. Distal iliotibial (IT) band syndrome is a disorder characterized by pain over the lateral aspect of the knee and is commonly diagnosed in a wide array of athletes, most frequently runners and cyclists. Most cases subside with conservative measures. Operative treatment is considered in chronic, recurrent, or refractory cases that persist for more than 6 months and include open or arthroscopic distal IT band lengthening, resection of the lateral synovial recess, transection of the posterior fibers of the IT band, and bursectomy. In this chapter, the endoscopic techniques are outlined.

Keywords

Knee · Cyst · Resection · Endoscopy · Posterior Arthroscopy · Loose bodies · Proximal tibiofibular joint Fibular head · Lateral collateral ligament · Biceps femoris tendon · Peroneal nerve · Iliotibial band syndrome · Iliotibial band tightness · Iliotibial band lengthening

The corresponding author of section 11.1 is Tun Hing Lui, Email: luithderek@yahoo.co.uk

The corresponding author of section 11.2 is Tun Hing Lui, Email: luithderek@yahoo.co.uk

The corresponding author of section 11.3 is Tun Hing Lui, Email: luithderek@yahoo.co.uk

The corresponding author of section 11.4 is Anthony J. Scillia, Email: scilliaa@sjhmc.org

L. Y. Cheng
Department of Orthopaedics and Traumatology, Queen Elizabeth Hospital, Hong Kong, China

T. H. Lui (✉)
Department of Orthopaedics and Traumatology, North District Hospital, Hong Kong, China

The Second Affiliated Hospital, Shenzhen University, Shenzhen, China

T. W. Chan
Department of Orthopaedics and Traumatology, Pamela Youde Nethersole Eastern Hospital, Chai Wan, Hong Kong SAR, China

I. M. Dávila Castrodad · M. J. Kraeutler · A. J. Scillia
St. Joseph's University Medical Center, Paterson, NJ, USA
e-mail: davilacasti@sjhmc.org; r_kraeutler@sjhmc.org; scilliaa@sjhmc.org

© The Author(s), under exclusive license to Springer Nature Singapore Pte Ltd. 2021
T. H. Lui (ed.), *Endoscopy of the Hip and Knee*, https://doi.org/10.1007/978-981-16-3488-8_11

11.1 Endoscopic Resection of Cysts of the Lateral Knee

Lok Yiu Cheng and Tun Hing Lui

11.1.1 Introduction

There are three anatomical layers to the lateral knee. The most superficial layer consists of the iliotibial band and the biceps femoris tendon. The second layer consists of the patellar retinaculum and patellofemoral ligament. The deepest layer includes the lateral collateral ligament, arcuate ligament, fabellofibular ligament, popliteofibular ligament, popliteus, and the knee joint capsule. The common peroneal nerve lies between the first and second layer. The inferior lateral geniculate artery is deep to the lateral collateral ligament.

Cystic or cyst-like lesions over lateral knee joint can be classified into intra-articular and extra-articular lesions. For intra-articular lesion, it can be further divided into ganglion cysts, synovial cysts, and meniscal cysts. Meniscal cyst was first described by Nicaise in 1883, and reported in detail by Ebner in 1904 [1, 2]. Meniscal cysts are more common in male patients between 20 and 30 years of age. Campbell et al. reported 4% incidence of meniscal cysts in 2572 knees with MRI performed, more commonly over medial side [3]. It is highly associated with meniscal tear, especially horizontal cleavage tear. Synovial fluid was trapped by a valve-like mechanism causing cystic formation. Myxoid degeneration was observed in histology [4, 5]. Terai et al. reported cyst formation occurred after meniscal repair with all-inside suture device [6].

For extra-articular lesion of the femorotibial joint, it includes ganglion cysts, iliotibial bursitis, bursitis underneath lateral collateral ligament, and lesions arising from proximal tibiofibular joint. Other non-cystic nor cyst-like lesions that occurred in lateral knee joint include localized nodular synovitis, hematoma, Morel-Lavallee lesion, abscess, hemangioma, peripheral nerve sheath tumor, and synovial sarcoma.

Most cysts of the lateral knee were asymptomatic. However, they can be presented with a palpable mass, knee pain, locking sensation, and decreased range of motion of the knee. Complications were reported in literature including infection, iliotibial band syndrome, and peroneal nerve compression [7–10]. Pisani described disappearance of the knee cystic swelling on flexion and reappearance on extension as a pathognomonic finding in patients with meniscal cysts [11].

Magnetic Resonance Imaging (MRI) is the choice of investigation in patients with cysts of the lateral knee. Not only it demonstrates the size, extent, and nature of the cystic lesion, it also allows evaluation of any associated intra-articular pathology, for example, meniscal cysts associated with meniscal tear, or ganglion with stalk connecting into knee joint. MRI is useful to study the relationship between the lesion and surrounding structures, facilitating subsequent surgical planning [3]. Ultrasound is an alternative of MRI, especially in patients with contraindications to MRI [12]. Ultrasound has the advantage of being both diagnostic and therapeutic. Ultrasound-guided aspiration and steroid injection can be performed. X-ray is a relatively less informative investigation for soft tissue pathologies. There was one reported case of lateral tibial plateau erosion on X-ray with a large lateral meniscal cyst [13].

In patients with symptomatic lateral knee cysts and failed conservative management, such as analgesics and physiotherapy, intervention can be considered. Percutaneous ultrasound-guided drainage with or without injection of steroids and local anesthetics has the advantage of being minimally invasive and simple [14]. MacMahon et al. reported a favorable outcome with ultrasound-guided aspiration of lateral knee cysts followed by injection of steroid and local anesthetic with no complications noted [15].

Surgical excision of meniscal cysts can be arthroscopic or open. Arthroscopically, cystotomy is performed to decompress the cyst, followed by debridement with shaver [16]. Howe et al. reported the use of arthroscopic internal marsupialization to decompress meniscal cysts [17]. Tudisco et al. described an outside-in technique for treatment of lateral meniscal cysts [18]. Apart from traditional anterolateral and anteromedial portals, Haklar et al. described the use of superomedial portal while Chen et al. reported the use of a direct inframeniscal portal for cyst decompression [19, 20].

These arthroscopic approaches are essentially intra-articular decompression of the cyst by resection of the valvular mechanism between the cyst and the knee joint. For posterolateral cysts, resection of the valvular mechanism by making a capsular defect at the posterolateral knee may damage the posterolateral complex causing knee instability. Moreover, it is difficult to make sure that all compartments of a multi-loculated cyst are effectively decompressed into the knee joint.

Open excision may be indicated if the cyst is large in size. Reagen et al. reported the use of Bruser incision for open cystectomy with 80% excellent-good results [21]. El-Assal et al. advocated open cystectomy if arthroscopy failed to decompress large multi-loculated cysts [22].

Treatment of lateral meniscal cysts should also address underlying meniscal tear if any. Arthroscopic examination of knee joint is important, lateral meniscal tear can be treated with partial meniscectomy or meniscal repair [16, 18–22]. Total meniscectomy is seldom performed as it may increase risks of late degenerative changes.

In lateral synovial cysts without any identifiable communication with the knee joint on MRI, Lui reported endoscopic resection using proximal tibiofibular arthroscopy portals as an alternative to classical knee arthroscopy [23]. It is especially useful for multi-loculated cysts and those cysts without identifiable communication with the knee joint [23]. The communication between the cyst and the knee joint is easier to be identified endoscopically than arthroscopically as the capsule would not be obscured by the lateral meniscus [23].

For ganglions arising from proximal tibiofibular joint, apart from surgical excision, Miskovsky et al. reported the option of proximal tibiofibular joint arthrodesis in a case of recurrent proximal tibiofibular joint ganglion despite repeated resection [24].

11.1.2 Indications

- Symptomatic cysts without identifiable communication with the knee joint
- Cysts associated with the proximal tibiofibular joint

11.1.3 Contraindications

- Solid tumor
- Associated intra-articular pathology, e.g. meniscal tear that need arthroscopic treatment, arthroscopic decompression of the cyst is preferred especially for simple cyst
- Extended posteriorly close to peroneal nerve or popliteal neurovascular bundles

11.1.4 Author Preferred Technique

11.1.4.1 Pre-operative Planning

Pre-operative magnetic resonance imaging (MRI) is essential for surgical planning. The relationship of the cyst to the peroneal nerve should be studied. Multi-loculation of the cyst should be noted and any associated intra-articular pathologies should be assessed.

The lateral knee extra-articular space can be divided into three zones. Zone 1 is posterior to the lateral collateral ligament. Zone 2 is at the level of the lateral collateral ligament. Zone 3 is anterior to the lateral collateral ligament. The location and size of the cyst should be determined in pre-operative MRI by studying which zone is involved (Fig. 11.1).

11.1.4.2 Patient Positioning

If only endoscopic resection of lateral knee cyst is planned, the patient is positioned laterally. If knee arthroscopy is planned for management of concomitant intra-articular pathologies, floppy lateral position is preferred so that the leg can be externally rotated to perform the knee arthroscopy

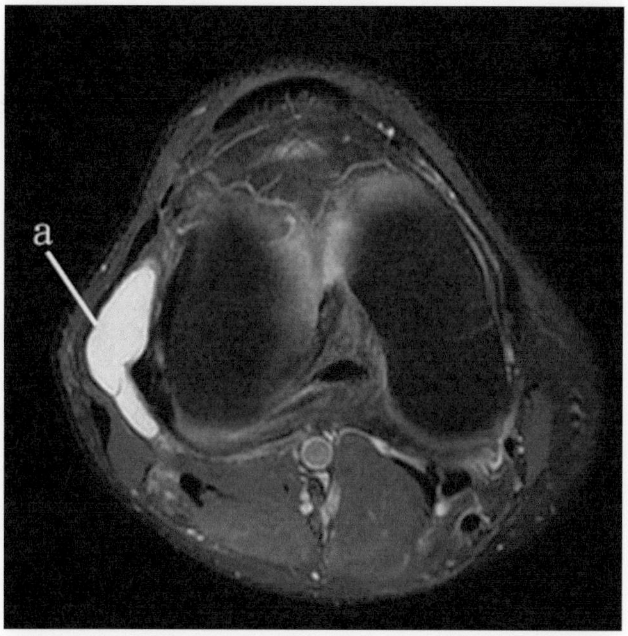

Fig. 11.1 Pre-operative magnetic resonance imaging identifies the span of the cyst (a) of the lateral knee

and internally rotated to perform the endoscopic cyst resection. During the endoscopic cyst resection, the knee is flexed in order to relax the peroneal nerve and displace it posteriorly away from the operative field [23].

A thigh tourniquet is applied to provide a bloodless operative field. A 4.0 mm, 30° arthroscope is used for endoscopic cyst resection. Fluid inflow is driven by gravity.

11.1.4.3 Portal Design

The procedure is performed via the anterior and posterior portals. The anterior portal is located at the anterior edge of the lateral collateral ligament and the posterior portal is located at the anterior edge of biceps femoris tendon. Both portals are at the level of lateral knee joint line (Fig. 11.2). These portals can also be used to access the lateral knee joint and the proximal tibiofibular joint.

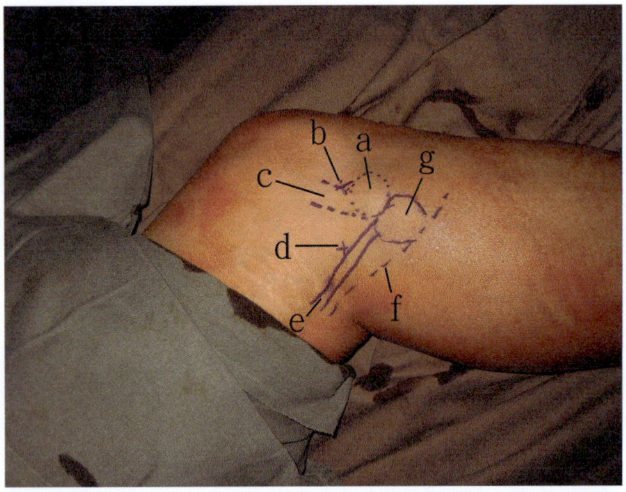

Fig. 11.2 The anterior portal is located at the anterior edge of the lateral collateral ligament and the posterior portal is located at the anterior edge of biceps femoris tendon. Both portals are at the level of lateral knee joint line. a: Cyst; b: anterior portal; c: lateral collateral ligament; d: posterior portal; e: biceps femoris tendon; f: peroneal nerve; g: fibular head

11.1.4.4 Step-by-Step Description of the Technique

- The anterior and posterior portals are interchangeable as the viewing and working portals.
- If the instrument needs to be inserted posteromedially via the anterior portal, the depth of insertion should be controlled and should not go beyond the anterior border of the biceps femoris tendon in order to avoid iatrogenic peroneal nerve injury (Fig. 11.3).

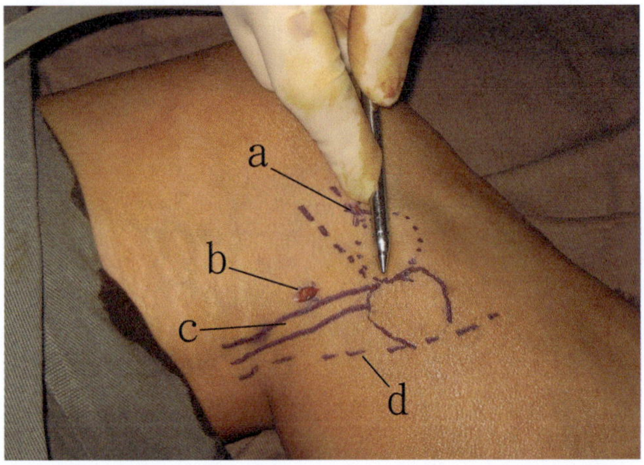

Fig. 11.3 If the instrument needs to be inserted posteromedially via the anterior portal, the depth of insertion should be controlled and should not go beyond the anterior border of the biceps femoris tendon in order to avoid iatrogenic peroneal nerve injury. a: Anterior portal; b: posterior portal; c: biceps femoris tendon; d: peroneal nerve

- The direction of insertion of the arthroscope and arthroscopic instrument into the portals should point medially (Fig. 11.4).
- The initial working space is the potential space deep to the lateral collateral ligament and anterior to the biceps femoris tendon.
- For resection of the cyst at zone 1 and zone 2, the anterior portal is the viewing portals and the posterior portal is the working portal (Fig. 11.5).
- During endoscopic cyst resection at zone 1, the stabilizing structures of the posterolateral complex including the popliteus tendon should be preserved. Resection of the cyst at the posterolateral knee corner must be performed under strict endoscopic visualization and the suction should be kept to a minimum in order to avoid injury to the peroneal nerve (Fig. 11.6).
- During endoscopic cyst resection at zone 2, the lateral collateral ligament and the biceps femoris tendon should

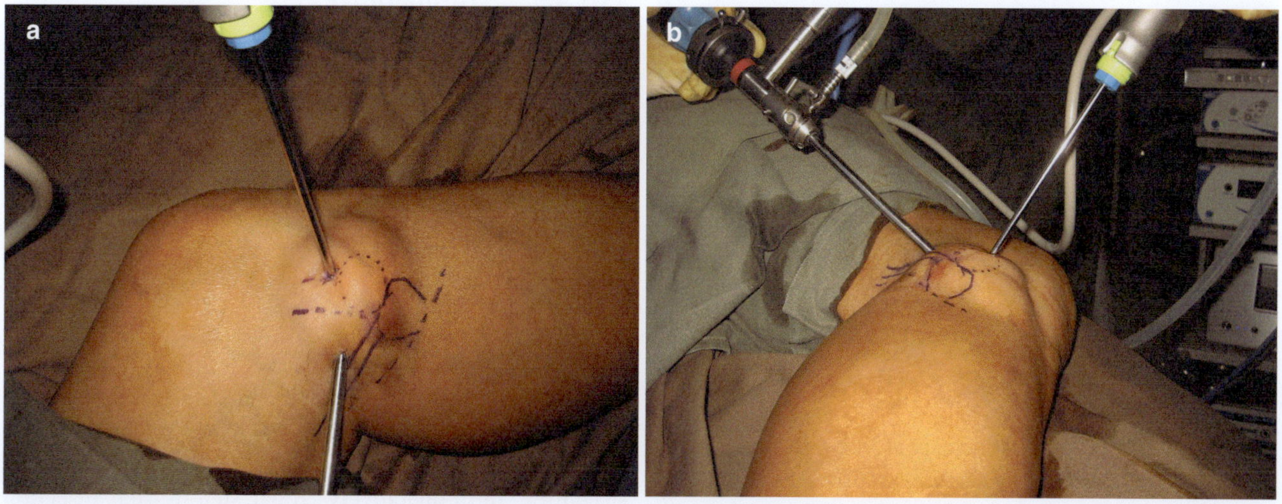

Fig. 11.4 (**a**) Endoscopic resection of the cyst of the lateral knee. (**b**) The direction of insertion of the arthroscope and arthroscopic instrument into the portals should point medially

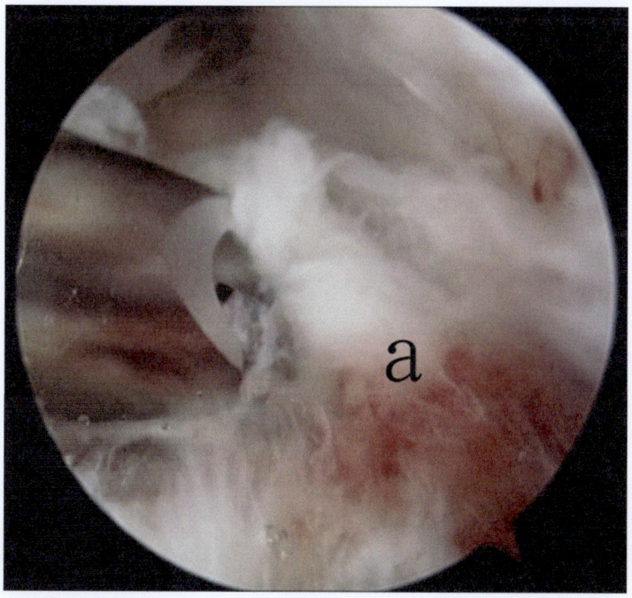

Fig. 11.5 Endoscopic view shows resection of the cyst wall (a) by an arthroscopic shaver

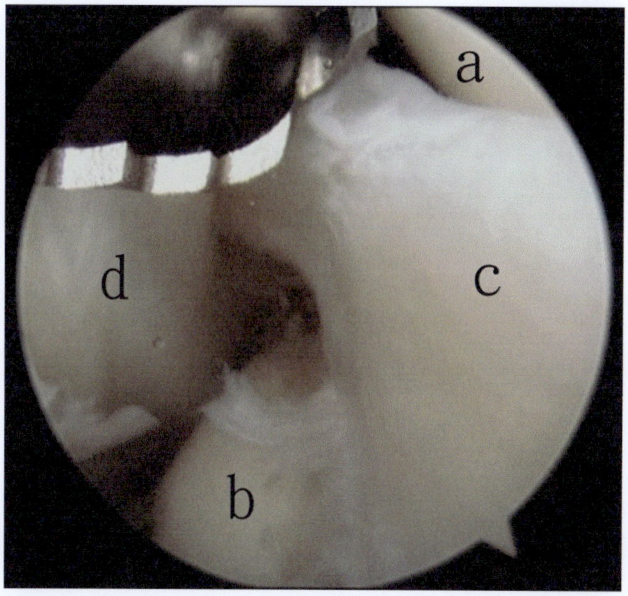

Fig. 11.6 During resection of the cyst at zone 1, a: the lateral femoral condyle, b: tibial plateau, c: lateral meniscus, and d: the popliteus tendon should be preserved

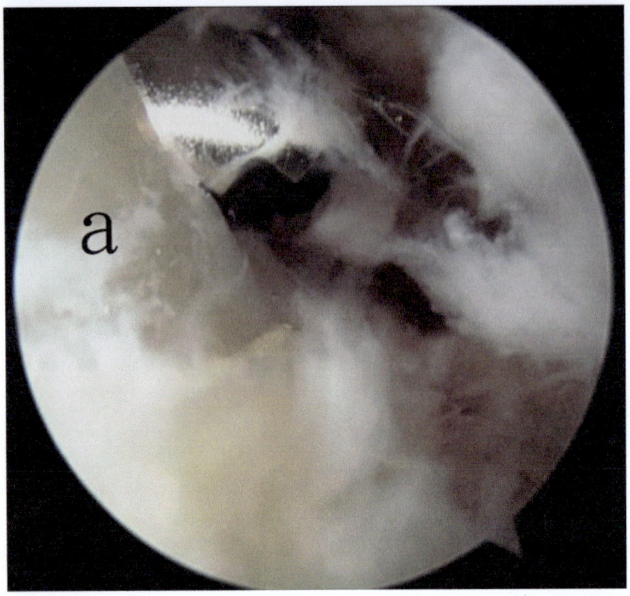

Fig. 11.7 During resection of the cyst at zone 2, a: the lateral collateral ligament is preserved

be preserved (Fig. 11.7). If debridement around the fibular head is needed, the anterior and posterior tibiofibular ligament should be respected.

- After completion of debridement at zone 1 and zone 2, the anterior and posterior portals are swap as the viewing and working portals and debridement of zone 3 is performed. If the debridement of zone 3 is needed to extend to the iliotibial band and the Gerdy's tubercle, the integrity of the iliotibial band should be preserved.
- The capsular attachments of the lateral meniscus should be preserved during debridement of all three zones.

11.1.4.5 Complications

- Injury to the lateral collateral ligament
- Injury to the biceps tendon
- Injury to the popliteal tendon
- Injury to the lateral capsule
- Injury to the lateral meniscus
- Injury to the peroneal nerve

11.1.4.6 Post-operative Care

Free mobilization of the knee joint is allowed after endoscopic cyst resection. If concomitant knee reconstruction procedure, e.g., meniscus repair is performed, the appropriate rehabilitation program should be followed.

11.1.5 Summary

Endoscopic resection of cyst of the knee is a feasible minimally invasive approach for symptomatic cystic lesion of the lateral knee. It is particularly useful for multi-loculated cysts. Pre-operative magnetic resonance imaging is important to confirm the diagnosis and study the multi-loculation of the cyst and its relationship to surrounding important structures. Intra-operatively, zonal step-by-step resection of the cyst can ensure complete cyst resection with preservation of surrounding tendons, ligaments, and neurovascular structures.

11.2 Endoscopic Creation of Posterolateral Portal of Posterior Knee Arthroscopy

Tze Wang Chan and Tun Hing Lui

11.2.1 Introduction

The posterior portion of the knee joint, which includes the tibial attachment of the posterior cruciate ligament (PCL) and the posterior horn of the menisci, has been called a "blind spot" because it is difficult to observe this area under arthroscopy through standard anterior portals. Posteromedial, posterolateral, and posterior transseptal portals have been developed for visualization and instrumentation of the posteromedial, and posterolateral compartments of the knee joint [25–29].

Transcondylar notch visualization, first described by Gillquist and Hagberg [30], can provide safe visualization of the posterior compartments. Visualization of the posterolateral compartment begins with the arthroscope in the anteromedial portal. The knee is flexed to 90° with a varus stress placed on the knee. The arthroscope is passed, under direct visualization, through the interval between anterior cruciate ligament and lateral femoral condyle into the posterolateral compartment. To facilitate transcondylar notch approach, Ahn and Ha advocated placement of anterolateral and anteromedial portals immediately adjacent to the borders of patellar tendon at 1 cm above the joint line [26].

The blind technique involves placement of a blunt obturator through the anteromedial portal to palpate the medial wall of lateral femoral condyle [27]. The obturator is then slowly advanced posteriorly until it gently pops through the interval between anterior cruciate ligament and lateral femoral condyle. The obturator is then replaced with the arthroscope to achieve visualization of the posterolateral compartment. To minimize trauma to intra-articular structures, a switching stick can be used as a guide to posterior compartment through the notch under direct visualization [31].

The soft spot for posterolateral portal is bounded by the lateral collateral ligament, iliotibial band, and biceps femoris tendon [32]. The light spot from the arthroscope in posterolateral compartment can guide the site and direction. A spinal needle is inserted to localize the optimal position. The entry site is just posterior to the lateral collateral ligament, anterior and superior to the biceps femoris. A superficial longitudinal incision through skin is followed by blunt dissection to penetrate the knee capsule. Plastic cannula may be used to facilitate instrument passage. When necessary two accessory portals in posterolateral soft spots can be established for more complex arthroscopic procedures [32].

Establishment of the posterolateral portal under arthroscopic visualization through the anterior portals may be difficult if the cruciate ligaments are intact, or if there was obstacle like a large loose body in the posterolateral compartment [33]. It can be done alternatively under endoscopic visualization, with the use of a lateral portal just anterior to the lateral collateral ligament at the level of lateral joint line [34].

11.2.2 Indications

1. Posterior loose bodies removal
2. Posterior compartment synovectomy
3. Arthroscopic reconstruction of the PCL
4. Meniscal procedure of the posterior horn
5. Resection of popliteal cyst
6. Posterior capsular release

11.2.3 Contraindications

- Ankylosed knee in extended position
- Active infection of the soft tissue envelops
- Marked fibrosis at the operative site, e.g., after previous operation
- Lack of expertise

11.2.4 Author Preferred Technique

11.2.4.1 Pre-operative Planning

The clinical examination and imaging findings should confirm the pathology locates at the posterior compartment of the knee joint.

11.2.4.2 Patient Positioning

- The patient is in supine position with the knee flexed.
- A thigh tourniquet is applied to provide a bloodless surgical field.
- A 30° 4.0 mm arthroscope is used for this procedure.
- Fluid inflow is driven by gravity and arthro-pump is not used in order to reduce the risk of extracapsular fluid extravasation.

11.2.4.3 Portal Design

- Lateral portal incision is made at the level of lateral joint line and anterior to the lateral collateral ligament. It can also serve as an arthroscopic portal for instrumentation of the posterolateral corner of the knee joint anterior to the popliteus tendon [23, 34, 35].

- Posterolateral portal is made at the lateral joint line level anterior to biceps femoris tendon (Fig. 11.8).

11.2.4.4 Step-by-Step Description of the Technique

- 4–5 mm incision is made at the lateral portal and posterolateral portal.
- With the lateral portal as the viewing portal and the posterolateral portal as the working portal, endoscopy of the potential space deep to the lateral collateral ligament is performed (Fig. 11.9).
- After minimal dissection, the posterolateral capsule can be seen.
- The soft spot at the posterolateral capsule between the lateral femoral condyle and tibial plateau just anterior to the lateral head of the gastrocnemius can be felt by the tip of a hemostat via the posterolateral portal.
- The capsule is perforated at the soft spot by the hemostat and this creates the posterolateral capsular portal (Fig. 11.10).

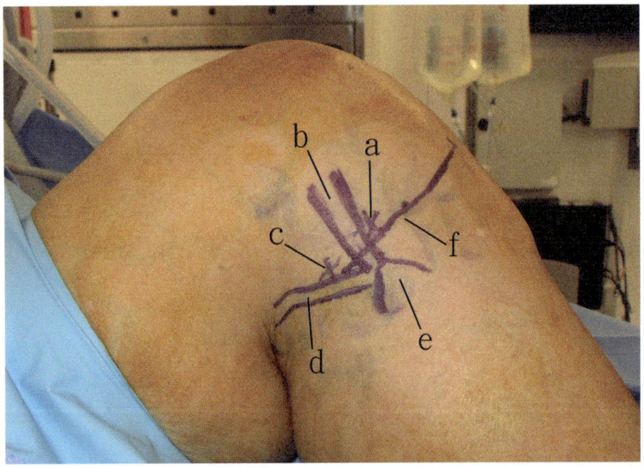

Fig. 11.8 Lateral portal is at the level of lateral joint line and anterior to the lateral collateral ligament. Posterolateral portal is at the lateral joint line level anterior to biceps femoris tendon. a: Lateral portal; b: lateral collateral ligament; c: posterolateral portal; d: biceps femoris tendon; e: fibular head; f: lateral tibial plateau

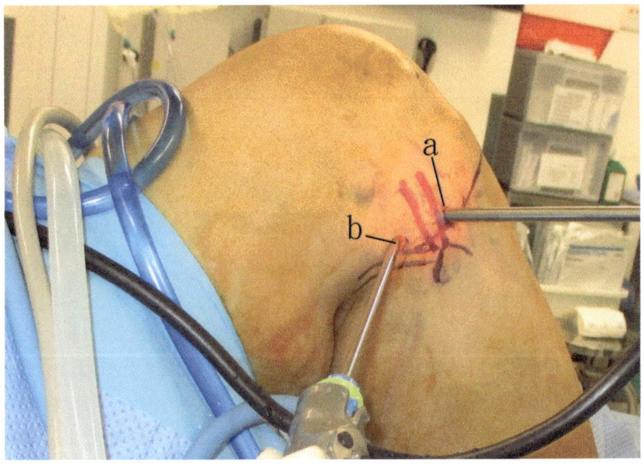

Fig. 11.9 With the lateral portal (a) as the viewing portal and the posterolateral portal (b) as the working portal, endoscopy of the potential space deep to the lateral collateral ligament is performed

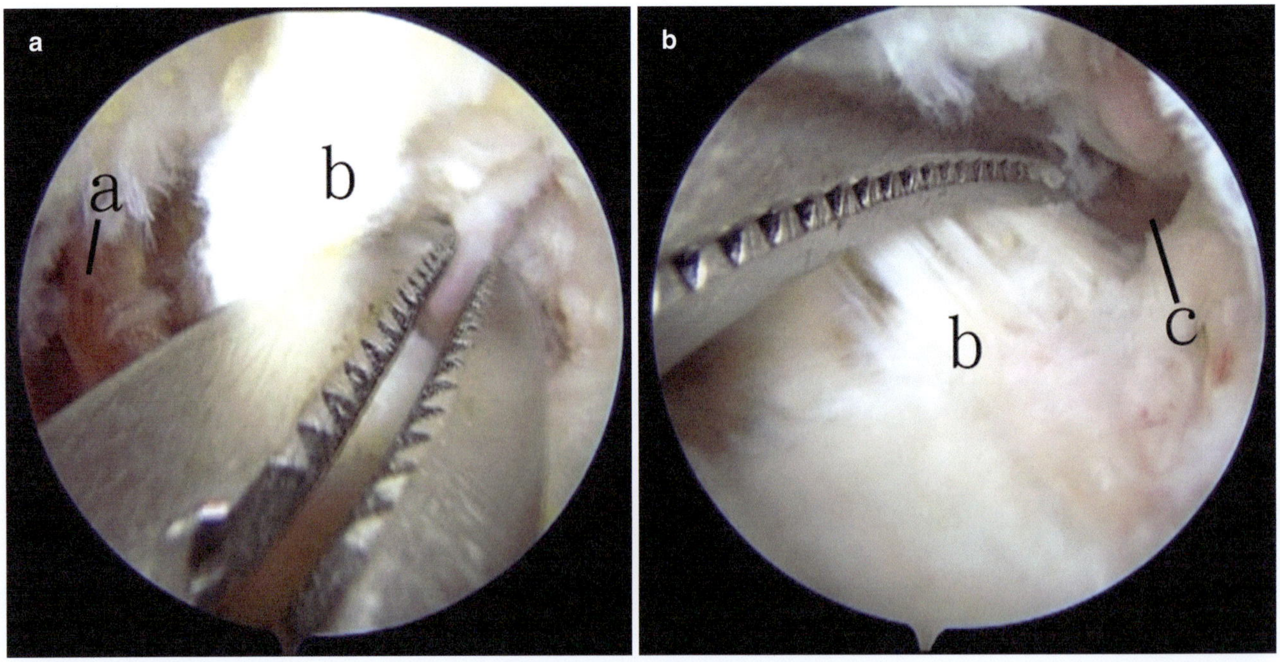

Fig. 11.10 (**a**) The posterolateral capsule is perforated at the soft spot by the hemostat and this creates the posterolateral capsular portal. (**b**) Close up view shows the posterolateral capsular portal. a: Lateral head of the gastrocnemius; b: posterolateral capsule; c: posterolateral capsular portal

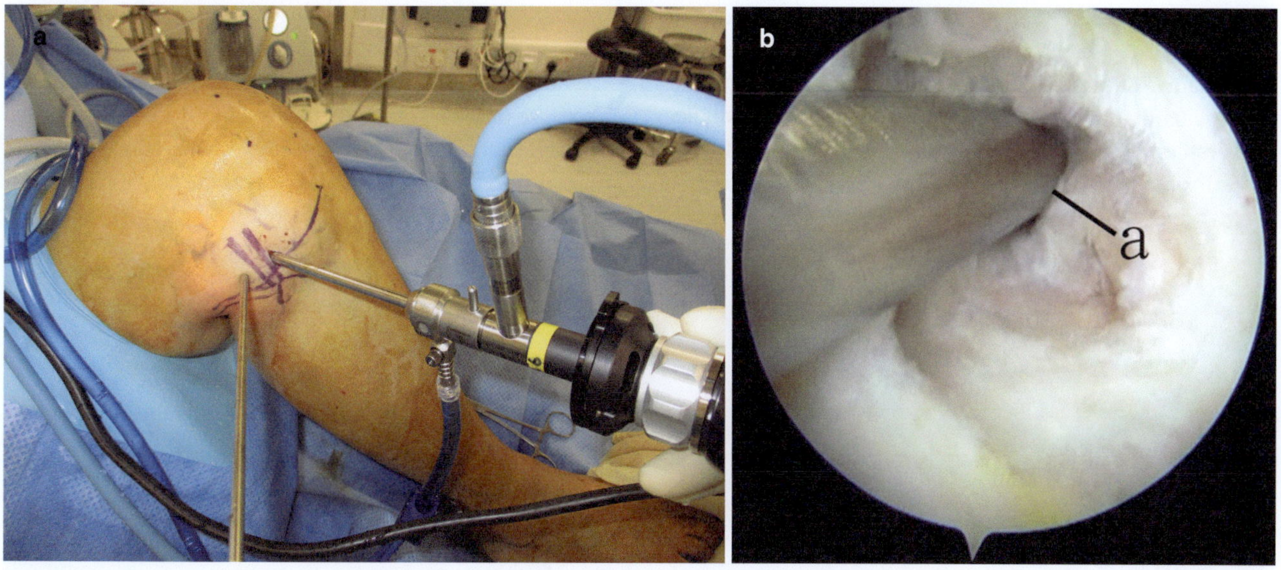

Fig. 11.11 (**a**, **b**) With the lateral portal as the viewing portal, a Wissinger rod is inserted via the posterolateral skin portal and posterolateral capsular portal (a)

- A Wissinger rod with the blunt conical tip can then be inserted into the posterolateral knee compartment via the posterolateral skin and capsular portals (Fig. 11.11).
- The arthroscopic cannula is inserted into the posterolateral compartment along the rod and the rod is replaced by the arthroscope.
- After confirming correct positioning of the scope in the posterolateral compartment by arthroscopic visualization, the scope is advanced medially until it touched the septum between the posteromedial and posterolateral compartments.
- The arthroscope is replaced by the Wissinger rod, keeping the cannula in situ.
- The septum above and behind the PCL is perforated by the rod close to the posterior femoral cortex and the posterior transseptal portal is created [36].
- The rod cannula is further advanced medially into the posteromedial compartment.
- The rod is removed again and replaced by the arthroscope and the correct positioning of the scope in the posteromedial compartment is confirmed by arthroscopic visualization.
- After that, the scope is advanced medially to the expected posteromedial capsular portal site.
- The expected posteromedial capsular portal is located just posterior to the medial femoral condyle, above the semimembranosus capsular fold and anterior to the gastrocnemius capsular fold. This corresponds to the medial soft spot at the posteromedial knee [27, 37].
- The arthroscope is advanced to this area and the long saphenous vein and the accompanied sartorial branch of the saphenous nerve are confirmed by transillumination that they are not at the posteromedial portal site.
- The scope is then replaced by the rod again and the posteromedial capsule is perforated by the rod and posteromedial portal incision is made over the tip of the rod.

- The posteromedial and posterolateral portals are coaxial portals (Fig. 11.12) and are interchangeable as the viewing and working portals for complete access to the posterolateral and posteromedial compartments of the knee. Complete synovectomy and removal of loose bodies are performed (Figs. 11.13, 11.14, and 11.15). Exchange of portals should be done by Wissinger rod technique (Fig. 11.16).
- Synovectomy of the posterolateral corner may be difficult because of the blockade by the tendon. Synovectomy of the posterolateral corner can be completed through the lateral portal with the posterolateral portal as the viewing portal.

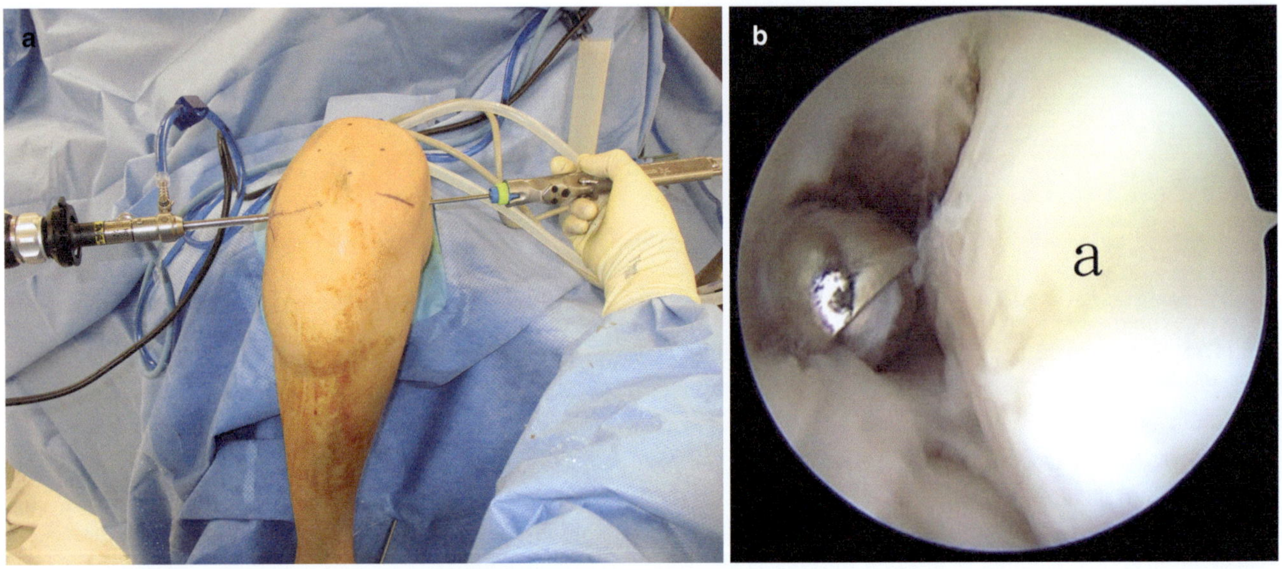

Fig. 11.12 (**a**, **b**) The posteromedial and posterolateral portals are coaxial portals. a: Femoral condyle

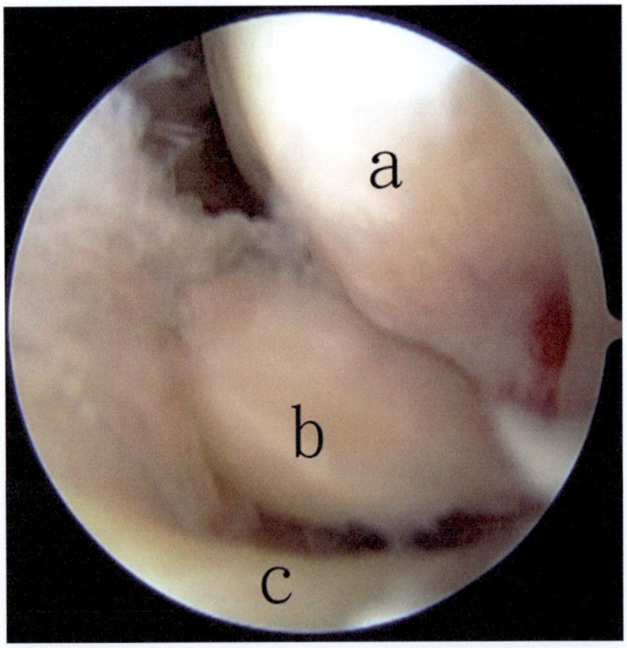

Fig. 11.13 Posterolateral portal is the viewing portal. Arthroscopic view of the posterolateral compartment of the knee. a: Lateral femoral condyle; b: Loose body; c: Lateral tibial plateau

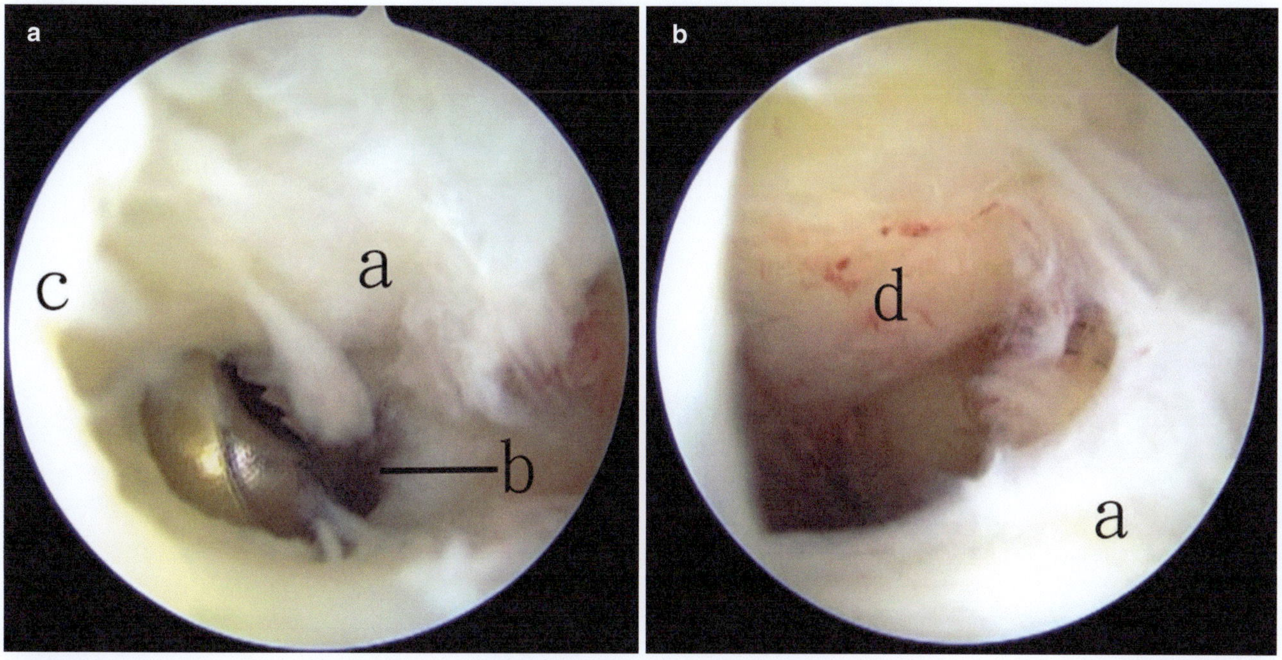

Fig. 11.14 Posterolateral portal is the viewing portal. (**a**) Enlargement of the septal fenestration by an arthroscopic shaver via the posteromedial portal. The shaver blade should face away from the posterior capsule. (**b**) Posteromedial compartment can be seen after enlargement of the septal fenestration. a: Septum between posteromedial and posterolateral compartments of the knee; b: septal fenestration; c: posterior capsule of the knee; d: posteromedial compartment

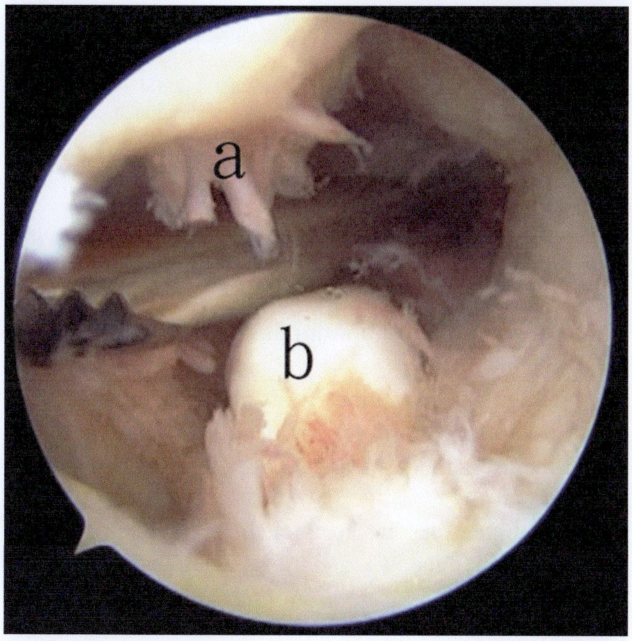

Fig. 11.15 Posterolateral portal is the viewing portal and posteromedial portal is the working portal. Arthroscopic view shows synovitis and loose body in the posteromedial compartment. a: Inflamed synovium; b: loose body

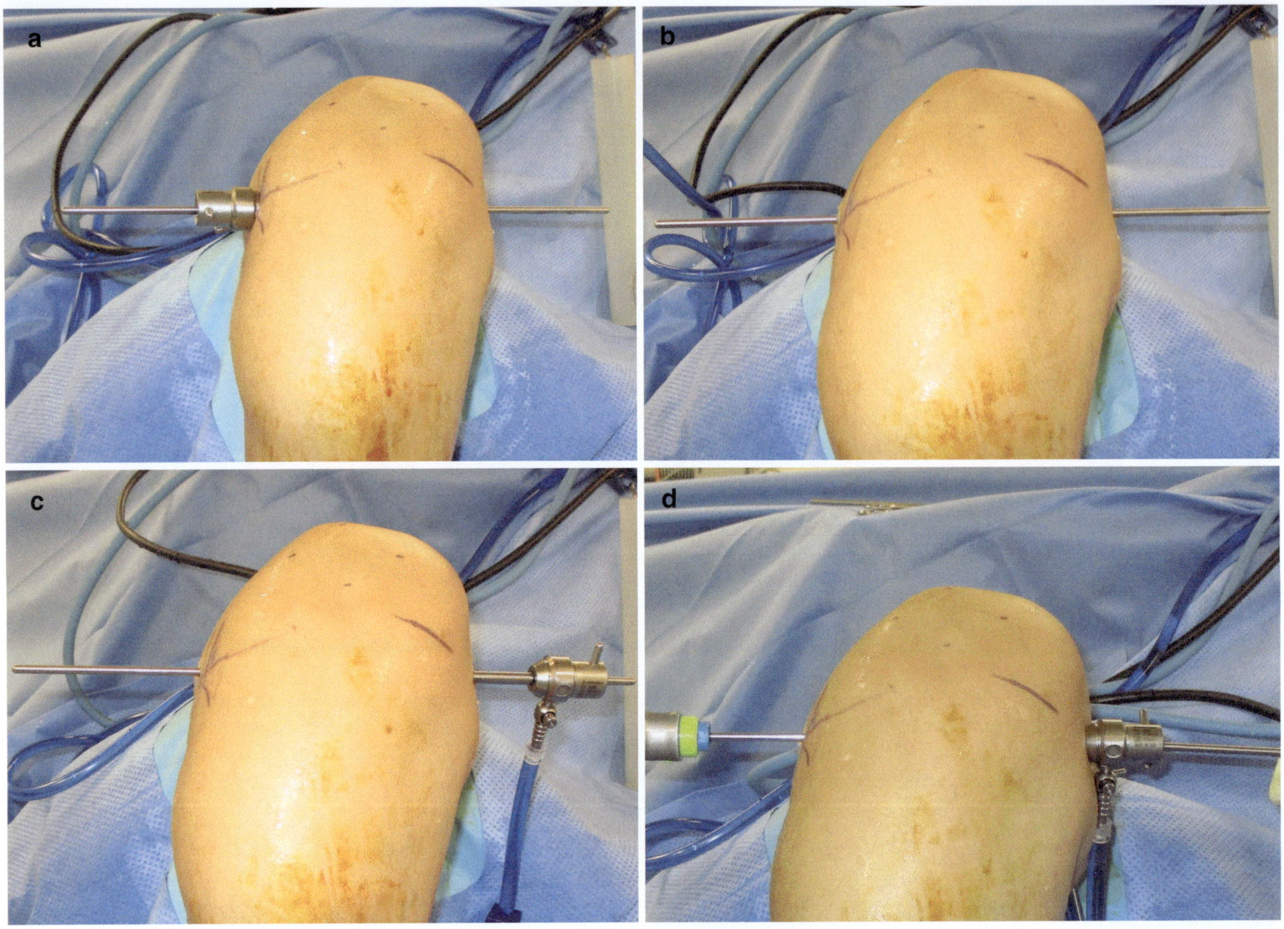

Fig. 11.16 Exchange of portals by Wissinger rod technique. (**a**) The arthroscope is replaced by the Wissinger rod with the cannula passing from posterolateral portal to posteromedial portal. (**b**) The cannula is removed leaving the rod in situ. (**c**) The cannula inserted along the rod via the posteromedial portal to the posterolateral portal. (**d**) The rod is replaced by the arthroscope. The cannula can serve as a conduit for insertion of both the arthroscope and shaver into the posterior knee compartment before the arthroscope incorporates into the cannula

11.2.4.5 Complications and Management

There is risk of iatrogenic injury to the surrounding neurovascular structures [27, 28]. The common peroneal nerve can be injured during the establishment of the posterolateral portal. The popliteal neurovascular bundle can be injured if the surgeon is working in proximity to the intercondylar septum or if the arthroscopic instrument slips extracapsular and posteriorly toward the neurovascular bundle [27, 28, 36].

The advantages of endoscopic creation of posterolateral portal include:

- The common peroneal nerve is protected by the biceps femoris tendon [27, 35].
- Endoscopic visualization allows creation of the posterolateral portal at the most posterior corner of the posterolateral capsule. This allow the portal to be far enough from the lateral femoral condyle so that instruments placed through this portal are never oriented in an anterior-to-posterior direction toward the popliteal neurovascular bundle [27].
- Endoscopic visualization avoids the Wissinger rod going extracapsular toward the popliteal neurovascular bundle during insertion.

The popliteal vessels lie immediately behind the tibial plateau, lateral to the PCL and the intercondylar septum [27, 28, 36]. If creation of the posterior transseptal portal is indicated, perforation of the septum from lateral to medial direction is less risky as the rod is moved away from the bundle. The shaver must always face anteriorly toward the knee joint and away from the popliteal neurovascular bundle. The risk of injury to the popliteal artery is greatest during resection of the inferior portion of the posterior septum [27].

11.2.4.6 Post-operative Care

The patient can have weight bearing walking as pain tolerated after synovectomy, loose bodies removal, or popliteal cyst excision. In patients with ligament reconstruction, meniscal repair, or chondroplasty, a period of protected weight bearing and limitation in knee range of motion would be required.

11.2.5 Summary

Lateral portal of the knee allows precise establishment of the posterolateral portal under endoscopic visualization. Structures and pathologies of the posterior compartment of the knee can be effectively approached via arthroscopy. Attention must be paid to avoid injury to neurovascular structures around posterior knee.

11.3 Endoscopic Approach to Proximal Tibiofibular Joint

Tze Wang Chan and Tun Hing Lui

11.3.1 Introduction

The proximal tibiofibular joint is an arthrodial sliding joint located between the lateral tibial condyle and the fibular head [38, 39]. There are two basic types of the joint including the horizontal type and the oblique type. The horizontal configuration is defined as <20° of inclination of joint surface in relation to the horizontal plane, and the oblique variation is defined as >20° of inclination of the joint surface in relation to the horizontal plane [38]. The oblique type was considered less stable because of less rotational mobility [40, 41]. The joint capsule is strengthened by the anterior and posterior ligaments. The anterior tibiofibular ligament is frequently fused intimately with the biceps femoris tendon [38, 42], while the posterior ligament is always well defined [42]. The posterior capsule consists of the popliteofibular ligament which runs from the fibular head to the popliteus tendon. Superiorly, the joint is supported by the lateral collateral ligament and the biceps femoris tendon. The rate of communication between the proximal tibiofibular joint and the knee in subpopliteal recess has been reported to be 10–63% [39, 43–45]. Because of this communication, the proximal tibiofibular joint might be considered as the fourth compartment of the knee to explain subtle knee problems [39, 45, 46].

The primary functions of the proximal tibiofibular joint are to dissipate torsional loads applied to the ankle, dissipate lateral tibial bending moments and tensile weight bearing [38]. The proximal tibiofibular joint demonstrates motion during knee flexion-extension, tibia rotation, and ankle dorsiflexion. The tibia and fibula move relative to one another at the proximal tibiofibular joint with coupled motion through the interosseus membrane and the distal tibiofibular syndesmosis [38, 43].

Various disorders of the joint have been reported including osteoarthrosis [46–48], rheumatic disease [49, 50], traumatic subluxation or dislocation [41, 42, 51, 52], ganglion or synovial cysts [53–57], synostosis [58, 59], synovial chondromatosis [60, 61], pigmented villonodular synovitis [35, 62], and hypomobility [63] of the joint. Peroneal nerve can be at risk with pathologies of the joint either by compressive effect or formation of intra-neural ganglion [64, 65]. Pathologies of the proximal tibiofibular joint should be kept in mind in the evaluation of lateral knee pain [40, 41, 45, 46, 50].

Open surgical approaches to the proximal tibiofibular joint may endanger the peroneal nerve, the anterior tibial artery, the popliteofibular ligament, and the lateral collateral ligament [39]. Endoscopic approach to proximal tibiofibular joint can reach adjacent capsulo-ligamentous structures including biceps femoris tendon, lateral collateral ligament, popliteofibular ligament, fibular head, and posterolateral corner of the knee. The anterior and posterior proximal tibiofibular ligaments can be identified at the anterior and posterior gutters of the proximal tibiofibular joint, respectively. The articular cartilage can be approached by resection of the capsule of the proximal tibiofibular joint with preservation of the ligaments [35, 66, 67].

11.3.2 Indications

1. Synovectomy
2. Ganglionectomy
3. Endoscopic assisted open reduction and internal fixation of an acutely dislocated or subluxed proximal tibiofibular joint
4. Endoscopic assisted proximal tibiofibular ligament and posterolateral complex reconstruction
5. Arthrodesis
6. Endoscopic resection of benign bone lesion of the fibular head
7. Endoscopic resection of the fibular head

11.3.3 Contraindications

- Active infection of the soft tissue envelop
- Severe soft tissue swelling or compromise
- Marked fibrosis at the operative site, e.g., after previous operation
- Lack of expertise

11.3.4 Author Preferred Technique

11.3.4.1 Pre-operative Planning

The symptoms should be confirmed to be coming from the proximal tibiofibular joint. Detailed history taking and clinical examination are essential to pinpoint the problem. Common physical signs include tenderness deep to fibular head and hamstring tightness [45]. Radiographs of the knee are useful to analyze the alignment and type of joint. Computed tomogram and magnetic resonance imaging are useful investigations to confirm the diagnosis and study the extent of involvement of various osteoarticular and soft tissue pathologies.

11.3.4.2 Patient Positioning

The patient is put in lateral position with a thigh tourniquet to provide a bloodless operative field. The knee is flexed during the procedure to relax the common peroneal nerve and displace the nerve away from the operative field. A 2.7 mm 30° arthroscope is used for this procedure. No arthro-pump is allowed in order to minimize the risk of nerve injury due to excessive fluid extravasation.

11.3.4.3 Portal Design

Proximal tibiofibular endoscopy is performed through the proximal anterior and posterior portals [35]. The proximal anterior portal is at the intersection between the anterior border of the lateral collateral ligament and the projection line of the posterior border of the fibular head. The proximal posterior portal was at the intersection between the anterior border of biceps femoris tendon and the projection line of the anterior border of the fibular head (Fig. 11.17).

The instruments should not go beyond the anterior border of the biceps femoral tendon in order to avoid injury to the common peroneal nerve (Fig. 11.18).

11.3.4.4 Step-by-Step Description of the Technique(s)

- 3–4 mm incisions are made at the proximal anterior and proximal posterior portals.
- The subcutaneous tissue is bluntly dissected down to the bones with a hemostat by "nick and spread" technique.
- The proximal anterior and proximal posterior portals are interchangeable as the viewing and working portals (Fig. 11.19).

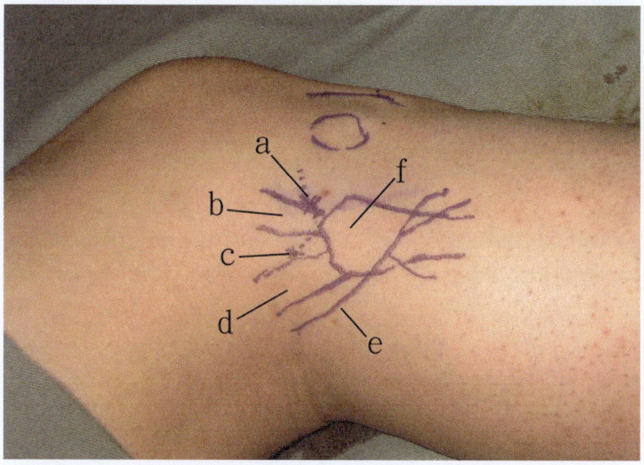

Fig. 11.17 Proximal tibiofibular endoscopy is performed through the proximal anterior and posterior portals. The proximal anterior portal is at the intersection between the anterior border of the lateral collateral ligament and the projection line of the posterior border of the fibular head. The proximal posterior portal was at the intersection between the anterior border of biceps femoris tendon and the projection line of the anterior border of the fibular head. a: Proximal anterior portal; b: lateral collateral ligament; c: proximal posterior portal; d: biceps femoris tendon; e: common peroneal nerve; f: fibular head

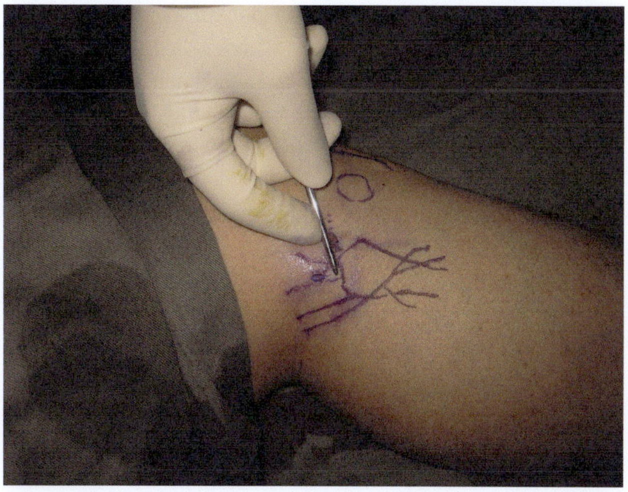

Fig. 11.18 The instrument inserted through the proximal anterior portal should not pass through the anterior border of the biceps femoris tendon

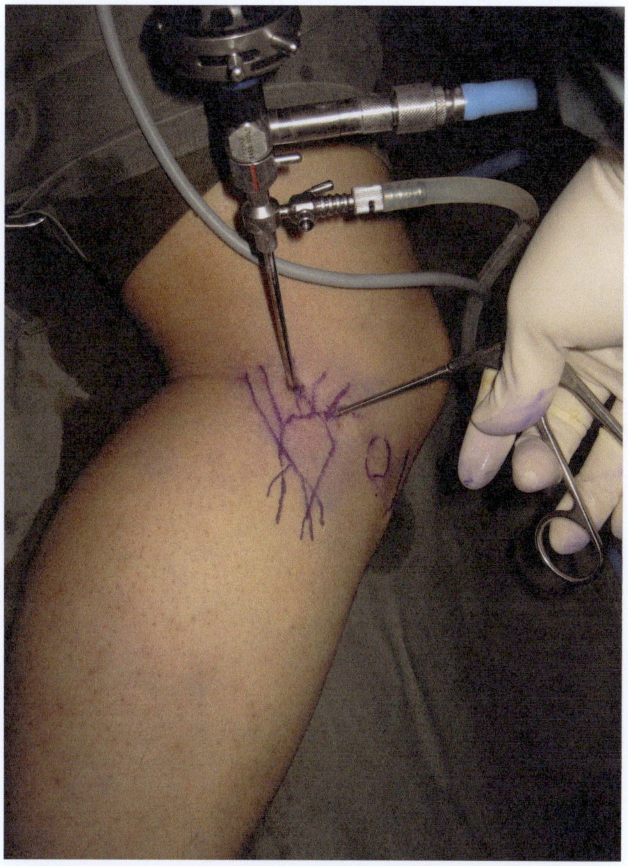

Fig. 11.19 Proximal tibiofibular arthroscopy is performed via the proximal anterior and proximal posterior portals

- The primary working area is the potential space just above the proximal tibiofibular joint which is deep to the lateral collateral ligament and anterior to the biceps femoris tendon. The arthroscopic instruments should point medially.
- After resection of the fatty tissue of the potential space, the lateral collateral ligament, the biceps femoris tendon, and the popliteofibular ligament can be identified.
- The posterolateral corner of the knee can also be reached through the proximal posterior portal.
- The anterior and posterior proximal tibiofibular ligaments can be identified at the anterior and posterior gutters of the joint, respectively.
- The capsule of the proximal tibiofibular joint between the anterior and posterior proximal tibiofibular ligaments is carefully resected with preservation of the ligaments. Intra-articular pathologies of the synovium and cartilage can be approached (Fig. 11.20).
- If this endoscopic is used to deal with bony pathologies of the fibular head, the portals can be placed a bit more distal to the usual positions in order to facilitate approach to the fibular head and avoid hindrance of instrumental mobility by the lateral thigh [67].

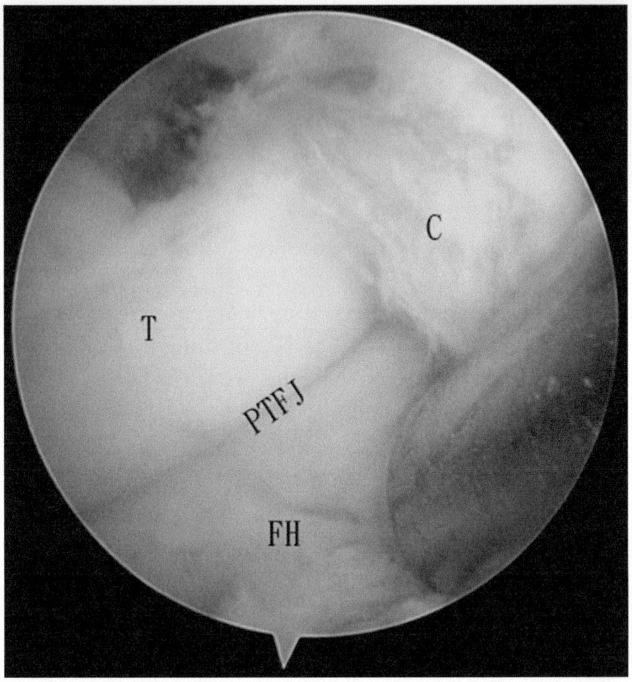

Fig. 11.20 Arthroscopic view shows that the proximal tibiofibular joint (PTFJ) between the proximal tibia (T) and fibular head (FH) is exposed after endoscopic resection of the dorsal capsule (C)

11.3.4.5 Complications and Management

The major risk of this procedure is injury to the common peroneal nerve. The precautions to reduce this complication include:

- Flex the knee during the procedure to relax the common peroneal nerve and displace it away from the operative field
- No arthro-pump is allowed
- Blunt dissection of soft tissue after making the portals should be directed medially
- Arthroscopic instruments should stay anterior to the biceps femoris tendon [35]

11.3.4.6 Post-operative Care

The patient can have weight bearing walking as pain tolerated after synovectomy or ganglionectomy. In patients with internal fixation, ligament reconstruction, or arthrodesis, a period of protected weight bearing and limitation in knee range of motion would be required.

11.3.5 Summary

Endoscopic approach to proximal tibiofibular joint is a feasible alternative to the open approaches. It allows access to the joint and adjacent important ligamentous structures. This may form the basis of further development of arthroscopic procedures of the joint and reconstruction of adjacent capsulo-ligamentous structure.

11.4 Endoscopic Iliotibial Band Lengthening for Distal Iliotibial Band Syndrome

Iciar M. Dávila Castrodad, Matthew J. Kraeutler, and Anthony J. Scillia

11.4.1 Introduction

- Distal iliotibial (IT) band syndrome is a disorder characterized by pain over the lateral aspect of the knee during loading of the lower extremity [68, 69]. This syndrome, which is considered to be one of overuse, was first described in 1975 by Lieutenant Commander James Renee [68]. The authors reported on 16 cases of IT band syndrome among a group of 1000 military recruits. Today, IT band syndrome is diagnosed in a wide array of athletes, most commonly runners and cyclists. This syndrome has been reported in up to 10% of patients with running-related injuries and 15% of cyclists who report problems at the knee [70, 71]. Other authors have reported this injury among skiers, hockey, basketball, and soccer players [72, 73].
- The IT band is a longitudinal fibrous sheath that runs along the lateral thigh. It is the distal fascial continuation of the tensor fascia lata. This band lies superficial to the vastus lateralis and inserts onto Gerdy's tubercle of the lateral tibial plateau [74, 75].
- As an extension of the tensor fascia lata, the IT band stabilizes the hip and also stabilizes the lateral aspect of the knee [76].
- Several theories exist regarding the etiology of the syndrome. Some authors suggest that constant knee flexion during activity leads to repetitive anterior and posterior motion of the IT band, friction on the lateral femoral condyle, and ultimately inflammation. Others believe the pain is derived from compression of the structures deep to the IT band including the richly innervated and vascularized adipose tissue, the bursa, and the lateral synovial recess [77–79]. There is little evidence to suggest that actual thickening, or pathological changes, of the band itself may be the root cause of the syndrome.
- Training, anatomical, and biomechanical risk factors have been associated with IT band syndrome. Improper footwear, changes in training regimen, high weekly mileage, and lack of recovery are several examples of training-related risk factors [80]. Leg-length inequalities, an increased angle of knee flexion, IT band tightness, and weakness of lower extremity muscle groups are considered some of the anatomic and biomechanical risk factors associated with its occurrence [75]. Multiple studies have specifically found hip abductor weakness and increased hip adduction in distal IT band patients [81–83]. When compared to controls, Noehren et al. [83] reported that female runners have been found to have increased hip adduction, knee internal rotation, and femoral external rotation while male runners exhibited increased knee adduction and hip internal rotation. Miller et al. [84] found that 8 of 16 runners with IT band syndrome demonstrated higher angles of knee flexion at heel strike and IT band strain following an exhaustive run.
- Patients with IT band dysfunction may present with lateral knee pain and swelling and can often report that the sharp pain subsides upon cessation of activities. On physical examination, there may be local tenderness at the lateral knee inferior to the epicondyle and superior to the joint line. Several maneuvers have been described to assess IT band status, though their diagnostic accuracy has not been thoroughly assessed. The Noble Compression Test is considered positive when lateral knee pain is reproduced as the knee extends from 90° to 30° [69]. The Ober test is also frequently performed as a measure of IT band tightness, which can range from minimal to maximal depending on the amount of passive adduction of the extremity from the lateral decubitus position [85].
- Given that IT band syndrome is a clinical diagnosis primarily based on patient history and, at times, physical examination findings, other diagnostic studies are not necessary. Radiographic films and magnetic resonance imaging (MRI) can be indicated to rule out osseous conditions or other soft tissue disorders of and around the knee joint. Previous studies have reported on the MRI findings of patients with IT band syndrome. Isusi et al. [86] found an area of high signal intensity deep to the IT band and lateral to the femoral condyle, osseous edema, and subchondral osseous erosion, and no changes to the IT band itself in two male patients diagnosed with IT band syndrome. Similarly, Nishimura et al. [87] found no changes to the integrity of the IT band, but reported local soft tissue inflammation and edema predominantly in its posterior fibers. Muhle et al. [88] evaluated 16 patients

with IT band syndrome and described MRI findings of signal intensity changes and localized fluid collections located medial to the IT band and lateral to the femoral condyle. In their series of six patients with IT band syndrome, Murphy et al. [89] found decreased signal abnormalities deep to the IT band adjacent to the femoral condyle. Ekman et al. [90] compared MRI findings between 7 patients with IT band syndrome and 10 age- and sex-matched controls. The authors identified fluid deep to the IT band in five of the seven patients. In contrast to other studies, they did find a significantly thicker IT band over the lateral femoral condyle. They went on to perform cadaveric dissection on 10 non-pathological knees and found evidence of a potential space, or bursa, between the knee capsule and the IT band. Anesthetic injection has also been used to aid in the diagnosis. Short-term improvement of lateral knee pain symptoms is both diagnostic and therapeutic following injection with corticosteroid.

- Sometimes the pain can radiate proximally along the length of the IT band leading to hip or thigh pain. This more proximal condition can be considered a form of snapping hip syndrome, which is characterized by an audible or palpable snapping during hip motion. IT band motion over the greater trochanter of the proximal femur is considered the primary cause for external, or extra-articular, hip snapping. In this case, treatment options include rest, activity modification, anti-inflammatory medications, and physical therapy. If conservative management fails, surgical treatments including IT band lengthening or release are performed [91].
- In the majority of cases, symptoms subside with conservative measures alone. These include rest, ice, activity and footwear modification, and physiotherapy including deep friction massages. Anti-inflammatory medication and local corticosteroid infiltration have also been described to reduce pain acutely [92, 93]. As symptoms subside, patients are progressed with stretching of the IT band, strengthening of hip abductors, neuromuscular retraining, and final return to regular activity [80].
- Operative treatment is considered in chronic, recurrent, or refractory cases that persist for more than 6 months. Resection of the lateral synovial recess, transection of the posterior fibers of the IT band, bursectomy, and IT band lengthening have been described with favorable results [78, 94–97].

11.4.2 Indications

Patients who have failed conservative measures for a period of 6 months, including rest, ice, activity and shoe wear modification, physiotherapy, anti-inflammatories, corticosteroids, stretching, strengthening, and corrective training.

11.4.3 Contraindications

Active infection and coagulopathy are contraindications for surgery.

11.4.4 Authors' Preferred Technique

11.4.4.1 Pre-operative Planning

- Arthroscopic IT band lengthening is considered after a failed course of conservative management, which is typically a minimum of 6 months.
- Required instrumentation includes a No. 11 blade scalpel, an arthroscopic camera, a spinal needle, an Arthrocare-1 wand (Smith & Nephew), Metzenbaum scissors (Smith & Nephew), and a small surgical instrument set.

11.4.4.2 Patient Positioning

- The patient is placed in a supine position with the affected knee in 30° of flexion to appropriately visualize the IT band. The lateral femoral condyle, the fibular head, and Gerdy's tubercle are identified and marked (Fig. 11.21).

11.4.4.3 Portal Design

- With a No. 11 blade scalpel, a proximal lateral portal is made at the midline of the IT band 10 cm proximal to the epicondyle and a trocar is inserted in the direction of the lateral femoral condyle. The arthroscopic camera is positioned and remains in the portal for the duration of the

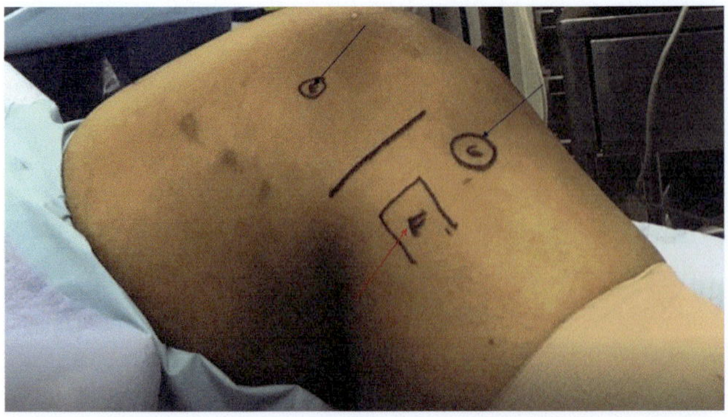

Fig. 11.21 The patient is placed in the supine position and the right knee is flexed to 30°. We have marked the lateral femoral epicondyle (black arrow), the head of the fibula (red arrow), and Gerdy's tubercle (blue arrow). Reprinted with permission from "Arthroscopy Techniques—Iliotibial Band Lengthening: An Arthroscopic Surgical Technique, 2017, In: 6(3):e785-e789"

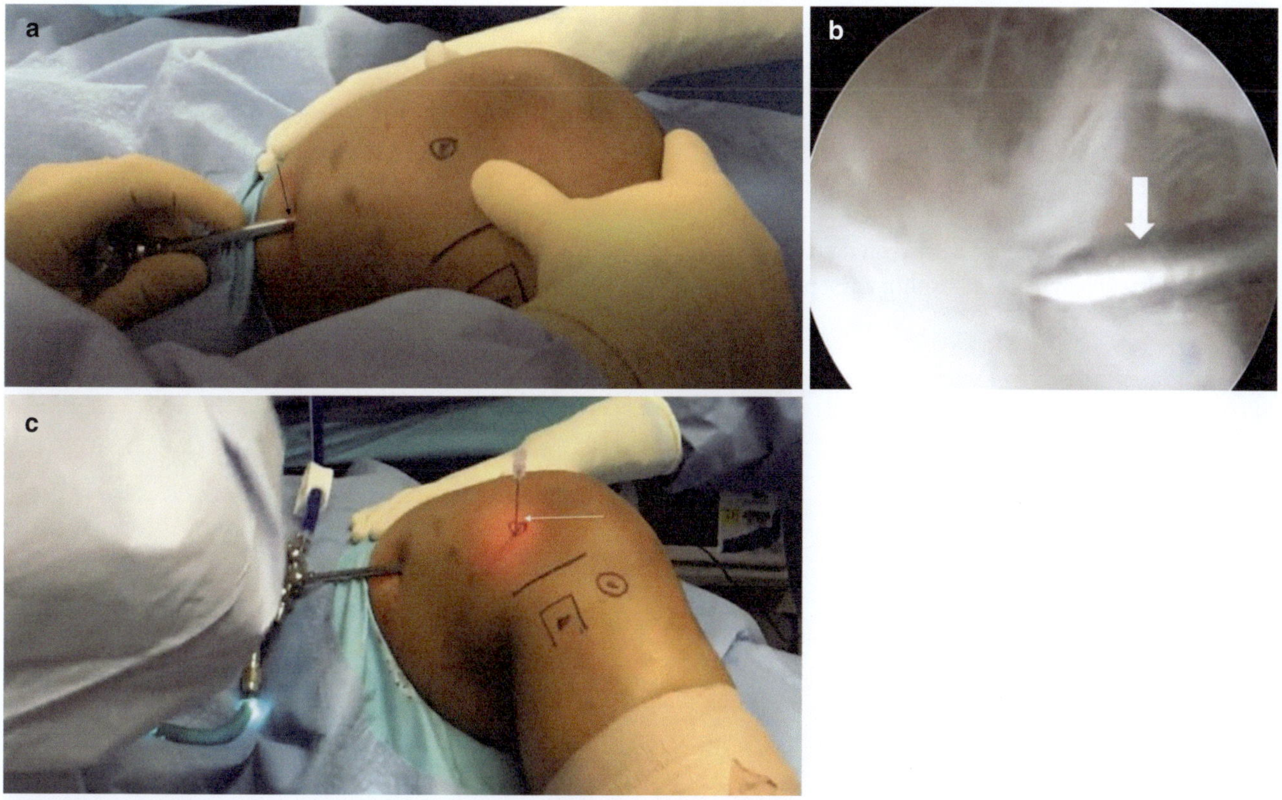

Fig. 11.22 (**a**) While the patient remains supine with the right knee flexed to 30°, the right proximal lateral portal is made using an 11-blade scalpel. The trochar (black arrow) is then inserted with angulation in the direction of the right lateral femoral condyle. The arthroscopic camera is inserted into this proximal portal and remains there for the duration of the procedure. Reprinted with permission from "Arthroscopy Techniques—Iliotibial Band Lengthening: An Arthroscopic Surgical Technique, 2017, In: 6(3):e785-e789". (**b**) and (**c**) A spinal needle (white arrow) is inserted directly over the right lateral femoral epicondyle. It is visualized by the arthroscopic camera, which is located in the right proximal portal. An 11-blade scalpel is used to create the working distal portal directly over the right lateral epicondyle. Reprinted with permission from "Arthroscopy Techniques—Iliotibial Band Lengthening: An Arthroscopic Surgical Technique, 2017, In: 6(3):e785-e789"

procedure (Fig. 11.22a). The insertion point for the distal lateral portal is visualized with a spinal needle, the portal is created with a No. 11 blade, and the IT band is incised longitudinally. The distal lateral portal should be over the lateral femoral epicondyle at the site of the pathology (Fig. 11.22b, c). The arthroscopic camera remains in the proximal lateral portal while the instrumentation will be inserted into the distal lateral portal.

11.4.4.4 Step-by-Step Description of the Technique

- With the shaver inserted through the distal lateral portal, a complete bursectomy is performed deep to the IT band to appropriately visualize the IT band (Fig. 11.23a). An Arthrocare-1 wand (Smith & Nephew, Austin, Texas) is used to achieve hemostasis (Fig. 11.23b).
- In order to create separation between the skin and the IT band, Metzenbaum scissors (Smith & Nephew) are used to spread the tissue over the IT band via the distal lateral portal (Fig. 11.24).
- IT band lengthening is then performed with the Metzenbaum scissors. Through the distal lateral portal, the scissors are inserted to incise the band 2–4 cm proximally, distally, anteriorly, and posteriorly from the point of initial insertion (Fig. 11.25a–d). The Arthrocare-1 wand is utilized to complete the lengthening with care to keep the overlying skin intact (Fig. 11.25e). A complete

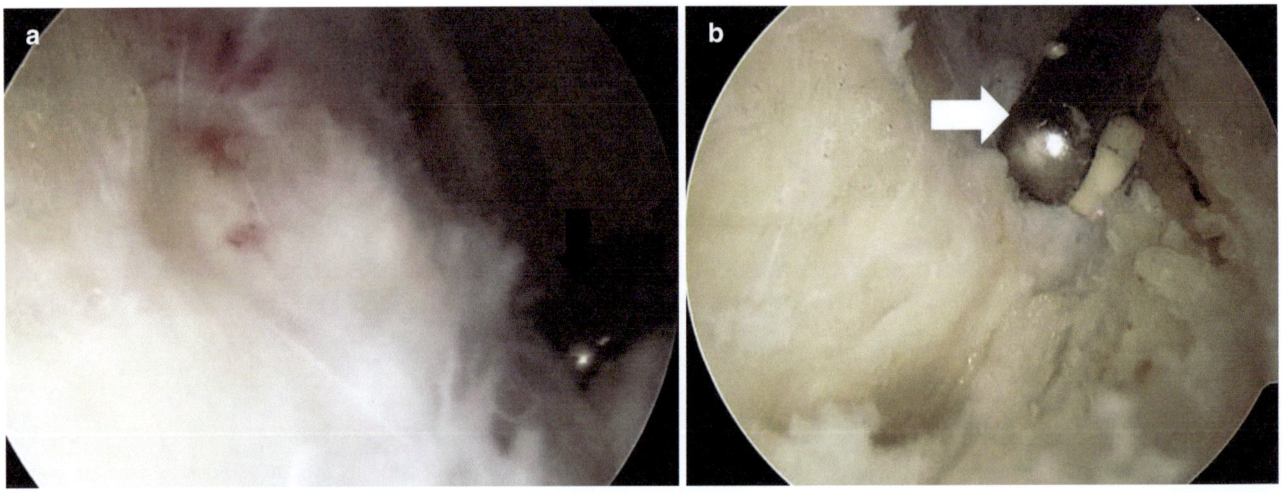

Fig. 11.23 (**a**) A bursectomy is then performed deep to the IT band using an arthroscopic shaver (Smith & Nephew, Austin, Texas) (black arrow) in the right distal lateral portal and the arthroscopic camera within the right proximal lateral portal. Reprinted with permission from "Arthroscopy Techniques—Iliotibial Band Lengthening: An Arthroscopic Surgical Technique, 2017, In: 6(3):e785-e789". (**b**) Once the bursectomy is completed with hemostasis being achieved using the Arthrocare-1 Wand (Smith & Nephew, Austin, Texas) (white arrow) within the right distal lateral portal. The camera remains within the proximal portal during this step. Reprinted with permission from "Arthroscopy Techniques—Iliotibial Band Lengthening: An Arthroscopic Surgical Technique, 2017, In: 6(3):e785-e789"

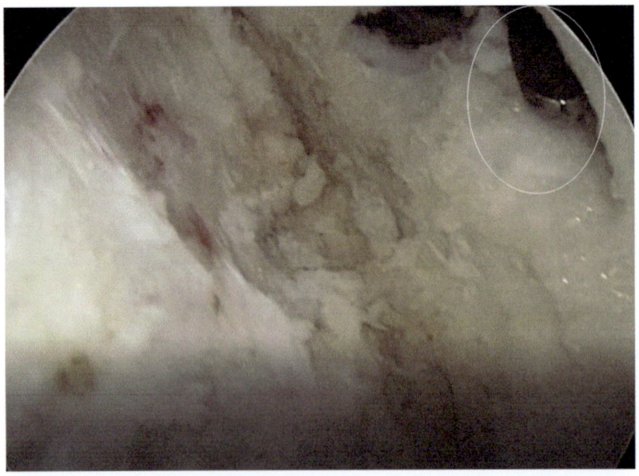

Fig. 11.24 Using the right distal lateral portal, Metzenbaum scissors (Smith & Nephew, Austin, Texas) (circle) are used to spread the tissue of the overlying skin of the IT band, thus protecting the skin during lengthening. Note visualization using the arthroscopic camera occurs via the proximal portal. Reprinted with permission from "Arthroscopy Techniques—Iliotibial Band Lengthening: An Arthroscopic Surgical Technique, 2017, In: 6(3):e785-e789"

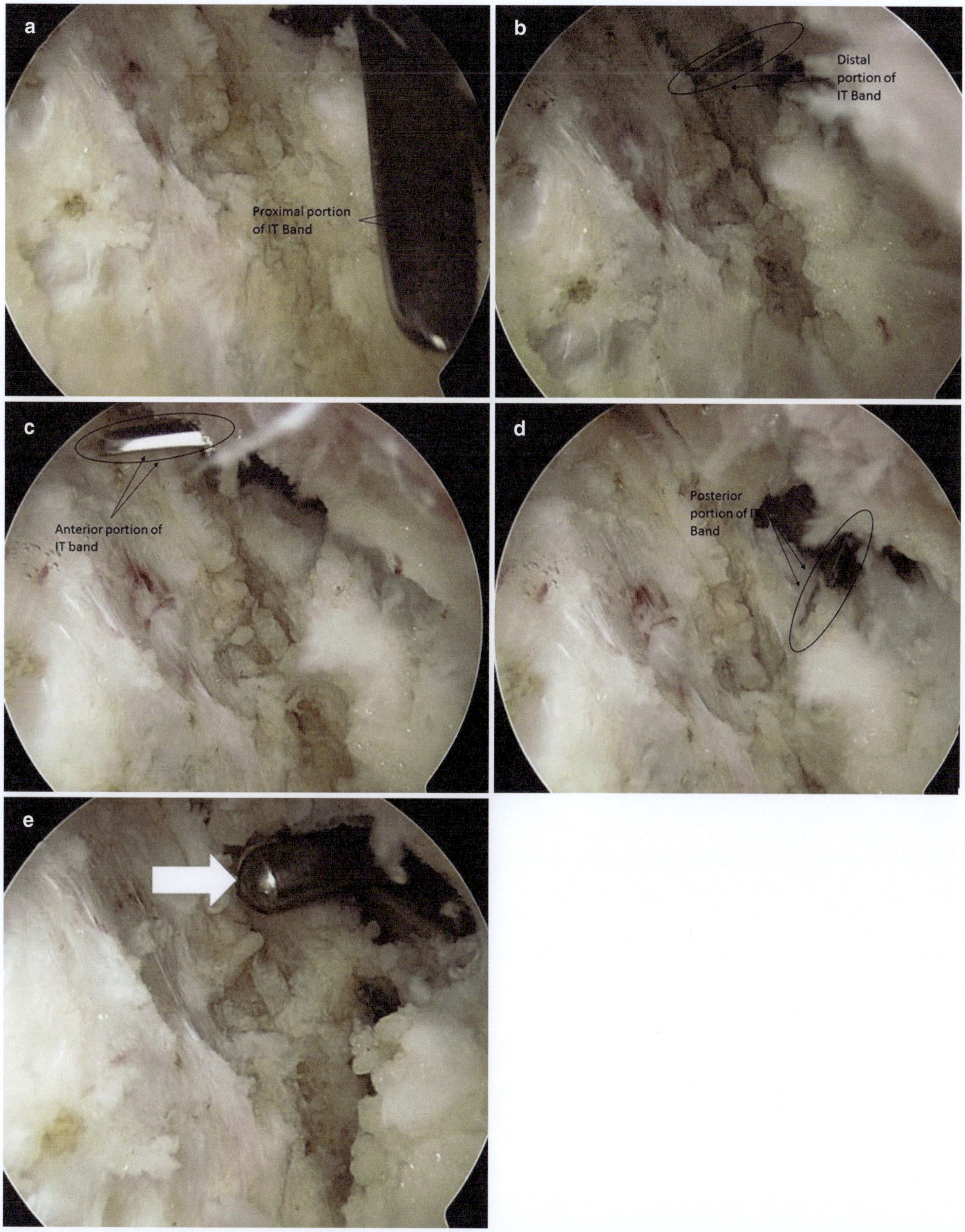

Fig. 11.25 (**a**)–(**d**) With the arthroscopic camera still within the right proximal portal, using the Metzenbaum scissors (circle) inserted into the distal lateral portal (Smith & Nephew, Austin, Texas), the lengthening is performed proximally (**a**), distally (**b**), anteriorly (**c**), and posteriorly (**d**) from its point of insertion at Gerdy's tubercle. Note that black arrows with labels are used to demonstrate the orientation at each dimension of the lengthening. Reprinted with permission from "Arthroscopy Techniques—Iliotibial Band Lengthening: An Arthroscopic Surgical Technique, 2017, In: 6(3):e785-e789". (**e**) The Arthrocare-1 Wand (Smith & Nephew, Austin, Texas) (white arrow) is inserted into the right distal portal is used to complete the lengthening with care taken not to damage the overlying skin. Note the arthroscopic camera remains in the right proximal portal for appropriate visualization. Reprinted with permission from "Arthroscopy Techniques—Iliotibial Band Lengthening: An Arthroscopic Surgical Technique, 2017, In: 6(3):e785-e789"

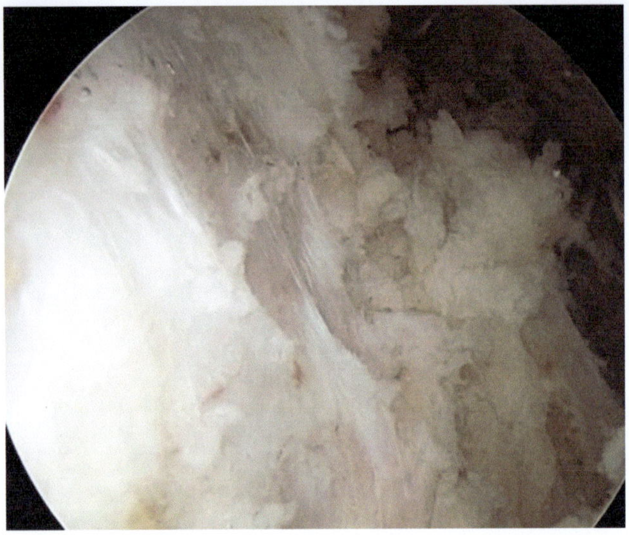

Fig. 11.26 A completed IT band lengthening. Reprinted with permission from "Arthroscopy Techniques—Iliotibial Band Lengthening: An Arthroscopic Surgical Technique, 2017, In: 6(3):e785-e789"

lengthening is necessary to minimize recurrence (Fig. 11.26).

11.4.4.5 Complications

- During the procedure, the overlying skin is at risk of damage without proper separation from the IT band. The risk of recurrence is possible in cases where complete lengthening (proximally, distally, anteriorly, posteriorly) is not achieved.

11.4.4.6 Post-operative Care

- Postoperatively, patients are weight bearing as tolerated with appropriate pain management. Soon after, patients begin physical therapy. Mild stretching and active range of motion exercises are performed. Gradual strengthening exercises are incorporated during rehabilitation with a focus on quadriceps, hamstring, and hip abductors.

11.4.4.7 Outcomes

- Both open and arthroscopic IT band lengthening have shown favorable outcomes. In their case series of 11 patients treated with open IT band lengthening, Hariri et al. demonstrated a significant improvement in pain scores at an average of 38 months postoperatively [78]. They also found that the Tegner activity scores in eight patients (73%) returned to or improved from their preinjury status. In another series of 36 athletes with refractory IT band syndrome, Michels et al. evaluated post-operative outcomes following a completely intra-articular arthroscopic IT band lengthening technique [95] and found that 100% of patients returned to running within 3 months.

11.4.5 Summary

Iliotibial (IT) band syndrome is characterized by lateral knee pain and is common among runners and cyclists. Conservative treatment is often sufficient, but in chronic, recurrent, or refractory cases operative treatment may be indicated.

References

1. Nicaise A. Ganglion articulaire du genou. Rev Chir. 1883;3:463–5.
2. Ebner A. Einfall von Ganglion am Kniegelenksmeniskus Münch. Med Wochenschr. 1904;51:1737–9.
3. Campbell SE, Sanders TG, Morrison WB. MR imaging of meniscal cysts. Am J Roentgenol. 2001;177(2):409–13.
4. Lantz B, Singer KM. Meniscal cysts. Clin Sports Med. 1990;9:707.
5. Barrie HJ. The pathogenesis and significance of meniscal cysts. J Bone Joint Surg. 1979;61:184–9.
6. Terai S, Hashimoto Y, Yamasaki S, Takahashi S, Shimada N, Nakamura H. Prevalence, development, and factors associated with cyst formation after meniscal repair with the all-inside suture device. Arch Orthop Trauma Surg. 2019;139(9):1261–8.
7. Wyss JF, Foye PM, Stitik TP. An infected, extruded lateral meniscal cyst as a cause of knee symptoms. Am J Phys Med Rehabil. 2010;89(3):175–6.
8. Costa M, Marshall T, Donell S, Phillips H. Knee synovial cyst presenting as iliotibial band friction syndrome. Knee. 2004;11(3):247–8.
9. Thompson A, Gallacher P, Rees R. Lateral meniscal cyst causing irreversible peroneal nerve palsy. J Foot Ankle Surg. 2013;52(4):505–7.
10. Jowett A, Johnston J, Gaillard F, Anderson S. Lateral meniscal cyst causing common peroneal palsy. Skelet Radiol. 2008;37(4):351–5.
11. Pisani A. Pathognomonic sign for cyst of the knee cartilage. Arch Surg. 1947;54(2):188.
12. Chen H. Diagnosis and treatment of a lateral meniscal cyst with musculoskeletal ultrasound. Case Rep Orthop. 2015;2015:1–3.
13. Al-Khateeb H, Ruiz A. Lateral meniscal cyst producing lesion of the tibial plateau and literature review. Int J Surg. 2008;6(5):412–4.
14. Dong F, Matthew A, Zhang L, Barrera CM, Xu J, Finkelstein ER, et al. Ultrasound guided aspiration of lateral parameniscal cysts causing iliotibial band friction syndrome. Biomed J Sci Tech Res. 2018;9(4).
15. MacMahon P, Brennan D, Duke D, Forde S, Eustace S. Ultrasound-guided percutaneous drainage of meniscal cysts: preliminary clinical experience. Clin Radiol. 2007;62(7):683–7.
16. Hulet C, Souquet D, Alexandre P, Locker B, Beguin J, Vielpeau C. Arthroscopic treatment of 105 lateral meniscal cysts with 5-year average follow-up. Arthroscopy. 2004;20(8):831–6.
17. Howe T, Koh J. Arthroscopic internal marsupialization of meniscal cysts. Knee. 2007;14(5):408–10.
18. Tudisco C, Meo A, Blasucci C, Ippolito E. Arthroscopic treatment of lateral meniscal cysts using an outside-in technique. Am J Sports Med. 2000;28(5):683–6.
19. Haklar U, Ayhan E, Ustundag S, Canbora K. A new arthroscopic technique for lateral parameniscal cyst decompression. Knee. 2014;21(1):126–8.
20. Chen D, Li Q, Sun Y, Qin J, Yao Y, Jiang Q. Arthroscopic management for the unstable inferior leaf of the lateral meniscus anterior horn and associated cysts through a direct inframeniscal portal: a retrospective study. Biomed Res Int. 2017;2017:9264907.
21. Reagan WD, Mcconkey J, Loomer R, Davidson R. Cysts of the lateral meniscus: arthroscopy versus arthroscopy plus open cystectomy. Arthroscopy. 1989;5(4):274–81.
22. El-Assal M, Mostafa M, Abdel-Aal A, El-Shafee M. Arthroscopy alone or in association with open cystectomy: in treatment of lateral meniscal cysts. Knee Surg Sports Traumatol Arthrosc. 2003;11(1):30–2.
23. Lui TH. Endoscopic resection of lateral synovial cyst of the knee. Arthrosc Tech. 2015;4(6):e815–8.
24. Miskovsky S, Kaeding C, Weis L, Pedroza A. Proximal tibiofibular joint ganglion cysts. Am J Sports Med. 2004;32(4):1022–8.
25. Ogilvie-Harris DJ, Biggs DJ, Mackay M, et al. Posterior portals for arthroscopic surgery of the knee. Arthroscopy. 1994;10(6):608–13.
26. Ahn JH, Ha CW. Posterior trans-septal portal for arthroscopic surgery of the knee joint. Arthroscopy. 2000;16(7):774–9.
27. Kramer DE, Bahk MS, Cascio BM, et al. Posterior knee arthroscopy: anatomy, technique, application. J Bone Joint Surg Am. 2006;88(Suppl 4):110–21.
28. Pace JL, Wahl CJ. Arthroscopy of the posterior knee compartments: neurovascular anatomic relationships during arthroscopic transverse capsulotomy. Arthroscopy. 2010;26(5):637–42. https://doi.org/10.1016/j.arthro.2009.09.009.
29. Ohishi T, Takahashi M, Suzuki D, et al. Arthroscopic approach to the posterior compartment of the knee using a posterior transseptal portal. World J Orthop. 2015;6(7):505.
30. Gillquist J, Hagberg G, Oretorp N. Arthroscopic visualization of the posteromedial compartment of the knee joint. Orthop Clin North Am. 1979;10(3):545–7.
31. Lee JY, Chia ZY, Jiang L, et al. A review of the Gillquist Maneuver: modifications for a safer and easily reproducible approach for knee transintercondylar notch posterior compartment arthroscopy. Arthrosc Tech. 2020;9(4):e435–8. https://doi.org/10.1016/j.eats.2019.11.014.
32. Dilworth B, Fehrenbacher V, Nyland J, et al. Lateral knee compartment portals: a cadaveric study defining a posterolateral viewing safety zone. Arthroscopy. 2018;34(7):2201–6. https://doi.org/10.1016/j.arthro.2018.02.006.
33. Dahuja A, Yang JH, Yoon JR, et al. Loose body as an obstacle for posterolateral arthroscopic portal formation in the knee joint. J Clin Orthop Trauma. 2016;7(3):212–4. https://doi.org/10.1016/j.jcot.2016.02.011.
34. Chai HL, Lui TH. Posterior knee loose bodies: treated by posterior knee arthroscopy. J Orthopaed Case Rep. 2017;7(2):57–61.
35. Lui TH. Arthroscopic treatment of pigmented villonodular synovitis of the proximal tibiofibular joint. Knee Surg Sports Traumatol Arthrosc. 2015;23(8):2278–82.
36. Louisia S, Charrois O, Beaufils P. Posterior "back and forth" approach in arthroscopic surgery on the posterior knee compartments. Arthroscopy. 2003;19(3):321–5.
37. McGinnis MD IV, Gonzalez R, Nyland J, et al. The posteromedial knee arthroscopy portal: a cadaveric study defining a safety zone for portal placement. Arthroscopy. 2011;27(8):1090–5. https://doi.org/10.1016/j.arthro.2011.02.031.
38. Ogden JA. The anatomy and function of the proximal tibiofibular joint. Clin Orthop Relat Res. 1974;101:186–91.
39. Espregueira-Mendes JD, da Silva MV. Anatomy of the proximal tibiofibular joint. Knee Surg Sports Traumatol Arthrosc. 2006;14(3):241–9.
40. Forster BB, Lee JS, Kelly S, et al. Proximal tibiofibular joint: an often-forgotten cause of lateral knee pain. AJR Am J Roentgenol. 2007;188(4):W359–66.
41. Semonian RH, Denlinger PM, Duggan RJ. Proximal tibiofibular subluxation relationship to lateral knee pain: a review of proximal tibiofibular joint pathologies. J Orthop Sports Phys Ther. 1995;21(5):248–57.
42. See A, Bear RR, Owens BD. Anatomic mapping for surgical reconstruction of the proximal tibiofibular ligaments. Orthopedics. 2013;36(1):e58–63.
43. Bozkurt M, Yilmaz E, Atlihan D, et al. The proximal tibiofibular joint. An anatomic study. Clin Orthop Rel Res. 2003;406:136–40.
44. Dirim B, Wangwinyuvirat M, Frank A, et al. Communication between the proximal tibiofibular joint and knee via the subpopliteal recess: MR arthrography with histologic correlation and stratigraphic dissection. Am J Roentgenol. 2008;191(2):W44–51. https://doi.org/10.2214/AJR.07.3406.

45. Bozkurt M, Yilmaz E, Akseki D, et al. The evaluation of the proximal tibiofibular joint for patients with lateral knee pain. Knee. 2004;11(4):307–12.
46. Sundaram K, Klare CM, Moschetti WE. Proximal tibiofibular osteoarthritis presenting as pain after total knee arthroplasty treated successfully with fusion of the proximal tibial-fibular joint. Arthroplast Today. 2018;4(2):139–42. https://doi.org/10.1016/j.artd.2018.02.006.
47. Boya H, Ozcan O, Oztekin HH. Radiological evaluation of the proximal tibiofibular joint in knees with severe primary osteoarthritis. Knee Surg Sports Traumatol Arthrosc. 2008;16(2):157–9.
48. Hirose J, Nishioka H, Nakamura E, et al. T1 and T2 mapping of the proximal tibiofibular joint in relation to aging and cartilage degeneration. Eur J Radiol. 2012;81:2776–82. https://doi.org/10.1016/j.ejrad.2011.11.019.
49. Canna SW, Chauvin NA, Burnham JM. A 17 year old with isolated proximal tibiofibular joint arthritis. Pediatr Rheumatol Online J. 2013;11(1):1. https://doi.org/10.1186/1546-0096-11-1.
50. Wakabayashi H, Nakamura T, Nishimura A, et al. Isolated proximal tibiofibular joint arthritis in a patient with juvenile idiopathic arthritis: a case report. Mod Rheumatol. 2018;28(1):203–6. https://doi.org/10.3109/14397595.2015.1083149.
51. Ogden JA. Subluxation and dislocation of the proximal tibiofibular joint. J Bone Joint Surg Am. 1974;56:145–54.
52. Kruckeberg BM, Cinque ME, Moatshe G, et al. Proximal tibiofibular joint instability and treatment approaches: a systematic review of the literature. Arthroscopy. 2017;33(9):1743–51. https://doi.org/10.1016/j.arthro.2017.03.027.
53. Miskovsky S, Kaeding C, Weis L. Proximal tibiofibular joint ganglion cysts: excision, recurrence, and joint arthrodesis. Am J Sports Med. 2004;32(4):1022–8.
54. Vatansever A, Bal E, Okcu G. Ganglion cysts of the proximal tibiofibular joint review of literature with three case reports. Arch Orthop Trauma Surg. 2006;126(9):637–40.
55. Lateur G, Pailhé R, Refaie R, et al. Ganglion cysts of the proximal tibiofibular articulation: the role of arthrodesis and combined partial fibula excision. Int Orthop. 2018;42(6):1233–9. https://doi.org/10.1007/s00264-017-3542-y.
56. Hersekli MA, Akpinar S, Demirors H, et al. Synovial cysts of proximal tibiofibular joint causing peroneal nerve palsy: report of three cases and review of the literature. Arch Orthop Trauma Surg. 2004;124:711–4.
57. Mortazavi SMJ, Farzan M, Asadollahi S. Proximal tibiofibular joint synovial cyst—one pathology with three different presentations. Knee Surg Sports Traumatol Arthrosc. 2006;14(9):875–9.
58. O'Dwyer KJ. Proximal tibio-fibular synostosis. A rare congenital anomaly. Acta Orthop Belg. 1991;57:204–8.
59. van Ooij B, van Ooij A, Morrenhof JW, van Dijk CN. Proximal tibiofibular synostosis as a possible cause of a pseudoradicular syndrome: a case report. Knee Surg Sports Traumatol Arthrosc. 2011;19(12):2115–8. https://doi.org/10.1007/s00167-010-1379-7.
60. Bozkurt M, Uğurlu M, Doğan M, et al. Synovial chondromatosis of four compartments of the knee: medial and lateral tibiofemoral spaces, patellofemoral joint and proximal tibiofibular joint. Knee Surg Sports Traumatol Arthrosc Jun. 2007;15(6):753–5.
61. Heybeli N, Ozcan M, Copuroglu C, et al. Isolated synovial chondromatosis of the proximal tibiofibular joint. Acta Orthop Traumatol Turc. 2009;43:448–52. https://doi.org/10.3944/AOTT.2009.448.
62. Ryan RS, Louis L, O'Connell JX, et al. Pigmented villonodular synovitis of the proximal tibiofibular joint. Australas Radiol. 2004;48(4):520–2.
63. Beazell JR, Grindstaff TL, Magrum EM, Wilder R. Treatment of lateral knee pain by addressing tibiofibular hypomobility in a recreational runner. N Am J Sports Phys Ther. 2009;4(1):21–8.
64. Alsahhaf A, Renno W. Ganglion cyst at the proximal tibiofibular joint in a patient with painless foot drop. Pain Physician. 2016;19(8):E1147–60.
65. Spinner RJ, Mokhtarzadeh A, Schiefer TK, et al. The clinicoanatomic explanation for tibial intraneural ganglion cysts arising from the superior tibiofibular joint. Skelet Radiol. 2007;36(4):281–92.
66. Chan TW, Lui TH. Proximal tibiofibular joint: an overview. J Orthop Trauma Rehabil. 2016;20(1):2–7. https://doi.org/10.1016/j.jotr.2014.12.002.
67. Lui TH. Endoscopic curettage of bone cyst of the fibular head. Arthrosc Tech. 2017;6(4):e1373–7.
68. Jiménez Díaz F, Gitto S, Sconfienza LM, Draghi F. Ultrasound of iliotibial band syndrome. J Ultrasound. 2020;23:379–85. https://doi.org/10.1007/s40477-020-00478-3.
69. Mellinger S, Neurohr GA. Evidence based treatment options for common knee injuries in runners. Ann Transl Med. 2019;7:S249. https://doi.org/10.21037/atm.2019.04.08.
70. Charles D, Rodgers C. A LITERATURE REVIEW AND CLINICAL COMMENTARY ON THE DEVELOPMENT OF ILIOTIBIAL BAND SYNDROME IN RUNNERS. Int J Sports Phys Ther. 2020;15:460–70.
71. Holmes JC, Pruitt AL, Whalen NJ. Iliotibial band syndrome in cyclists. Am J Sports Med. 1993;21:419–24. https://doi.org/10.1177/036354659302100316.
72. Devan M, Pescatello L, Faghri P, Anderson J. A prospective study of overuse knee injuries among female athletes with muscle imbalances and structural abnormalities. J Athl Train. 2004;39:263–7.
73. Lucas CA. Iliotibial band friction syndrome as exhibited in athletes. J Athl Train. 1992;27:250–2.
74. Hadeed A, Tapscott DC. Iliotibial Band friction syndrome – PubMed. In: StatPearls. https://pubmed.ncbi.nlm.nih.gov/31194342/. Accessed 25 Aug 2020.
75. Lavine R. Iliotibial band friction syndrome. Curr Rev Musculoskelet Med. 2010;3:18–22.
76. Peabody T, Bordoni B. Anatomy, bony pelvis and lower limb, fascia lata. 2020.
77. Fairclough J, Hayashi K, Toumi H, et al. The functional anatomy of the iliotibial band during flexion and extension of the knee: implications for understanding iliotibial band syndrome. J Anat. 2006;208:309–16. https://doi.org/10.1111/j.1469-7580.2006.00531.x.
78. Hariri S, Savidge ET, Reinold MM, et al. Treatment of recalcitrant iliotibial band friction syndrome with open iliotibial band bursectomy: indications, technique, and clinical outcomes. Am J Sports Med. 2009;37:1417–24. https://doi.org/10.1177/0363546509332039.
79. Nemeth WC, Sanders BL. The lateral synovial recess of the knee: anatomy and role in chronic iliotibial band friction syndrome. Arthroscopy. 1996;12:574–80. https://doi.org/10.1016/S0749-8063(96)90197-8.
80. McKay J, Maffulli N, Aicale R, Taunton J. Iliotibial band syndrome rehabilitation in female runners: a pilot randomized study. J Orthop Surg Res. 2020;15:188. https://doi.org/10.1186/s13018-020-01713-7.
81. Fredericson M, Cookingham CL, Chaudhari AM, et al. Hip abductor weakness in distance runners with iliotibial band syndrome. Clin J Sport Med. 2000;10:169–75. https://doi.org/10.1097/00042752-200007000-00004.
82. Macmahon JM, Chaudhari AM, Andriacchi TP. BIOMECHANICAL INJURY PREDICTORS FOR MARATHON RUNNERS: STRIDING TOWARDS ILIOTIBIAL BAND SYNDROME INJURY PREVENTION. 2000.
83. Noehren B, Davis I, Hamill J. ASB Clinical Biomechanics Award Winner 2006. Prospective study of the biomechanical factors asso-

ciated with iliotibial band syndrome. Clin Biomech. 2007;22:951–6. https://doi.org/10.1016/j.clinbiomech.2007.07.001.
84. Miller RH, Lowry JL, Meardon SA, Gillette JC. Lower extremity mechanics of iliotibial band syndrome during an exhaustive run. Gait Posture. 2007;26:407–13. https://doi.org/10.1016/j.gaitpost.2006.10.007.
85. Gajdosik RL, Sandler MM, Marr HL. Influence of knee positions and gender on the Ober test for length of the iliotibial band. Clin Biomech. 2003;18:77–9. https://doi.org/10.1016/S0268-0033(02)00168-7.
86. Isusi Fontán M, Oleaga L, Campo M, Grande D. MRI findings in iliotibial band friction syndrome: a report of two cases. Radiologia. 2007;49:433–5. https://doi.org/10.1016/S0033-8338(07)73816-X.
87. Nishimura G, Yamato M, Tamai K, et al. MR findings in iliotibial band syndrome. Skelet Radiol. 1997;26:533–7. https://doi.org/10.1007/s002560050281.
88. Muhle C, Ahn JM, Yeh LR, et al. Iliotibial band friction syndrome: MR imaging findings in 16 patients and MR arthrographic study of six cadaveric knees. Radiology. 1999;212:103–10. https://doi.org/10.1148/radiology.212.1.r99jl29103.
89. Murphy BJ, Hechtman KS, Uribe JW, et al. Iliotibial band friction syndrome: MR imaging findings. Radiology. 1992;185:569–71. https://doi.org/10.1148/radiology.185.2.1410374.
90. Ekman EF, Pope T, Martin DF, Curl WW. Magnetic resonance imaging of iliotibial band syndrome. Am J Sports Med. 1994;22:851–4. https://doi.org/10.1177/036354659402200619.
91. Pierce TP, Kurowicki J, Issa K, et al. External snapping hip: a systematic review of outcomes following surgical intervention: external snapping hip systematic review. HIP Int. 2018;28:468–72.
92. Gunter P, Schwellnus MP. Local corticosteroid injection in iliotibial band friction syndrome in runners: a randomised controlled trial. Br J Sports Med. 2004;38:269–72. https://doi.org/10.1136/bjsm.2003.000283.
93. Schwellnus M, Theunissen L, Noakes T, Reinach S. Anti-inflammatory and combined anti-inflammatory/analgesic medication in the early management of iliotibial band friction syndrome. A clinical trial. South African Med J. 1991;79:602–6.
94. Drogset JO, Rossvoll I, Grøntvedt T. Surgical treatment of iliotibial band friction syndrome: a retrospective study of 45 patients. Scand J Med Sci Sports. 1999;9:296–8. https://doi.org/10.1111/j.1600-0838.1999.tb00249.x.
95. Michels F, Jambou S, Allard M, et al. An arthroscopic technique to treat the iliotibial band syndrome. Knee Surg Sports Traumatol Arthrosc. 2009;17:233–6. https://doi.org/10.1007/s00167-008-0660-5.
96. Pierce TP, Mease SJ, Issa K, et al. Iliotibial band lengthening: an arthroscopic surgical technique. Arthrosc Tech. 2017;6:e785–9. https://doi.org/10.1016/j.eats.2017.02.010.
97. Walbron P, Jacquot A, Geoffroy JM, et al. Iliotibial band friction syndrome: an original technique of digastric release of the iliotibial band from Gerdy's tubercle. Orthop Traumatol Surg Res. 2018;104:1209–13. https://doi.org/10.1016/j.otsr.2018.08.013.

Posterior Knee Endoscopy

12

Tun Hing Lui, Adrian Góralczyk, Konrad Malinowski, Lukas Rasulić, Milan Lepić, Rui Yang, and Yi Long

Abstract

Popliteal cyst is a common condition of popliteal region and usually coexists with intra-articular pathologies. Typically it is an extension of the natural gastrocnemius-semimembranosus bursa caused by one-way joint fluid leakage to the bursa through existing valvular mechanism. If symptomatic, the popliteal cyst should be treated surgically. The most effective treatment involves correction of intra-articular pathologies, elimination of the valvular mechanism, and excision of cystic walls. In this chapter we present an arthroscopic technique of typical popliteal cyst treatment addressing each step of pathophysiological pathway of cyst formation.

The sural nerve is the most commonly used donor nerve in peripheral nerve and brachial plexus surgery. The grafts may reach up to 40 cm in length from one sided sural nerve harvest depending on the leg size. Graft harvesting procedure results in an acceptable donor site deficit, but the incision extending over the whole lower leg may both compromise cosmetic appearances and predispose subsequent regional complications. Endoscopic harvest preserves the best of both worlds, maintaining the small incision, with complete graft extraction and preservation.

The outside-in method is widely performed for suturing the anterior horn of the lateral meniscus, however, it has some disadvantages including skin incision and superficial knots. The all-inside devices were hard to be applied in anterior half of lateral meniscus (AHLM) due to the limited angle under arthroscopy. The safe Larai portal is developed as a feasible alternative to repair tears of the AHLM by all-inside devices under direct arthroscopic visualization.

The corresponding author of section 12.1 is Konrad Malinowski, Email: konrad.malinowski@artromedical.pl
The corresponding author of section 12.2 is Lukas Rasulić, Email: lukas.rasulic@gmail.com
The corresponding author of section 12.3 is Rui Yang, Email: yangr@mail.sysu.edu.cn

T. H. Lui (✉)
Department of Orthopaedics and Traumatology, North District Hospital, Hong Kong, China

The Second Affiliated Hospital, Shenzhen University, Shenzhen, China

A. Góralczyk
Ortim Orthopedic Clinic, Bialystok, Poland
e-mail: a.goralczyk1@spzoz-bielsk.pl

K. Malinowski
Artromedical Orthopedic Clinic, Belchatow, Poland
e-mail: konrad.malinowski@artromedical.pl

L. Rasulić
Faculty of Medicine, University of Belgrade, Belgrade, Serbia

Department of Peripheral Nerve Surgery, Functional Neurosurgery and Pain Management Surgery, Clinic for Neurosurgery, Clinical Center of Serbia, Belgrade, Serbia

M. Lepić
Faculty of Medicine, University of Belgrade, Belgrade, Serbia

Medical Faculty of the Military Medical Academy, University of Defence, Belgrade, Serbia

Clinic for Neurosurgery, Military Medical Academy, Belgrade, Serbia

R. Yang · Y. Long
Department of Orthopedics, Sun Yat-sen Memorial Hospital, Sun Yat-sen University, Guangzhou, Guangdong, China
e-mail: yangr@mail.sysu.edu.cn

© The Author(s), under exclusive license to Springer Nature Singapore Pte Ltd. 2021
T. H. Lui (ed.), *Endoscopy of the Hip and Knee*, https://doi.org/10.1007/978-981-16-3488-8_12

Keywords

Popliteal cyst · Baker's cyst · Endoscopy · Valvular mechanism · Fluid overproduction · Cyst excision Peripheral nerve · Brachial plexus · Nerve repair · Sural nerve · Larai portal · All-inside · Arthroscopy · Anterior half of lateral meniscus · Meniscus tear

12.1 Endoscopic Treatment of Popliteal Cysts

Adrian Góralczyk and Konrad Malinowski

12.1.1 Introduction

A popliteal cyst, commonly called Baker's cyst, is a frequent pathology meet in everyday orthopedic practice. Affected patients usually complain on symptoms as posterior knee pain, knee stiffness, limited knee flexion at the end of the day or palpable mass, and feeling of fullness in the popliteal region, depending on the size and location of the cyst [1, 2]. However, it is important to remember that in adults almost all popliteal cysts are secondary and thus should be treated rather as an indicator of intra-articular pathologies than the disease itself [2]. In fact, the popliteal cyst usually is an enlargement of a natural gastrocnemius-semimembranosus bursa located in the posteromedial part of the knee [3]. The pathomechanism of its development is well-investigated and two main factors, namely excessive joint fluid production and valvular mechanism in the posteromedial joint capsule play the key roles in this process [2–4]. Common knee pathologies as meniscal tears, chondral lesions, or different types of instabilities are observed in as much as 94% of patients with popliteal cysts [5, 6]. All of them are responsible for an overproduction of synovial fluid and increase in an intra-articular pressure which lead to fluid extravasation to gastrocnemius-semimembranosus bursa through the existing in almost a half of population natural connection in the posteromedial capsule [7]. Further, the posteromedial fold that in most cases works as a valve allows only for a unidirectional fluid flow to the bursa during knee extension and precludes its evacuation during knee flexion [7]. To summarize, *synovial fluid overproduction, increased intra-articular pressure, and valvular mechanism allowing for unidirectional fluid flow are responsible for development and enlargement of popliteal cyst leading to symptoms.*

Conservative treatment involving fluid evacuation, intra-articular or intra-cystic steroids injections, or sclerotherapy is just a temporary solution and is not effective, especially in case of osteoarthritic changes [3, 8]. Surgical treatment is a gold standard of popliteal cyst management and many surgical techniques were developed for addressing this pathology. Open surgical procedures are associated with extensive approach, high risk of important anatomical structures injuries, potential risk of wound complications, prolonged recovery time and provide an unacceptable risk of cyst recurrence [1, 4, 5]. One of the main reasons of ineffectiveness of classic surgeries has been explained in the literature through the lack of addressing concomitant intra-articular pathologies involved in cyst development [9]. The importance of managing articular lesions concurrently with treatment of the cyst itself has been broadly outlined in the literature and thus, arthroscopic techniques have become the treatment of choice [3, 5, 6, 9, 10]. On the other hand, elimination of only the intra-articular lesions appears to be not enough to resolve the problem with popliteal cyst [5]. Arthroscopy allows for concomitant pathologies treatment, provides easy access to cyst decompression, and is characterized with minimal invasiveness and fast recovery [11, 12]. The controversies appear around the method of dealing with valvular mechanism. Whereas some authors suggest that valvular mechanism should be corrected by closing the posteromedial fold, others favor broad opening of the posteromedial fold that allows to re-establish the natural bidirectional fluid flow between the knee joint and gastrocnemius-semimembranosus bursa [1, 5]. We support the second approach because the data suggests that valvular-closing surgeries provide lower success rate (84.6% vs 96.7%), higher recurrence rate due to persistent high pressure in the cyst and finally, the connection between the knee joint and bursa is a normal anatomical variant [5, 7, 9, 13]. The last point of a broad discussion is whether ones should excise or not the cyst walls. The literature suggests that cyst walls excision may be associated with lower rate of recurrence (0 vs 8%), higher rate of overall success (98.2% vs 94.7%), but also with more intraoperative and postoperative complications (6.5% vs 1.6%) and longer operative time [4, 9, 14]. However, it is suggested that cyst wall excision should be popularized especially among the experienced and skilled knee surgeons [9]. To summarize, *the most up-to-date data evidence that the most effective management on popliteal cyst is an arthroscopic treatment of concomitant intra-articular pathologies with opening of the valvular mechanism and cystic walls excision* [3, 7–19].

Based on a 17-years experience in arthro/endoscopic treatment of popliteal cysts of the senior author (K.M) we support the approach to address the whole pathophysiological pathway of popliteal cyst development. In our opinion that is only way to treat our patients effectively. In this chapter we present a simple, safe, and effective technique of typical popliteal cyst arthroscopic treatment with valvular mechanism opening and cyst wall excision. We also show how to manage with demanding, atypical popliteal cysts. At the end we present some pearls and pitfalls which facilitate effective and safe maneuvering in the "dark side of the knee."

12.1.2 Indications

Presented procedure is indicated for symptomatic popliteal cysts diagnosed with clinical and radiological examination (Fig. 12.1).

12.1.3 Contraindications

The procedure should not be performed in case of cysts which are not typical "popliteal" ones: an aneurysm, a varicose, cysts developed in location other than gastrocnemius-semimembranosus bursa, as well as in patients with limited knee flexion below 80–90° and unacceptable general risk of surgery.

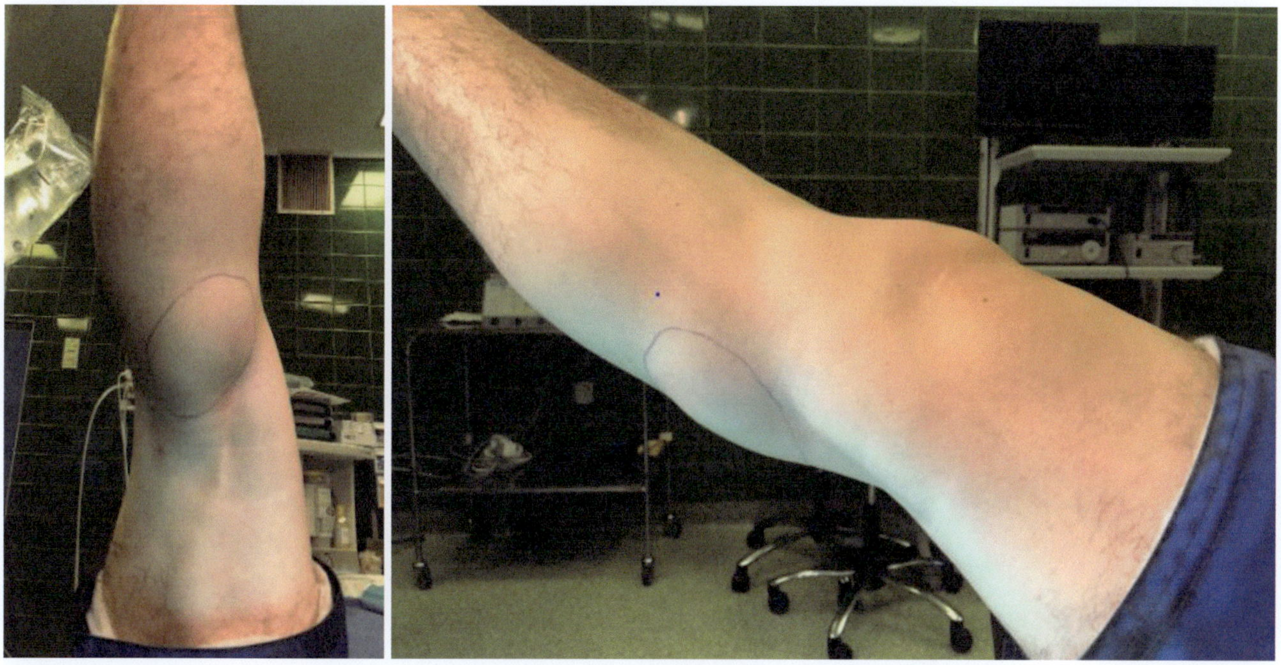

Fig. 12.1 Typical clinically symptomatic cyst in the popliteal region of the right knee

12.1.4 Author Preferred Technique

12.1.4.1 Preoperative Planning

Each patient scheduled for an arthroscopic treatment of popliteal cyst should have an MRI performed to diagnose concomitant intra-articular lesions and to determine the main features of the cyst. One should focus on the size of the cyst, its connection with the joint cavity, its location-neighborhood of popliteal neurovascular bundle, and other important muscular and tendinous structures (Fig. 12.2). It allows to plan adequate arthroscopic portals placement and exclude atypical cysts, which could be contraindications for surgery. If any doubt occurs, Doppler ultrasound exam may be helpful to determine the position of lateral wall of the cyst in relation

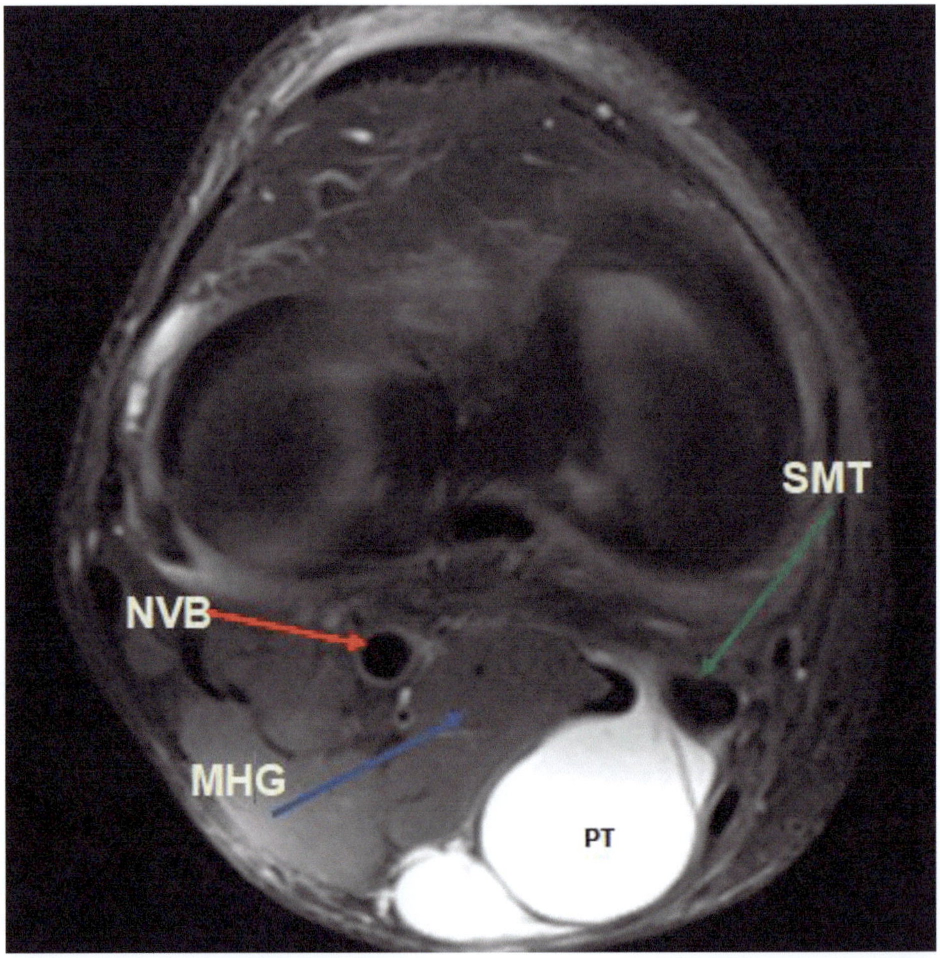

Fig. 12.2 Axial MRI scan of the right knee. Popliteal cyst (PT) with connection to the knee joint. The cyst is located typically between the medial head of gastrocnemius (MHG) and semimembranosus (SMT). Note that the lateral wall of popliteal cyst is separated from popliteal neurovascular bundle (NVB) by the medial head of gastrocnemius

to popliteal neurovascular bundle (Fig. 12.3). Remember that *typical popliteal cyst should be well separated from the popliteal neurovascular bundle with medial head of gastrocnemius.*

12.1.4.2 Patient Positioning

For typical popliteal cysts the patient is positioned supine with the knee placed in a leg support that it is possible to flex the knee above 90°. A non-sterile thigh tourniquet is placed

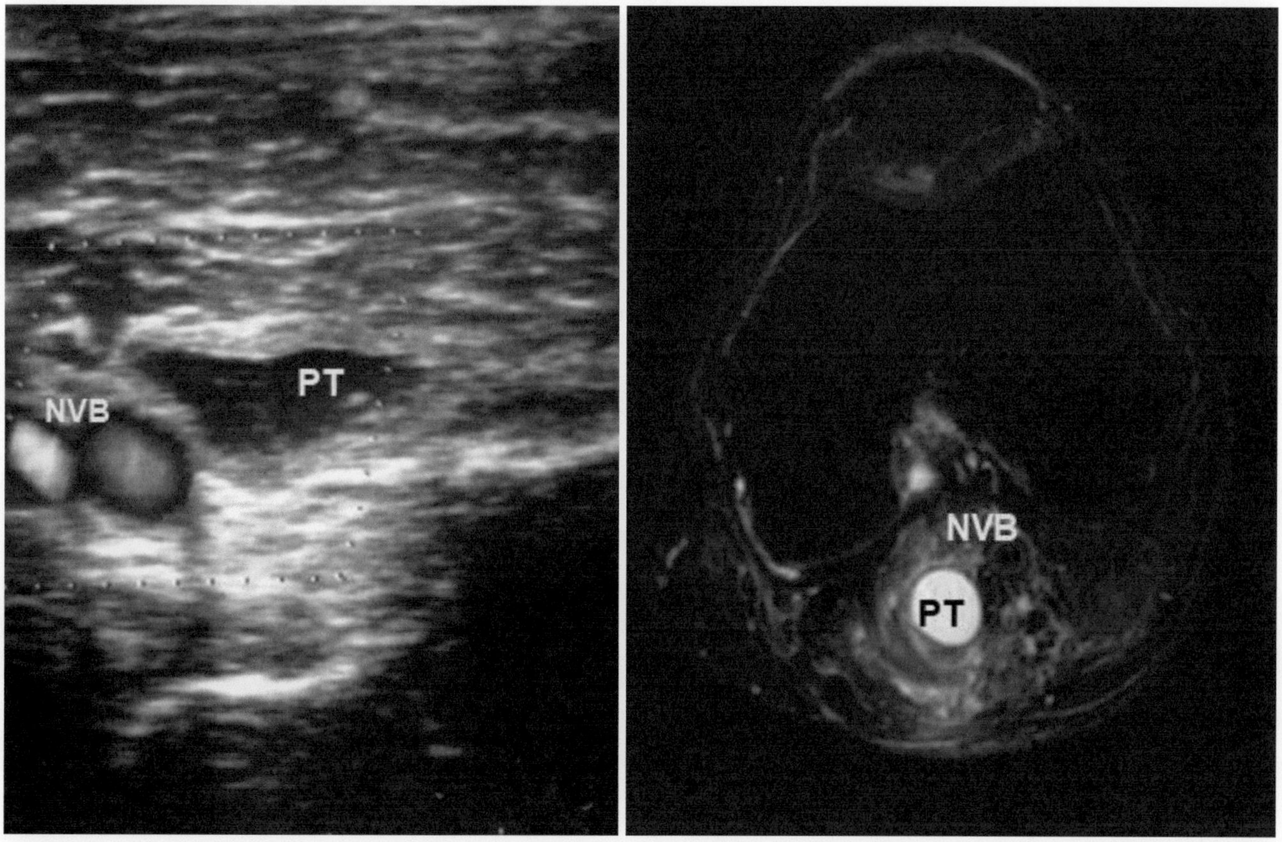

Fig. 12.3 Ultrasound examination (left) and axial MRI scan (right) of the popliteal cyst (PT). The lateral wall of the cyst is located in a close proximity to the popliteal neurovascular bundle (NVB). Atypical location of the cyst is visible on MRI

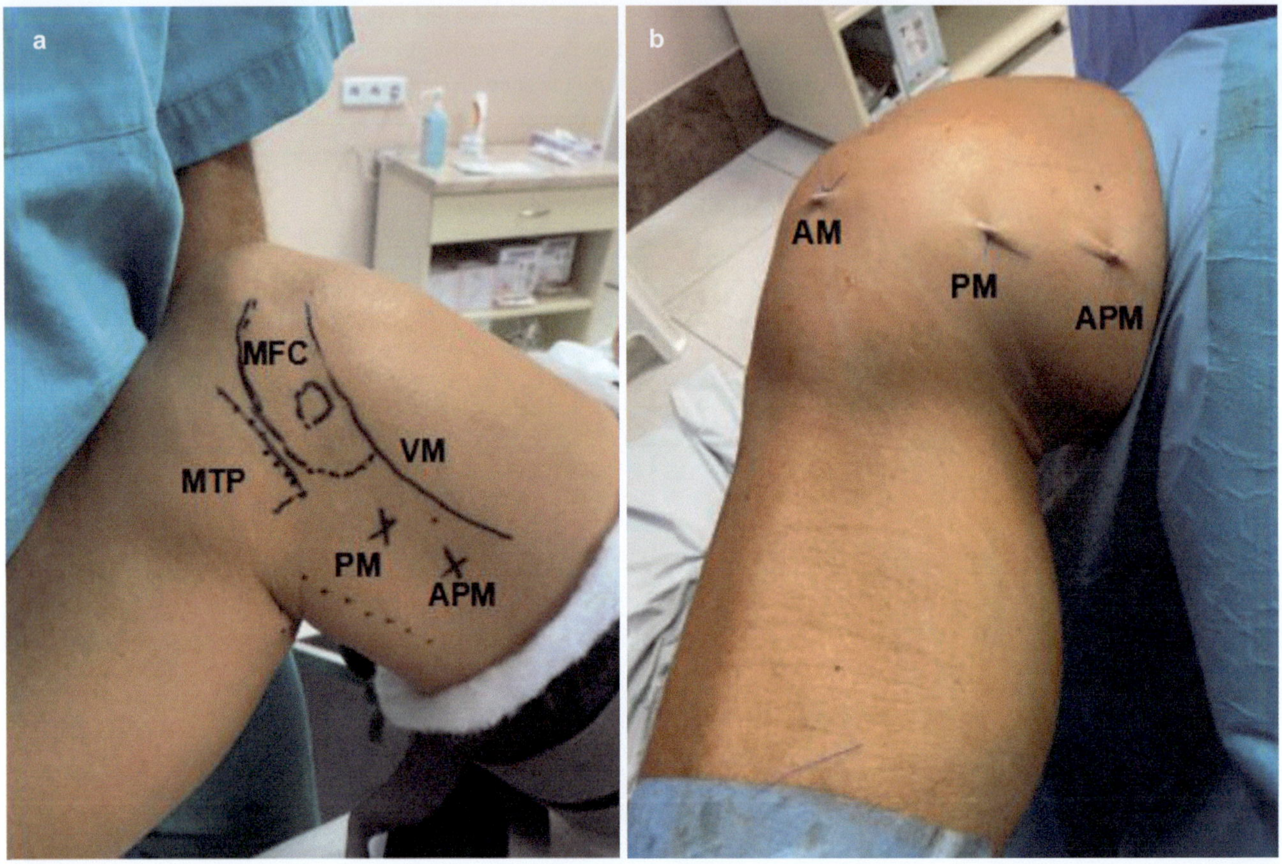

Fig. 12.4 (**a**) The right knee before surgery. The positions of posteromedial (PM) portal and additional posteromedial (APM) portal are located between the vastus medialis (VM, solid line) and hamstrings tendons (dashed line) 3–7 cm proximal to the medial joint line. *MFC* medial femoral condyle, *MTP* medial tibial plateau. (**b**) The medial side of the right knee after surgery. The positions of anteromedial (AM), posteromedial (PM), and additional posteromedial (APM) portals are presented

high at the thigh and inflated to avoid excessive bleeding and disrupted visualization through the procedure. The knee is prepared and draped in a sterile fashion (Fig. 12.4). For atypical popliteal cysts which are large, descends to the calf, or lie adjacently to the popliteal neurovascular bundle the patient may be positioned prone when all intra-articular procedures are finished. The procedure is performed under regional or general anesthesia.

12.1.4.3 Diagnostic Arthroscopy and Treatment of Concomitant Intra-articular Pathologies

The diagnostic arthroscopy is performed through standard anterolateral and anteromedial portals. If concomitant intra-articular lesions exist, they should be treated at first. If the cyst is addressed before intra-articular pathologies, the risk of fluid extravasation into the cyst and, theoretically, risk of compartment syndrome development increases. *Pay attention to properly diagnose and treat concomitant lesions. If left untreated, the chance for resolve the popliteal cysts decreases.*

12.1.4.4 Typical Popliteal Cyst Treatment

At the beginning of the "popliteal" part of the procedure the arthroscope should be placed in the posteromedial compartment of the knee. To do it, the so-called trans-notch maneuver is performed. With the knee in a slight flexion a mild valgus stress is applied and the arthroscope introduced through the anterolateral portal is pushed through the space between posterior cruciate ligament (PCL) superiorly, lateral wall of medial femoral condyle (MFC) medially, and posterior horn of medial meniscus (MM) inferiorly, to the posteromedial compartment (Fig. 12.5). The rest of procedure is performed with the knee flexed to 90°. In cases of typical connection between the knee joint and gastrocnemius-semimembranosus bursa, posteromedial fold and medial border of tendinous part of gastrocnemius should be visualized (Fig. 12.6). The entrance to the cyst is usually located just behind the fold, between the medial margin of the medial head of gastrocnemius and the lateral margin of the semimembranosus. The valve and the entrance to the cyst should be identified percutaneously using a spinal needle (Fig. 12.6). In the next step the posteromedial portal is created under visual control just above the posteromedial fold, 5–8 mm medially to the medial margin of medial head of gastrocnemius. Transillumination may be helpful to determine the position of saphenous vein and nerve to avoid their injury during portal formation. Under visual control the shaver and radiofrequency probe are sequentially introduced through posteromedial portal and used to excise the posteromedial fold and other tissue that

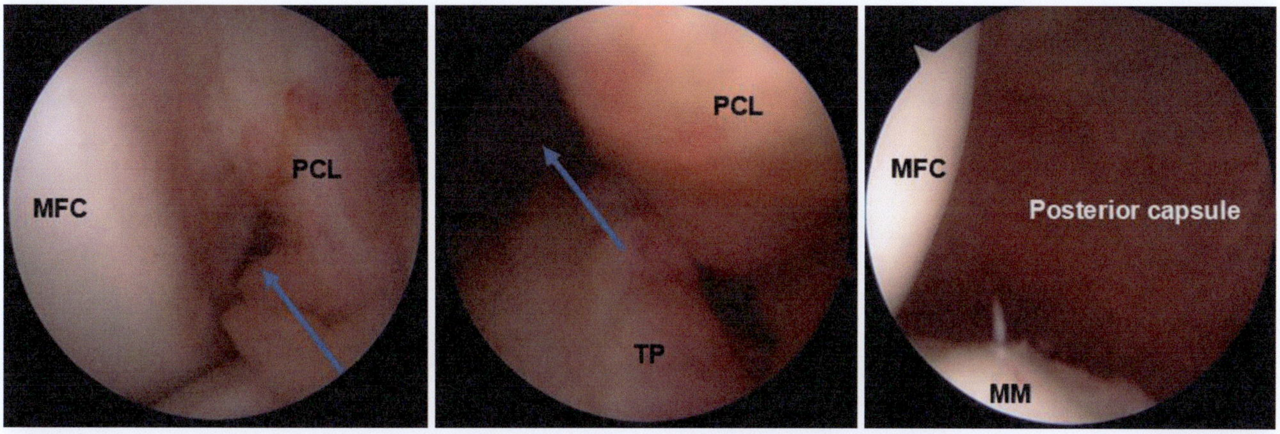

Fig. 12.5 Arthroscopic view from anterolateral portal in the left knee. Following steps of "trans-notch" maneuver. With the knee in a slight flexion a mild valgus stress is applied and the arthroscope introduced through the anterolateral portal is pushed through the space between posterior cruciate ligament (PCL) superiorly, lateral wall of medial femoral condyle (MFC) medially, and posterior horn of medial meniscus (MM) inferiorly, to the posteromedial compartment. The blue arrow determines a proper course of arthroscope. *TP* tibial plateau

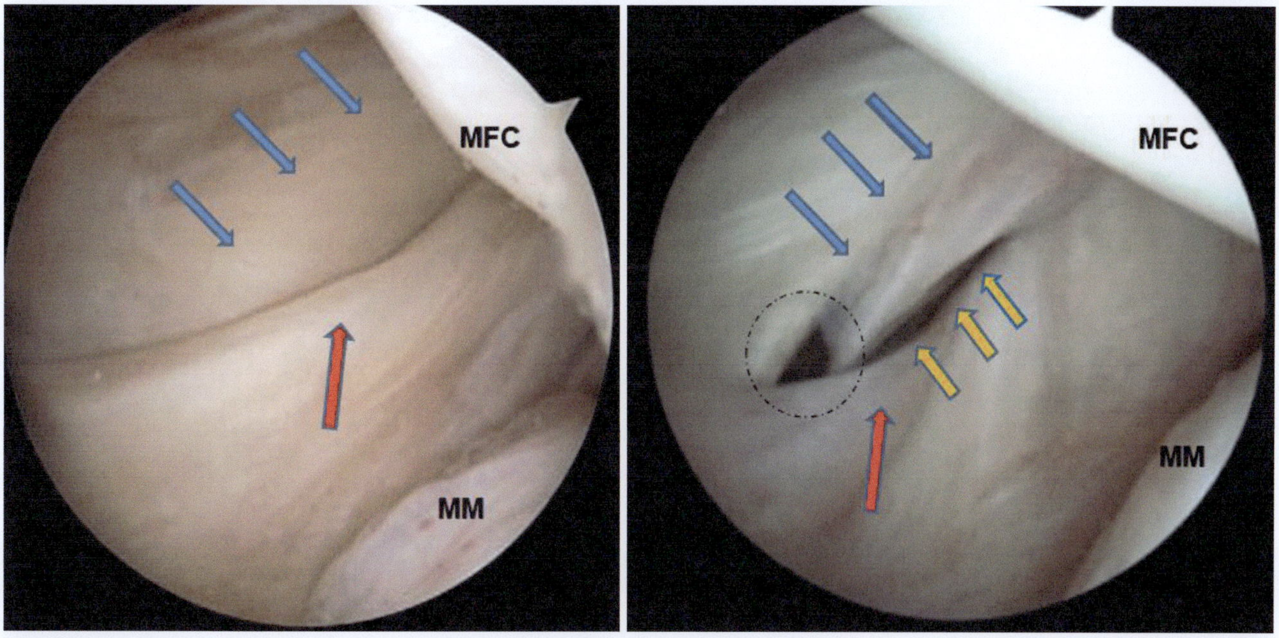

Fig. 12.6 Arthroscopic view from the anterolateral viewing portal after trans-notch maneuver in the right knee. Posteromedial compartment. The entrance to the cyst (black dotted circle) is usually located just behind the posteromedial fold (red arrow), medially to the course of medial head of gastrocnemius (blue arrows). The needle (yellow arrows) pierced through skin may be helpful to depress posteromedial synovial fold to determine the cyst entrance. *MFC* medial femoral condyle, *MM* medial meniscus

could act as a valve to enlarge the communication between the cyst and the joint and to restore the bidirectional fluid flow (Fig. 12.7). It is extremely important to keep the working side of instruments directed anteriorly and medially, away from popliteal neurovascular bundle and not to use an aggressive shaver tip. In the last step of procedure, the arthroscope is pushed forward inside the cyst. The shaver is introduced subcutaneously through posteromedial portal, carefully moved dorsally along the medial wall of the cyst with the visual control of the position of its tip, introduced to the cyst through the medial wall and used to excise it (Fig. 12.8). Other walls are also resected using the shaver. At

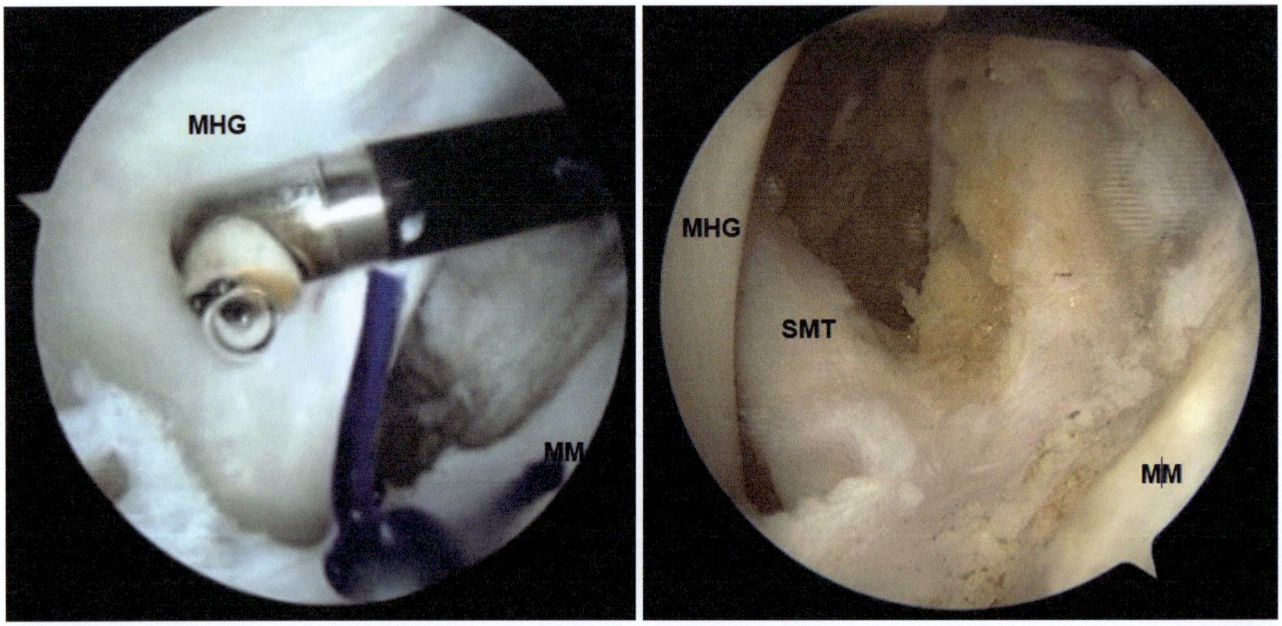

Fig. 12.7 Arthroscopic view from the anterolateral viewing portal in the right knee. Posteromedial compartment. Radiofrequency probe is used to remove posteromedial fold and all soft tissue limiting bidirectional fluid flow between the popliteal cyst and the knee joint. On the right the bidirectional fluid flow has been restored. *MHG* medial head of gastrocnemius, *SMT* semimembranosus tendon, *MM* medial meniscus (on the left after repair the RAMP lesion)

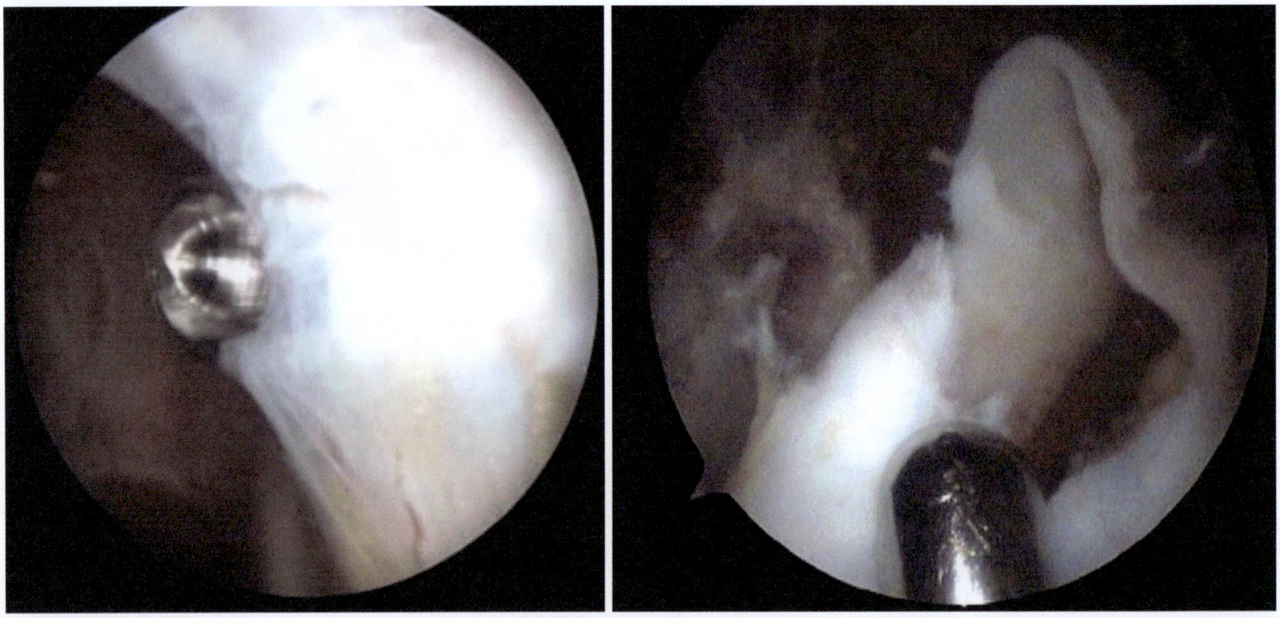

Fig. 12.8 Arthroscopic view from the anterolateral viewing portal in the right knee. Arthroscope inside the popliteal cyst. The shaver introduced through posteromedial portal subcutaneously is used to remove cystic walls. Note that the non-aggressive tip of the shaver is directed away from popliteal neurovascular bundle

the end of the procedure, the arthroscope is moved back and the bidirectional fluid flow is inspected. Each tissue which may limit unrestricted fluid flow should be removed with shaver or radiofrequency probe.

Sometimes the posteromedial fold and the entrance to the cyst are not clearly visible, but the existence of popliteal cyst is known based on preoperative imaging. In this situation the posteromedial portal should be placed 5–8 mm medially to the medial margin of the medial head of gastrocnemius just above the level of posterior horn of MM. The shaver and radiofrequency probe should be introduced and used to carefully excise the posterior joint capsule vertically, just medial to tendinous margin of medial head of gastrocnemius and lateral to the semimembranosus tendon, where the entrance to the cyst is usually located. The dissection should be continued along the course of gastrocnemius. The walls of the cyst should be removed as presented previously.

12.1.4.5 Tips for Managing Difficult Popliteal Cysts [20]

Large popliteal cyst extending to the thigh

If the cyst is large and extends to the thigh an additional posteromedial portal may be created to facilitate its excision. It is located in the "soft spot" 3–7 cm proximal to the posteromedial portal above the hamstrings and below the vastus medialis. The switching stick is introduced straight to the cyst through posteromedial portal to determine the direction for further work with the shaver. The arthroscope is inserted to the cyst through additional posteromedial portal over the switching stick inserted again under direct visualization. The shaver and radiofrequency probe are used to excise the cystic walls and resect the valvular mechanism limiting the unrestricted bidirectional fluid flow (Fig. 12.9). In such a procedure when two posteromedial portals are used, the surgeon is partially turned away from the monitor. To make this situation more comfortable one could move the monitor to the head or affected side of the patient and make a maximal abduction of the leg.

Popliteal cyst caused by posterior medial meniscus pathology

If the popliteal cysts seem to have a connection with the cyst of posterior horn of MM and the body of meniscus looks like empty inside, based on the preoperative imaging, both pathologies may be treated at once. With the arthroscope introduced through the anterolateral portal, the scalpel is inserted through the anteromedial portal and used to open inner margin of MM body horizontally. Then the shaver and hook probe are used to enlarge the tunnel in the MM what provides bidirectional fluid flow between the popliteal cyst

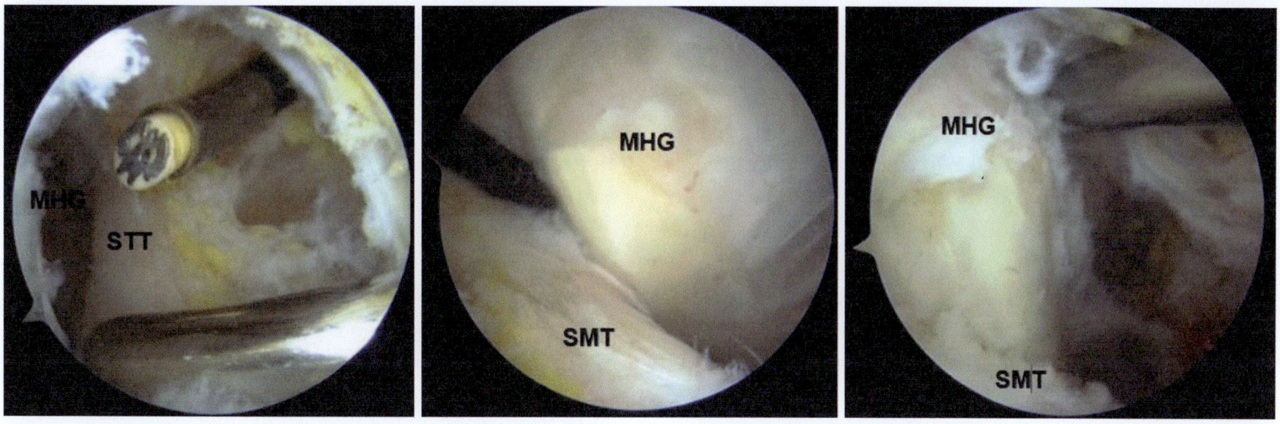

Fig. 12.9 The technique of two posteromedial portals in the right knee. Arthroscopic view from an anterolateral viewing portal (on the left), from an additional posteromedial portal (in the middle) and from the posteromedial portal (on the right). All these portals may be interchangeably used to introduced arthroscope, radiofrequency probe, and switching stick. *MHG* medial head of gastrocnemius, *STT* semitendinosus tendon, *SMT* semimembranosus tendon

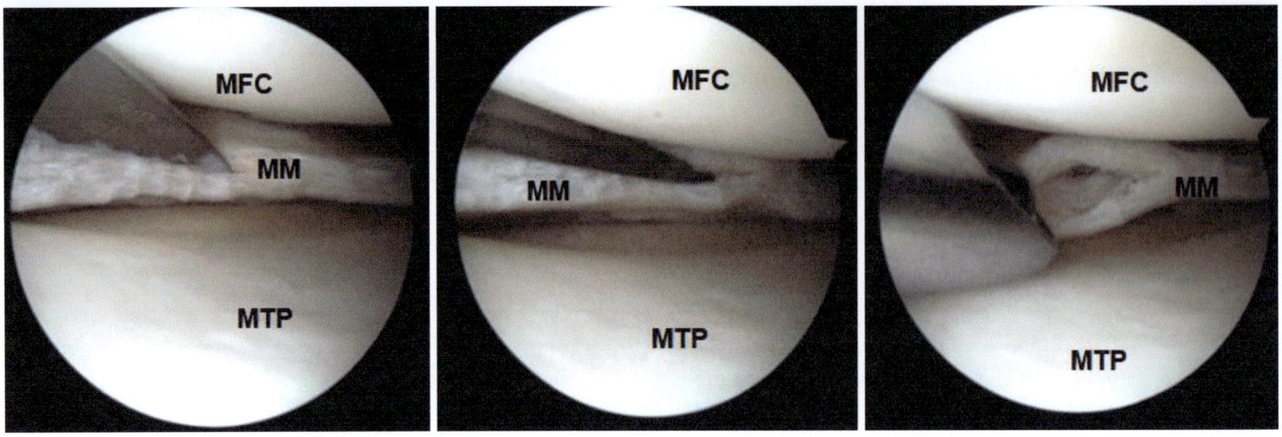

Fig. 12.10 The view from the anterolateral portal in the left knee. Modified Sansone-De Ponti technique. Simultaneous treatment of popliteal cyst and the cyst of posterior horn of medial meniscus (MM). The horizontal incision is made in the body of the meniscus. The shaver is used to enlarge the tunnel, what decompresses both cysts. *MFC* medial femoral condyle, *MTP* medial tibial plateau

and the joint cavity. One could remove meniscal cyst thorough this trans-meniscal approach (Fig. 12.10).

Large popliteal cyst descending to the calf

If the popliteal cyst is large and descends to the calf, a special approach is required. The patient should be positioned prone. The ultrasound imaging should be used to determine the cyst and mark its boundaries. Then, at the medial side of lower boundary of the cyst a small skin incision is performed, the subcutaneous tissue is dissected bluntly, and the scope is introduced between the skin and cystic wall. Then the lateral portal is created under visual control. The needle is advanced percutaneously to the cyst until the fluid leakage is observed. It confirms the proper direction of the portal. Then the transcystic portals are made and the shaver is used to excise cystic walls under direct arthroscopic control.

The same approach or two posteromedial portal technique may be utilized to treat popliteal cyst which lateral wall lies close the popliteal neurovascular bundle. However, a resection of the deep part of the lateral wall of this kind of cyst may be very dangerous and finally, it does not improve significantly clinical results.

12.1.4.6 Complications and Management

Maneuvering in the posteromedial compartment of the knee may lead to some serious and minor complications.

- Injury to popliteal neurovascular bundle
- To avoid it, use a non-aggressive tip of the shaver, always have the tip of the shaver visualized and directed anteriorly and medially, away from popliteal neurovascular structures. You can also resign from excising the lateral wall of the cyst, to make the procedure safer. Always check orientation of the scope because the landmarks are less obvious in popliteal space. Palpation and feeling of the instruments through the skin is very helpful. The neurovascular bundle in our procedure should be separated from the cyst by the muscle belly of medial head of gastrocnemius and some loose adipose tissue around. An old orthopedic sentence says: “Do not touch a red and yellow tissue if you want to stay out of trouble”. When the injury to the popliteal neurovascular bundle occurs, the consultation of vascular surgeon may be needed.
- Injury to saphenous nerve and vein
- To avoid it, use a transillumination and keep the knee in 90° of flexion when creating the posteromedial portals.
- Compartment syndrome in the calf
- It is a theoretical complication, which may occur. To avoid it, treat concomitant intra-articular lesions at first, and then start to manage with popliteal cyst. Carefully check arthroscopic pump pressure and regularly assess a calf condition manually.
- Popliteal hematoma
- It usually occurs when an aggressive shaver tip is used to remove cyst walls lying on muscle bellies which are accidentally scratched or some minor subcutaneous veins are damaged. To avoid this, do not touch a “red” part of muscles, use a non-aggressive shaver’s tips, and coagulate all bleeding points before you finish. This minor complication usually resolves over time. Cold compresses and vascular agents may be helpful to accelerate this process.
- Infection
- That is not an isolated problem and occurs along with joint infection. As in any case of arthroscopic surgery, an antibiotic prophylaxis and sterile conditions are applied to avoid this complication.

12.1.4.7 Postoperative Care

The special rehabilitation protocol for popliteal cyst treatment does not exist. The rehabilitation is determined by the main intra-articular pathology which caused popliteal cyst development and was treated simultaneously with the cyst.

To avoid postoperative contracture it is recommended to gain a free range of motion in the range of 0–90° on the first postoperative day.

12.1.5 Outcome

The senior author (K.M) in the last 17 years treated more than 1000 cases of patients with popliteal cysts. Since 2006–2012, 136 cases met our restricted inclusion criteria for simple technique of endoscopic typical popliteal cyst excision. 111 of them were available on follow-up. The surgical procedure involves treatment of intra-articular lesions, correction of valvular mechanism and cyst walls excision using single posteromedial portal in supine position. The patients were observed at 6, 12 months postoperatively and then once a year. The average follow-up was 37 months (6–71). The recurrence of the cyst was observed in 14 patients (12.3%), but in 12 of them the cyst was completely asymptomatic and found only in the ultrasound examination as a slit or small residual extension of gastrocnemius-semimembranosus bursa. The recurrence was strongly associated with severe cartilage lesions and residual instabilities, which could not be effectively addressed during primary surgery. In this study group no serious complications were observed. Transient complications involve calf swelling (9), popliteal hematoma (6), sensory deficit (2), superficial soft tissue infection (1), superficial vein damage (1).

12.1.6 Summary

- Popliteal cyst is usually an extension of natural gastrocnemius-semimembranosus bursa which lies in the posteromedial part of the knee. In most cases it is associated with concomitant intra-articular lesions.
- Popliteal cyst develops when intra-articular pressure increases due to joint fluid overproduction and the fluid leaks into the bursa through the valvular mechanism localized in the posteromedial capsule, which allows only for a unidirectional fluid flow.
- The most effective surgical technique for addressing the popliteal cyst involves an arthroscopic treatment of intra-articular lesions with correction of valvular mechanism, which restores a bidirectional fluid flow followed with excision of cystic walls.
- Maneuvering in the posteromedial compartment of the knee may be dangerous and to avoid complications some specific rules for using arthroscopic instruments must be applied.

Table 12.1 summarizes complex approach to treatment of popliteal cyst [20]. Used from *Arthroscopy Techniques*. It is an open access book published by Elsevier.

Table 12.1 Complex approach to treatment of popliteal cysts (Reprint from K. Malinowski et. al, Possible Approaches to Endoscopic Treatment of Popliteal Cysts: From the Basics to Troublesome Cases. *Arthrosc Tech*. 2019;8(4):e375-e382)

Pearls		
Step		
1	Preoperative magnetic resonance imaging (MRI)	Assess the location of popliteal cyst, valvular mechanism, position of the popliteal cyst against popliteal neurovascular bundle. The regular popliteal cyst should be well separated from the neurovascular bundle with medial head of gastrocnemius muscle. Identify intra-articular lesions and treatment possibilities.
2	Preoperative ultrasound examination	Do it when the popliteal cyst is large and there is a need of additional posteromedial and popliteal portals creation. Draw safe area on the skin.
3	Arthroscopy	Treat concomitant intra-articular lesions and the popliteal cyst with communication-enlargement surgery.
4	*Match the approach to the type of the cyst*	
	Typical popliteal cyst in gastrocnemius-semimembranosus bursa with visible valvular mechanism	Patient position: supine. Viewing portal: anterolateral with trans-notch maneuver. Working portal: posteromedial portal
	The popliteal cyst without visible connection with the joint. Large popliteal cyst ascending to the thigh. The popliteal cyst close to the popliteal neurovascular bundle on the thigh	Patient position: supine Viewing portal: anteromedial portal with trans-notch maneuver, then additional posteromedial portal. Working portal: posteromedial portal
	The popliteal cyst without connection with the joint caused by pathology of posterior part of medial meniscus	Patient position: supine Viewing portal: anterolateral Working portal: anteromedial
	Large popliteal cyst descends to the calf. The popliteal cyst more central close to the popliteal neurovascular bundle on the calf	Patient position: prone Viewing portal: medial popliteal Working portal: lateral popliteal
Pitfalls		
1) Using aggressive shaver for cyst wall removal		
2) Directing tip of working instrument toward neurovascular bundle		
3) Resecting muscle fibers or loose connective tissue		
4) Working without correct visibility		
5) Losing control of working depth and direction		
6) Losing anatomic position of the scope		
7) Resecting tissue too lateral from the medial border of gastrocnemius		
8) Leaving part of posteromedial fold or any tissues that could impair bidirectional fluid flow		

12.2 Endoscopic Harvest of Sural Nerve Graft

Lukas Rasulić and Milan Lepić

12.2.1 Introduction

Sural nerve is the most frequently used donor nerve in peripheral nerve and brachial plexus reconstruction procedures, as well as in orthopedic surgery, for iatrogenic and associated peripheral nerve injuries [21, 22]. Open surgery for sural nerve harvesting is usually done by making an incision over the whole length, or a series of small incisions along the pathway of the nerve. Both procedures have their advantages and flaws: while the long incision is related to extensive scarring, the series of incisions usually does not provide enough visualization and may be related to inadvertent damage, whereby the latter procedure was introduced only lately and requires further corroboration [23]. The imperfections of the open method served as a platform for an interesting application of endoscope in peripheral nerve surgery. The method for endoscopic sural nerve harvesting was first introduced by Kobayashi et al. in 1995 [24], and since then the technique has passed through many stages of improvement The procedure usually lasts no longer than 25 min, and with the latest technique it requires only one skin incision of 12 mm [25].

12.2.2 Anatomical and Physiological Considerations

Except for unmyelinated autonomic fibers, the sural nerve is a purely sensory nerve, providing cutaneous innervation. It is typically formed through the union of the lateral and medial sural cutaneous nerves, which originate from the common fibular (branch of the peroneal nerve) and tibial nerves. Rarely, the sural nerve is formed solely from the tibial nerve (medial sural cutaneous nerve) and even less commonly from the peroneal (lateral sural cutaneous nerve) [26].

The medial sural cutaneous nerve passes between the two heads of the gastrocnemius muscle, and runs through the deep fascia of the posterior compartment of the leg. At the midcalf level it conjures with the peroneal communicating branch and a lateral sural cutaneous nerve from the peroneal nerve. The nerve passes lateral to the calcaneal tendon, near the short saphenous vein, along the lateral border of the Achilles tendon and posterior to the lateral malleolus and the calcaneus. There, the nerve provides sensory supply to the posterior and lateral skin of the distal third of the leg, before passing distally along the lateral side of the foot and the little toe, to supply the overlying skin. The nerve anastomoses with the superficial fibular nerve on the dorsum of the foot [27]. Figure 12.11 illustrates the anatomy of the sural nerve(s).

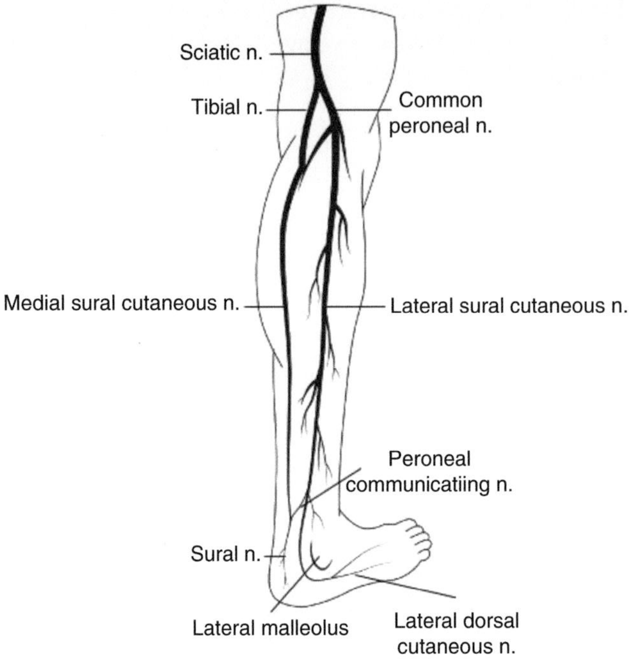

Fig. 12.11 The sural nerve anatomy

12.2.3 Indications

Grafts from the sural nerve are considered the most appropriate for the use in peripheral nerve and brachial plexus surgery. Whenever the nervous tissue defect (nerve gap) is longer than 1–2 cm, the graft is needed to achieve the distal end for direct repair, as well as in nerve transfers, when donor nerve length is not sufficient for the coaptation with the target nerve.

Short grafts have better reinnervation potential. A single piece long graft may be divided into a few pieces, shorter in length, which may be used to adequately match the donor and target nerves thickness when appropriate. The use of up to eight pieces was reported when using the viable C5 nerve root, four to repair the musculocutaneous nerve and the other four to repair the axillary nerve [28].

12.2.4 Contraindications and Limitations

General limitations and contraindications applying to the peripheral nervous system reconstructive procedures apply to the use of sural nerve grafts as well.

Timing is important. The denervated muscle atrophies and develops fibrosis, losing its contraction capacity and reinnervation potential through the vanishing of functional units. Motor reinnervation procedure in the absence of functional motor units in the target muscle is redundant [29].

The most common specific contraindication for the use of a sural nerve graft is the presence of peripheral neuropathy, compromising the sensation of the lower extremity. This pathological state raises concerns for the sural nerve harvest, primarily due to the donor site morbidity, which may cause more severe complications, and secondarily due to the questionable viability and nerve soundness.

Patients with previous surgery or trauma involving the posterior aspect of the leg within the sural nerve pathway should be investigated for possible damage and nerve indemnity.

Some authors consider the nerve defect longer than 6 cm as a threshold for the use of a vascular graft; although debatable, this should be taken into account in the decision-making process. In these circumstances, free vascularized nerve grafts are preferred over traditional nerve grafts. Another indication for the free vascularized nerve graft is for the patients considered to have poor regional vascularization, as well as those with significant scarring and fibrosis [31].

12.2.5 Surgical Procedure

12.2.5.1 Preoperative Considerations

Although the sural nerve harvest is usually only a small part of a complex reconstructive procedure, the functional sacrifice in a previously healthy region is subject to a serious medico-legal arrangement. The procedure must be explained to the patient and a family member in detail. Even though the donor site morbidity (anesthesia of the lateral calf and dorsum of the foot) may recover in the future, understanding that it may be a permanent sacrifice is of utmost importance.

12.2.5.2 Equipment

The endoscopic procedure is not demanding in terms of equipment, as there is no dedicated system for the sural nerve harvesting. Apart from the rigid endoscopes, flexible instruments are usually utilized, and there is also a recently introduced technique with the endoscopic system primarily designed for greater saphenous vein harvesting [25].

The application of this system in sural nerve harvesting procedure is even less complicated than is the case for its primary purpose (vein graft harvesting), due to the lack of bleeding, the toughness of the nerve in comparison to the vein, the resistance to the minor force, and potential adherence of the vein. The system uses a bisector rotating carriage with a large profile cutting toggle and C-Ring slider to separate the nerve, with a common CO_2 insufflation, and a 0-degree 5-mm camera [25].

12.2.5.3 Technique

As a rule, patients are positioned to the prone position for the sural nerve harvesting procedure. Exceptionally, endoscopic harvesting can also be performed from a supine position.

Before the patient is prepared and draped, it is essential to mark the landmarks and outline the sural nerve for the endoscopic procedure. The most reliable starting point to locate the nerve is at the classic spot, posterior to the lateral malleolus approximately half way between the malleolus and the Achilles tendon.

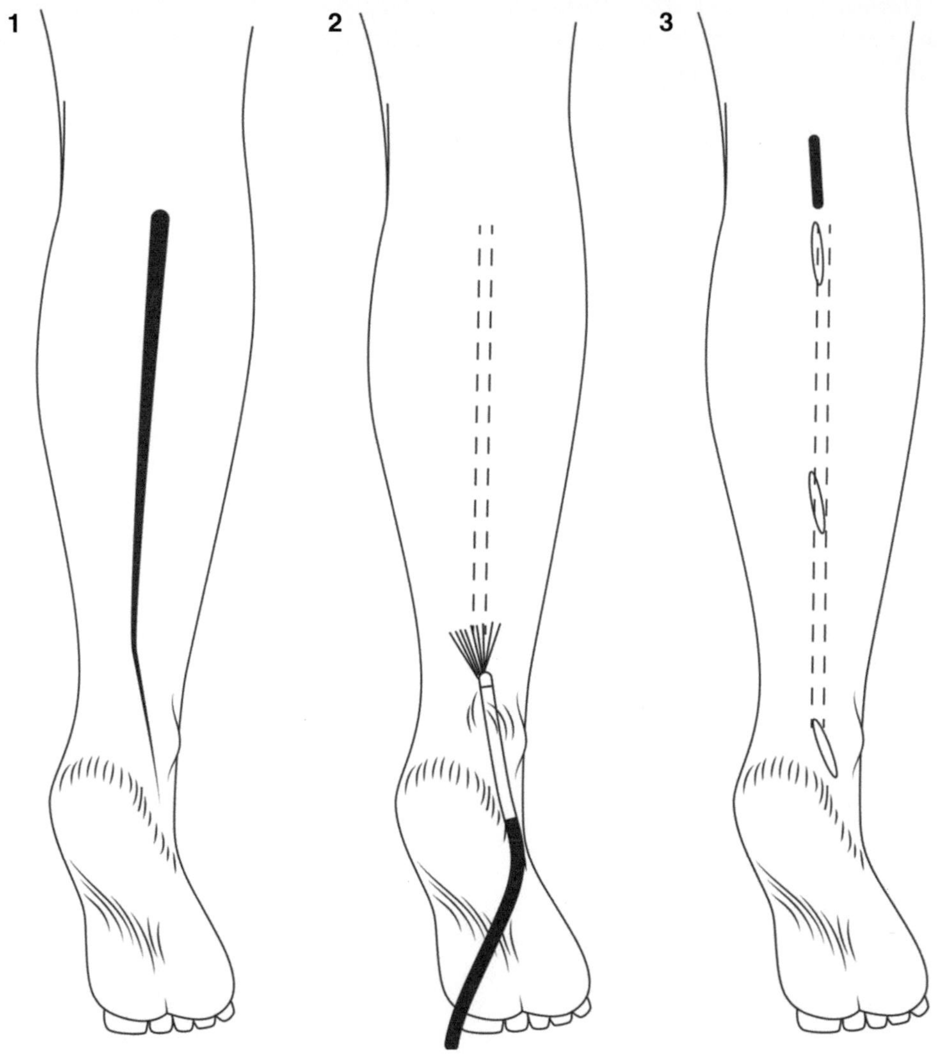

Fig. 12.12 Classical endoscopic sural nerve harvesting procedure. (1) Outlining the sural nerve on the skin. (2) Introduction of the endoscope through the incision at the starting point. (3) Harvested graft through three incisions

Classical endoscopic procedure (Fig. 12.12) is performed with the introduction of the endoscope through the 2 cm vertical incision at the starting point, along the outlined pathway to reach the length of the endoscope. Another incision is made, and the sural nerve is marked, before the procedure is repeated. Depending on the length of the endoscope, 3–4 incisions are needed to harvest the full-length sural nerve graft. The sural nerve is then resected and pulled out, and the incisions are closed. This technique allows for better bleeding control than when using a vein stripper [32].

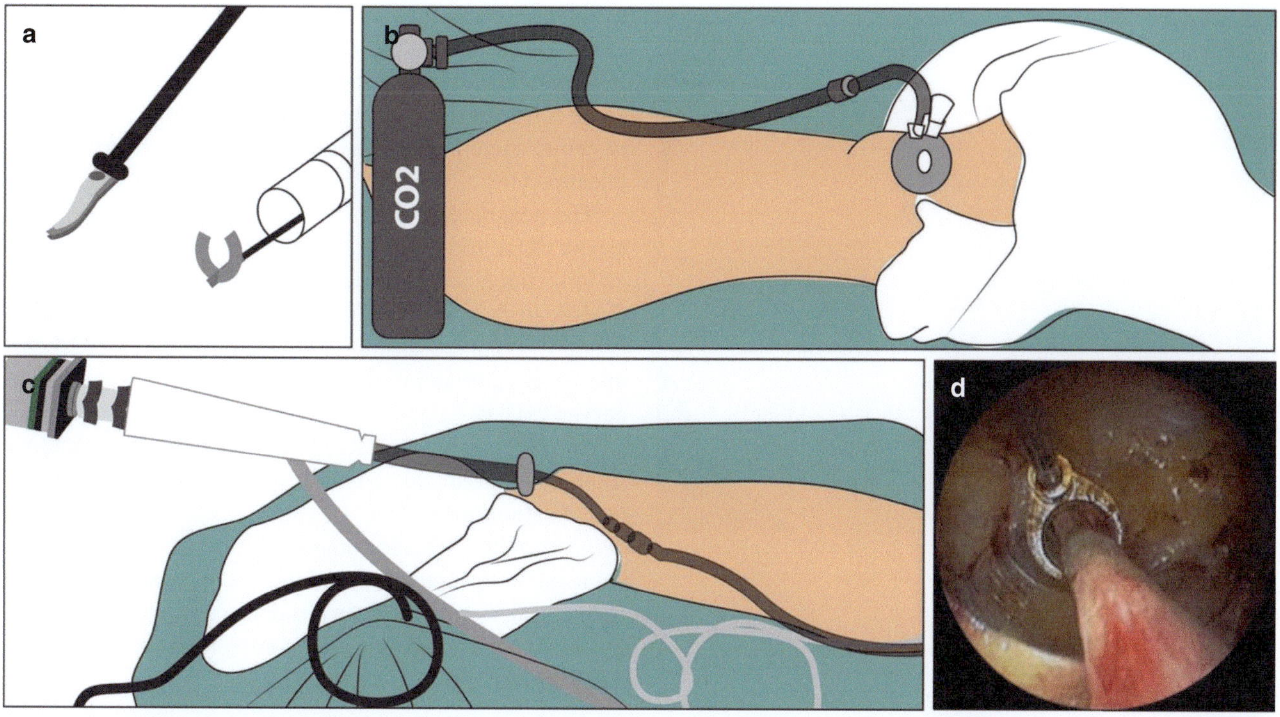

Fig. 12.13 Sural nerve harvesting using the greater saphenous vein graft endoscopic system

The procedure using the greater saphenous vein graft endoscopic system (Fig. 12.13) is performed through a 12 mm vertical incision at the starting point. The sural nerve is identified and dissected proximally to prepare for the insufflation and dissection. A 12 mm trocar is inserted to create a seal for CO_2 insufflation through the side port. The dissector with conical tip is introduced for initial dissection, before CO_2 insufflation to 12 mmHg to expand the tunnel.

Guided with the camera, the dissector is advanced along the four surface sides of the sural nerve at the desired length, with careful dissection of all branches. The conical tip dissector is then replaced with a bipolar bisector. The C ring is advanced along the nerve, to allow for branches identification and retraction, before cauterizing and cutting with the bipolar bisector. It is important to keep the distance of at least 2 mm between the bipolar bisector and the sural nerve graft to prevent thermal damage. The graft is separated with scissors, while the distal and proximal stumps are coagulated to prevent neuroma formation.

Hemostasis is achieved with the bipolar bisector, and the equipment and the graft are pulled out before the incisions are closed.

12.2.6 Advantages and Disadvantages

The strongest advantage of the sural nerve graft harvesting procedure with the use of endoscope is that it allows for the

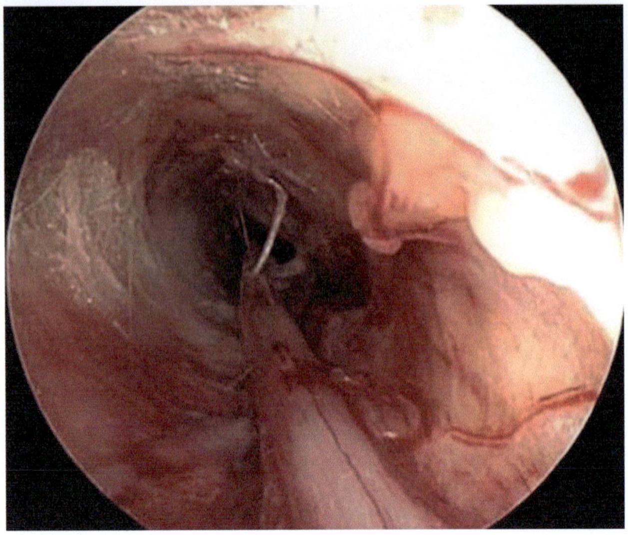

Fig. 12.14 Endoscopic visualization of the sural nerve (at 6 o'clock position)

intraprocedural visualization of the nerve for its viability and deflects an injury (Fig. 12.14). Also, it is done through a small incision, nevertheless allowing for complete nerve harvesting.

For many patients, especially young women, a long incision is not an option, since it only adds to the overall trauma of the nerve repair procedure. In particular, the presence of scars on the leg must be discussed ahead of the procedure.

Hemostasis is the most common limitation of the endoscopic procedures, but both presented methods deal well with this issue.

The most important unavoidable disadvantage is a relatively steep learning curve, which requires experienced endoscopic hands. Hence, for the surgeons switching from the open to the endoscopic approach, a supplementation with the cadaver lab training is a recommended way to go.

12.2.7 Complications

The general surgical complications are also common to the sural nerve harvesting procedures (poor wound healing and hypertrophic scarring). However, their probability is significantly lower with endoscopic techniques.

A painful neuroma at the site of nerve proximal section is a rare complication after sural nerve harvesting, and it is suggested to cauterize the proximal stump to prevent this complication [33].

The postoperative anesthesia of the dorsum and lateral aspect of the foot is a consequence rather than the complication. Some patients, however, may experience a hard time dealing with the sensory deficit. The pertinent anesthesia is expected to improve over a period of 1–2 years due to the collateral sprouting of the adjacent sensory nerves [31].

As they are unavoidable, these general complications should be considered natural history rather than procedural complications per se.

A procedure-specific complication occurs when the graft intended for the use with functional sacrifice at the donor site is damaged, especially when this damage remains unnoticed, in which case it might seriously compromise the whole complex reconstructive procedure.

12.2.8 Conclusion

The sural nerves grafts are probably the best possible option to use in peripheral nerve and brachial plexus reconstructive procedures. Both open and endoscopic harvesting procedures are still developing, each with its own imperfections.

The two endoscopic techniques presented have advantages over open surgery in terms of complete nerves visualization, mobilization, and adequate hemostasis. Providing a minimally invasive approach, with one or a few small incisions, the endoscopic techniques reduce common surgical complications and yield a far better cosmetic effect. Nevertheless, open surgery remains the most commonly used method, and is still a predominant standard for the graft harvesting in referential surgical centers worldwide.

12.3 Arthroscopic Management for the Anterior Half of Lateral Meniscus Through the Larai Portal

Rui Yang and Yi Long

Currently, the outside-in method is widely performed for suturing the anterior horn of the lateral meniscus, however, it has disadvantages in that an 1–2 cm long skin incision and knots tied subcutaneously over the capsule are needed [30, 34–38]. The all-inside method would overcome all these drawbacks. However, due to the limited angle under arthroscopy, it is difficult to suture the anterior half of lateral meniscus (AHLM) in tears by all-inside devices [39, 40]. Furthermore, it is much more challenging for arthroscopic surgeons to visualize and resect the inferior leaf of the AHLM through routine arthroscopic portals, especially the tears involved the anterior horn of the lateral discoid meniscus [41–43].

We proposed the Larai portal to observe the lesions and facilitate the application of all-inside devices in AHLM. We describe the portal "Larai" due to the following main points: (a) Lateral. This portal is established for lateral meniscus; (b) All-round. This portal can be acted as a working portal or viewing portal to observe and treat various tears extending to the AHLM; (c) All-inside. The portal permits all-inside instruments to pass through, providing a broader application for all-inside meniscal suture technique. The establishment of the Larai portal during the arthroscopy is performed in the figure of four position around the level of the knee joint line. The trajectory passes through the posterior septum from posteromedial to posterolateral compartments of the knee, and closely adjoins the posterolateral margin of the posterior cruciate ligament (PCL) to lateral compartment of the knee joint. The main surgical steps are as follows.

Surgery is performed in the supine position under combined spinal-epidural anesthesia. Routine diagnostic arthroscopy is performed using the standard anterolateral (AL) and anteromedial (AM) portals. If injuries to the AHLM are diagnosed based on preoperative local findings and imaging examination or arthroscopic examination, the Larai portal can be established. The knee is placed in the "figure of four" position with a 90° knee flexion to open the lateral compartment. First, a 1.0 mm long puncture needle is inserted from a point 1–2 cm lateral to the edge of the patellar tendon, closely adjoined to posterolateral margin of posterior cruciate ligament (PCL) under arthroscopic visualization, and pierced through the medial skin of distal thigh. Second, the trajectory was broadened from the medial skin of distal thigh along the indwelled long puncture needle by a 3.5 mm cannulated switching stick with blunt end. Third, the long puncture needle is pulled out after the tip of switching stick reached the lateral compartment of knee under arthroscopic visualization. Next, the slotted cannula inserted into the articular cavity along the switching stick, locating behind it with the slot toward to the front. The switching stick is then retrieved but the slotted cannula is maintained in the trajectory until the arthroscopic procedure is finished. At last, the AHLM can be observed, resected, or repaired as needed through this protecting cannula (Fig. 12.15).

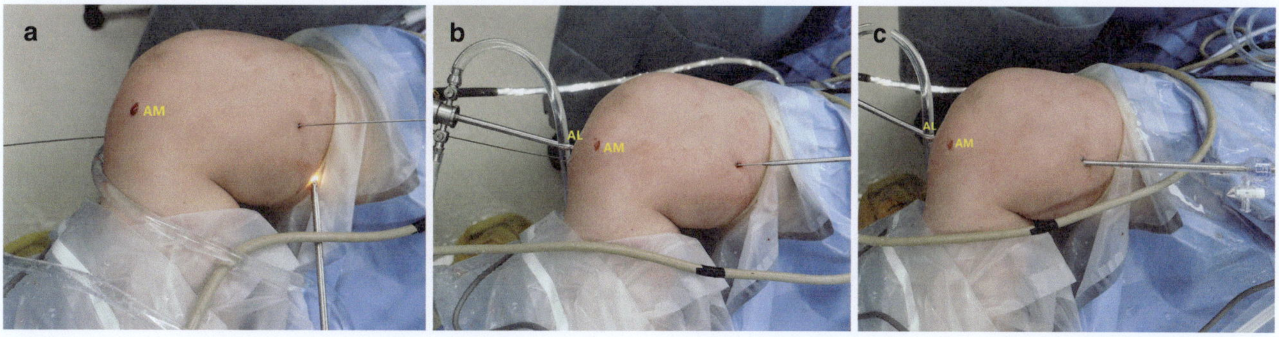

Fig. 12.15 The procedure of the Larai portal. (**a**) Inserting the 1.0 mm long puncture needle. (**b**) Broadening the trajectory by a 3.5 mm inner hollow core switching stick. (**c**) Inserting the slotted cannula along the switching stick. (**d**) Inserting the endoscope through the protecting cannula. (**e**) View from the Larai portal: the AHLM is trimmed by punch forceps through AL. (**f**) View from the AM: the AHLM is repaired by the FasT-Fix 360 system (Smith & Nephew, Andover, MA) through Larai portal. *AHLM* anterior half of lateral meniscus, *AL* anterolateral portal, *AM* anteromedial portal

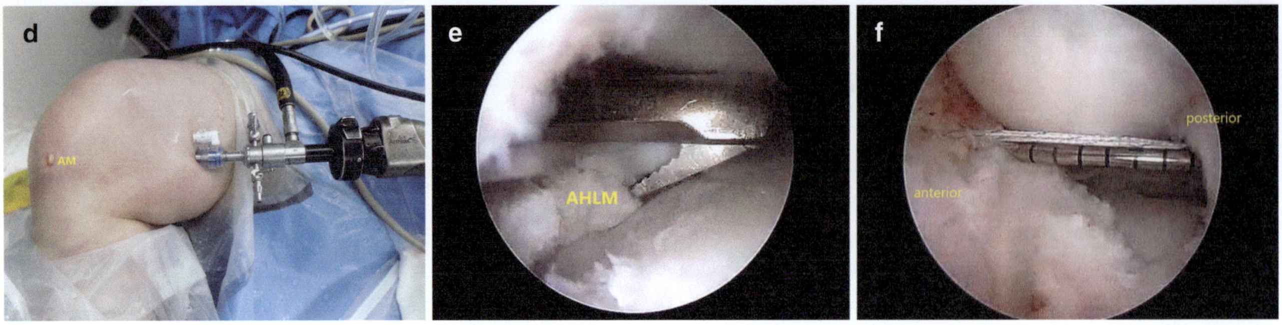

Fig. 12.15 (continued)

Some authors developed the all-inside methods that enables simple suture of the injury to the anterior horn of the meniscus through routine arthroscopic portal without using a specific instrument [44–47]. Meanwhile, various additional portals were proposed and described to visualize and resect the inferior leaf of the AHLM, including inframeniscal, lateral patellofemoral axillary, high anteromedial, or far anteromedial portal [48–52]. However, it is still insufficient to observe the deep-seated inferior leaf of the anterior horn meniscus and potentially increased risk of meniscus injury during the procedure. In addition, surgeons can hardly perform all-inside repair of the meniscal tears extending to the AHLM through these additional portals. The Larai portal which is a new portal permitting arthroscopic instruments to pass through from posteromedial side of the knee joint and provide a new route for all-inside repair of the AHLM tear under direct arthroscopic visualization.

Acknowledgments None

Funding disclosure None

Conflict of interest The authors have nothing to disclose, nor conflicts of interest related to this article, and the contents of this manuscript have not been previously published.

References

1. Frush TJ, Noyes FR. Baker's cyst: diagnostic and surgical considerations. Sports Health. 2015;7(4):359–65.
2. Cao Y, Jones G, Han W, et al. Popliteal cysts and subgastrocnemius bursitis are associated with knee symptoms and structural abnormalities in older adults: a cross-sectional study. Arthritis Res Ther. 2014;16(2):R59.
3. Herman AM, Marzo JM. Popliteal cysts: a current review. Orthopedics. 2014;37(8):e678–84.
4. Han JH, Bae JH, Nha KW, et al. Arthroscopic treatment of popliteal cysts with and without cystectomy: a systematic review and meta-analysis. Knee Surg Relat Res. 2019;31(2):103–12.
5. Zhou XN, Li B, Wang JS, Bai LH. Surgical treatment of popliteal cyst: a systematic review and meta-analysis. J Orthop Surg Res. 2016;11:22.
6. Rupp S, Seil R, Jochum P, Kohn D. Popliteal cysts in adults. Prevalence, associated intraarticular lesions, and results after arthroscopic treatment. Am J Sports Med. 2002;30(1):112–5.
7. Lie CW, Ng TP. Arthroscopic treatment of popliteal cyst. Hong Kong Med J. 2011;17(3):180–3.
8. Jiang J, Ni L. Arthroscopic internal drainage and cystectomy of popliteal cyst in knee osteoarthritis. J Orthop Surg Res. 2017;12(1):182.
9. Su C, Kuang SD, Zhao X, Li YS, Xiong YL, Gao SG. Clinical outcome of arthroscopic internal drainage of popliteal cysts with or without cyst wall resection. BMC Musculoskelet Disord. 2020;21(1):440.
10. Ohishi T, Takahashi M, Suzuki D, et al. Treatment of popliteal cysts via arthroscopic enlargement of unidirectional valvular slits. Mod Rheumatol. 2015;25(5):772–8.
11. Ahn JH, Yoo JC, Lee SH, Lee YS. Arthroscopic cystectomy for popliteal cysts through the posteromedial cystic portal. Arthroscopy. 2007;23(5):559.e1–4.
12. Pankaj A, Chahar D, Pathrot D. Arthroscopic management of popliteal cysts. Indian J Orthop. 2016;50(2):154–8.
13. Takahashi M, Nagano A. Arthroscopic treatment of popliteal cyst and visualization of its cavity through the posterior portal of the knee. Arthroscopy. 2005;21(5):638.
14. Cho JH. Clinical results of direct arthroscopic excision of popliteal cyst using a posteromedial portal. Knee Surg Relat Res. 2012;24(4):235–40.
15. Ahn JH, Lee SH, Yoo JC, Chang MJ, Park YS. Arthroscopic treatment of popliteal cysts: clinical and magnetic resonance imaging results. Arthroscopy. 2010;26(10):1340–7.
16. Ko S, Ahn J. Popliteal cystoscopic excisional debridement and removal of capsular fold of valvular mechanism of large recurrent popliteal cyst. Arthroscopy. 2004;20(1):37–44.
17. Liebensteiner MC, Thaler M, Putzer D, Wurm A, Nogler M. Arthroskopische Operation der Baker-Zyste: Operationstechnik. Videobeitrag [Arthroscopic procedure for Baker's cysts: surgical technique. Video article]. Orthopade. 2015;44(10):803–5.
18. Kongmalai P, Chernchujit B. Arthroscopic treatment of popliteal cyst: a direct posterior portal by inside-out technique for intracystic debridement. Arthrosc Tech. 2015;4(2):e143–8.
19. Vaishya R, Krishnan M, Vijay V, Agarwal AK. Arthroscopic management of popliteal cyst: comments and concerns. Indian J Orthop. 2017;51(2):229.
20. Malinowski K, Hermanowicz K, Góralczyk A, et al. Possible approaches to endoscopic treatment of popliteal cysts: from the basics to troublesome cases. Arthrosc Tech. 2019;8(4):e375–82.
21. Rasulic L, Savic A, Vitosevic F, Samardzic M, Zivkovic B, Micovic M, et al. Iatrogenic peripheral nerve injuries-surgical treatment and outcome: 10 years' experience. World Neurosurg. 2017;103:841–51.e6. https://doi.org/10.1016/j.wneu.2017.04.099.
22. Rasulic L, Cinara I, Samardzic M, Savic A, Zivkovic B, Vitosevic F, et al. Nerve injuries of the upper extremity associated with vascular trauma-surgical treatment and outcome. Neurosurg Rev. 2017;40(2):241–9. https://doi.org/10.1007/s10143-016-0755-2.
23. Cinal H, Barin EZ, Kara M, Karaduman H, Cengiz IZ, Tan O, et al. A new method to harvest the sural nerve graft. Eurasian J Med. 2020;52(1):12–5. https://doi.org/10.5152/eurasianjmed.2019.19102.
24. Kobayashi S, Akizuki T, Sakai Y, Ohmori K. Harvest of sural nerve grafts using the endoscope. Ann Plast Surg. 1995;35(3):249–53. https://doi.org/10.1097/00000637-199509000-00005.
25. Park SB, Cheshier S, Michaels D, Murovic JA, Kim DH. Endoscopic harvesting of the sural nerve graft: technical note. Neurosurgery. 2006;58(1 Suppl):ONS-E180; discussion ONS-E. https://doi.org/10.1227/01.NEU.0000193527.31749.2F.
26. Riedl O, Frey M. Anatomy of the sural nerve: cadaver study and literature review. Plast Reconstr Surg. 2013;131(4):802–10. https://doi.org/10.1097/PRS.0b013e3182818cd4.
27. Craig A. Chapter 48 – Nerve compression/entrapment sites of the lower limb. In: Tubbs RS, Rizk E, Shoja MM, Loukas M, Barbaro N, Spinner RJ, editors. Nerves and nerve injuries. San Diego, CA: Academic Press; 2015. p. 755–70.
28. Rasulic L, Savic A, Lepic M, Kovacevic V, Vitosevic F, Novakovic N, et al. Viable C5 and C6 proximal stump use in reconstructive surgery of the adult brachial plexus traction injuries. Neurosurgery. 2020;86(3):400–9. https://doi.org/10.1093/neuros/nyz179.
29. Rasulić L, Simić V, Savić A, Lepić M, Kovačević V, Puzović V, et al. The role of arm volumes evaluation in the functional outcome and patient satisfaction following surgical repair of the brachial plexus traumatic injuries. Neurological Res. 2020.
30. Silberberg MJ, Nilo FA, Gimenez M, Muina RJ. Outside-in single-lasso loop technique for meniscal repair: fast, economic, and reproducible. Arthrosc Tech. [Journal Article]. 2018;7(11):e1191–6.
31. Butler DP, Johal KS, Wicks CE, Grobbelaar AO. Objective sensory and functional outcomes at the donor site following endoscopic-assisted sural nerve harvest. J Plast Reconstr Aesthet Surg. 2017;70(5):659–65. https://doi.org/10.1016/j.bjps.2017.02.022.
32. Mobbs R. Peripheral nerve endoscopy: a cadaveric study. 2002.
33. Brunelli GA. Prevention of damage caused by sural nerve withdrawal for nerve grafting. Hand Surg. 2002;7(2):163–6. https://doi.org/10.1142/s0218810402001138.
34. Serrano PM, Amorim-Barbosa T, Santos SM, Sousa R. Alternative method of outside-in meniscal repair for anterior horn tears. Open Access J Sports Med. [Journal Article]. 2018;9:167–70.
35. Menge TJ, Dean CS, Chahla J, Mitchell JJ, LaPrade RF. Anterior horn meniscal repair using an outside-in suture technique. Arthrosc Techn. 2016;5(5):e1111–6.
36. Thompson SM, Spalding T, Church S. A novel and cheap method of outside-in meniscal repair for anterior horn tears. Arthrosc Techn. 2014;3(2):e233–5.
37. Dave LY, Caborn DN. Outside-in meniscus repair: the last 25 years. Sports Med Arthrosc Rev. [Journal Article; Review]. 2012;20(2):77–85.
38. Vinyard TR, Wolf BR. Meniscal repair: outside-in repair. Clin Sports Med. [Journal Article; Review]. 2012;31(1):33–48.
39. Alentorn-Geli E, Choi J, Stuart J, Toth A, Garrett W, Taylor D, et al. Inside-out or outside-in suturing should not be considered the standard repair method for radial tears of the midbody of the lateral meniscus: a systematic review and meta-analysis of biomechanical studies. J Knee Surg. 2016;29(07):604–12.
40. Elmallah R, Jones LC, Malloch L, Barrett GR. A meta-analysis of arthroscopic meniscal repair: inside-out versus outside-in versus all-inside techniques. J Knee Surg. 2019;32(08):750–7.
41. Na SI, Woo MS, Lee JM, Kim MK. A new surgical technique of arthroscopic partial meniscectomy for unstable inferior leaf of the

anterior horn in a horizontal tear of lateral meniscus. Knee Surg Relat Res. 2013;25(3):147–9.
42. Muniandy M, Rajagopal S, Tahir S. Arthroscopic all-inside repair of tear of the anterior horn of discoid lateral meniscus. Surg J. 2019;05(01):e35–7.
43. Chen D, Li Q, Sun Y, Qin J, Yao Y, Jiang Q. Arthroscopic management for the unstable inferior leaf of the lateral meniscus anterior horn and associated cysts through a direct inframeniscal portal: a retrospective study. Biomed Res Int. 2017;2017:1–7.
44. Kan H, Arai Y, Nakagawa S, Inoue H, Fujii Y, Fujiwara H, et al. All-inside meniscus repair method for injury of the margin of the anterior segment of the meniscus. Arthrosc Techn. 2018;7(3):e215–8.
45. Wang Z, Xiong Y, Tang X, Li Q, Zhang Z, Li J, et al. An arthroscopic repair technique for meniscal tear using a needle and suture: outside-in transfer all-inside repair. BMC Musculoskel Dis. 2019;20(1).
46. Cho J. Arthroscopic all-inside repair of anterior horn tears of the lateral meniscus using a spinal needle. Knee Surg Sports Traumatol Arthrosc. 2008;16(7):683–6.
47. Lee CK, Suh JT, Yoo CI, Cho HL. Arthroscopic all-inside repair techniques of lateral meniscus anterior horn tear: a technical note. Knee Surg Sports Traumatol Arthrosc. [Journal Article; Review]. 2007;15(11):1335–9.
48. Kim J, Bin S, Kim E. Inframeniscal portal for horizontal tears of the meniscus. Arthrosc J Arthrosc Relat Surg. 2009;25(3):269–73.
49. Choi N, Victoroff BN. Anterior horn tears of the lateral meniscus in soccer players. Arthrosc J Arthrosc Relat Surg. 2006;22(5):484–8.
50. Kim SJ, Jung KA, Kim JM, Kwun JD, Baek SH, Han JN. Arthroscopic all-inside repair of tears of the anterior horn of the lateral meniscus. Arthroscopy. [Journal Article]. 2005;21(11):1399.
51. Kim SJ, Park IS. Arthroscopic resection for the unstable inferior leaf of anterior horn in the horizontal tear of a lateral meniscus. Arthroscopy. [Journal Article; Technical Report]. 2004;20 Suppl 2:146–8.
52. Kim SJ, Kim HJ. High portal: practical philosophy for positioning portals in knee arthroscopy. Arthroscopy. [Journal Article]. 2001;17(3):333–7.

Bone Endoscopy Around the Knee: Navigation Endoscopic Assisted Tumor (NEAT) Surgery for Benign Bone Tumors Around the Knee

13

Kwok Chuen Wong, Hiu Woo Lau, Wang Kei Chiu, and Shekhar Madhukar Kumta

Abstract

We describe a novel technique, Navigation and Endoscopic Assisted Tumor (NEAT) surgery in patients with benign bone tumors. The technique combines the advantages of both bone endoscopy and navigation guidance. It enables surgeons to perform intra-lesional tumor curettage in selected benign bone tumors in minimal access with less surgical trauma. The curettage procedure and the tumor cavity not only can be visualized with an endoscope but also can be assessed for tumor clearance with real-time feedback of navigation information on the preoperative CT images. It is particularly useful in benign bone tumors at difficultly accessed locations or tumors with irregular bone cavity and internal septae. The technique may avoid excessive bone removal to minimize the risk of fracture while preserving normal bone for better limb function. An initial learning curve, the facilities required, and a lack of long-term clinical results are some obstacles to its widespread use.

Keywords

Bone endoscopy · Navigation · Benign bone tumors NEAT · Tumor curettage

13.1 Introduction

- Benign bone tumors frequently occur in the knee region, namely distal femur and proximal tibia. They are more common in pediatric and young adults. Diagnosis includes simple bone cyst, aneurysmal bone cyst, fibrous dysplasia, enchondroma, chondroblastoma, and giant cell tumor of bone. Progressive bone destruction in chondroblastoma and giant cell tumor of bone at the juxta-articular locations often lead to bone pain, may even result in fracture or deformity due to weakened bone or damage of articular cartilage with secondary osteoarthritis [1, 2].
- Given that the tumors are benign and the patients are in a young, active population, intra-lesional curettage is the mainstay of the surgical treatment. Tumor removal prevents further bone destruction, and yet preserves surrounding normal bone for joint function.
- The conventional tumor curettage in chondroblastoma and giant cell tumor of bones requires large surgical exposure. A cortical window is created over the tumor, usually reaching the peripheral edge of the tumor so that it is wide enough to visualize the tumor cavity for tumor clearance. Inadequate tumor removal accounts for the high rate of recurrence that was reported to be between 10–35% in Chondroblastoma [3] and 18–53% in giant cell tumor of bones [4, 5]. Also, the bigger the cortical window is made, the weaker is the weight-bearing and juxta-articular bone of the knee joint. It may compromise early post-operative recovery or has a risk of fracture.
- To address the potential undesirable effects of the conventional technique, endoscopic guided tumor curettage was reported in the surgical management of benign bone tumors [6–9]. The reports suggested that endoscopically guided curettage not only had the benefit of minimal access with less surgical trauma but also allowed visualization of the curettage procedure. The intramedullary cavity could be better assessed under direct and magnified endoscopic visualization in contrast to the open technique under naked eyes. Better visualization might facilitate complete tumor removal with less local tumor recurrence. Also, the endoscopic technique might avoid excessive curettage and minimize cartilage damage or risk of fracture [8, 10].

K. C. Wong (✉) · H. W. Lau · W. K. Chiu
Department of Orthopaedics and Traumatology, Prince of Wales Hospital, Hong Kong, SAR, China
e-mail: skcwong@cuhk.edu.hk

S. M. Kumta
Department of Orthopaedics and Traumatology, Prince of Wales Hospital, The Chinese University of Hong Kong, Hong Kong, SAR, China

© The Author(s), under exclusive license to Springer Nature Singapore Pte Ltd. 2021
T. H. Lui (ed.), *Endoscopy of the Hip and Knee*, https://doi.org/10.1007/978-981-16-3488-8_13

- The endoscopic approach often requires an intraoperative 2D fluoroscopic image to locate the bone tumor, guide the site of the cortical window, and position the operating instruments. 2D images may not provide adequate bone information for the guidance if the tumors have complex geometry, multi-loculated components with internal calcified septae, or in a difficult accessed location such as distal radius, proximal femur, or pelvis. A modified method, Navigation Endoscopic Assisted tumor (NEAT) surgery, was reported [11]. A computer navigation system that has been applied in orthopedic tumor resection [12] was used in addition to endoscopic tumor curettage. The navigation system allows surgeons to get an instant and real-time visual feedback of the patients' anatomy by referencing to the preoperative images about the spatial orientation of the extent of the tumor. Therefore, the NEAT surgery combines the advantages of navigation and endoscopic techniques to orientate and visualize the tumor cavity during the curettage procedure in a minimal access manner. It may facilitate adequate tumor clearance with the potential of minimizing tumor recurrence.
- This chapter is to describe the details of the tumor curettage using the NEAT technique in a patient with chondromyxoid fibroma of the distal femur.

13.2 Indications

- Biopsy-proven benign bone tumors (such as giant cell tumor of bone, enchondroma, chondromyxoid fibroma, aneurysmal bone cyst).
- Benign bone tumors at the difficult access locations (such as distal radius, proximal femur, pelvis).
- Benign bone tumors having multi-loculated components with internal septae, irregular peripheral bony borders, or close to articular cartilage at the subchondral bone, in which endoscopic curettage alone is difficult to ensure tumor clearance or avoid damage of the cartilage.
- Denosumab-treated giant cell tumor of bone in which newly formed internal calcification makes the curettage difficult to ensure tumor clearance.

13.3 Contra-indications

- Malignant bone tumors

13.4 Author Preferred Technique

13.4.1 Preoperative Planning

- Preoperative plain radiograph, CT, and MR examinations of the knee were performed to delineate the extent of the tumor (Fig. 13.1a, b). The CT images were acquired at the same setting when the patient underwent a CT-guided tissue biopsy. Axial CT images (slices with 0.625 mm thickness) of the knee were obtained using a 16-detector scanner (General Electric LightSpeed, Milwaukee, WI).
- The image datasets in Digital Imaging and Communications in Medicine (DICOM) format were imported into the CT-based navigation system (VectorVision, BrainLAB, iPlan Spine 2.0.1, Feldkirchen, Germany). The images were reformatted into different views. The extent of the bone tumor was mapped, and a

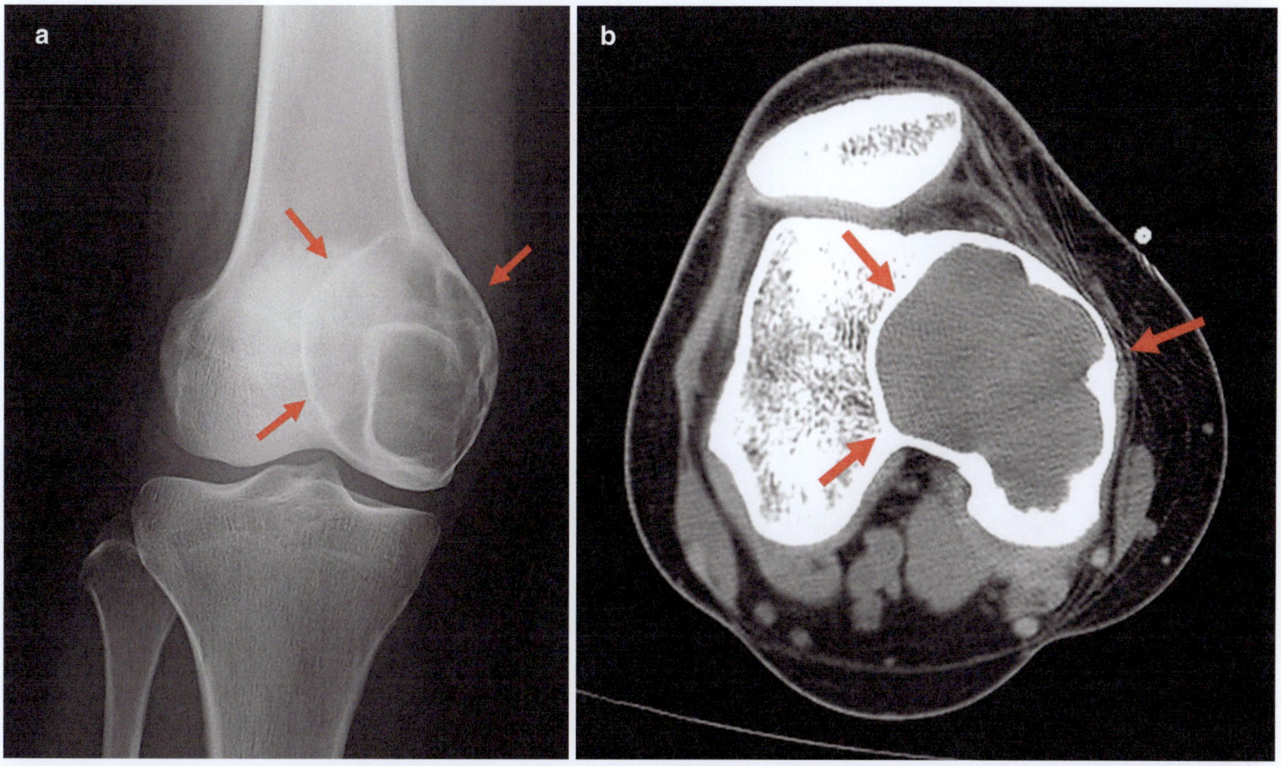

Fig. 13.1 (**a**) The plain radiograph (anteroposterior view) of the right knee shows a mildly expansile osteolytic lesion with a well-defined sclerotic border at the medial condyle of the right femur in a 30-year-old patient. (**b**) The axial view of CT images of the same patient shows the osteolytic lesion at the medial femoral condyle with thinning of the cortex, close to the subchondral bone of the knee joint, and some irregularities of the inner tumor cavity. The CT-guided biopsy confirmed a benign bone tumor with the histological diagnosis of a chondromyxoid fibroma

3D tumor model was generated (Fig. 13.2a). The sites of endoscopic portals were planned in the navigation system so that the entire tumor cavity could be reached and curetted by instruments (Fig. 13.2b–d).

- Required instruments: a shoulder arthroscope (30° lens, 4 mmS.W.A.; Karl Storz, Tuttlingen, Germany); curettes, high-speed bone burr, and a CT-based navigation system with the navigation trackers and probe.

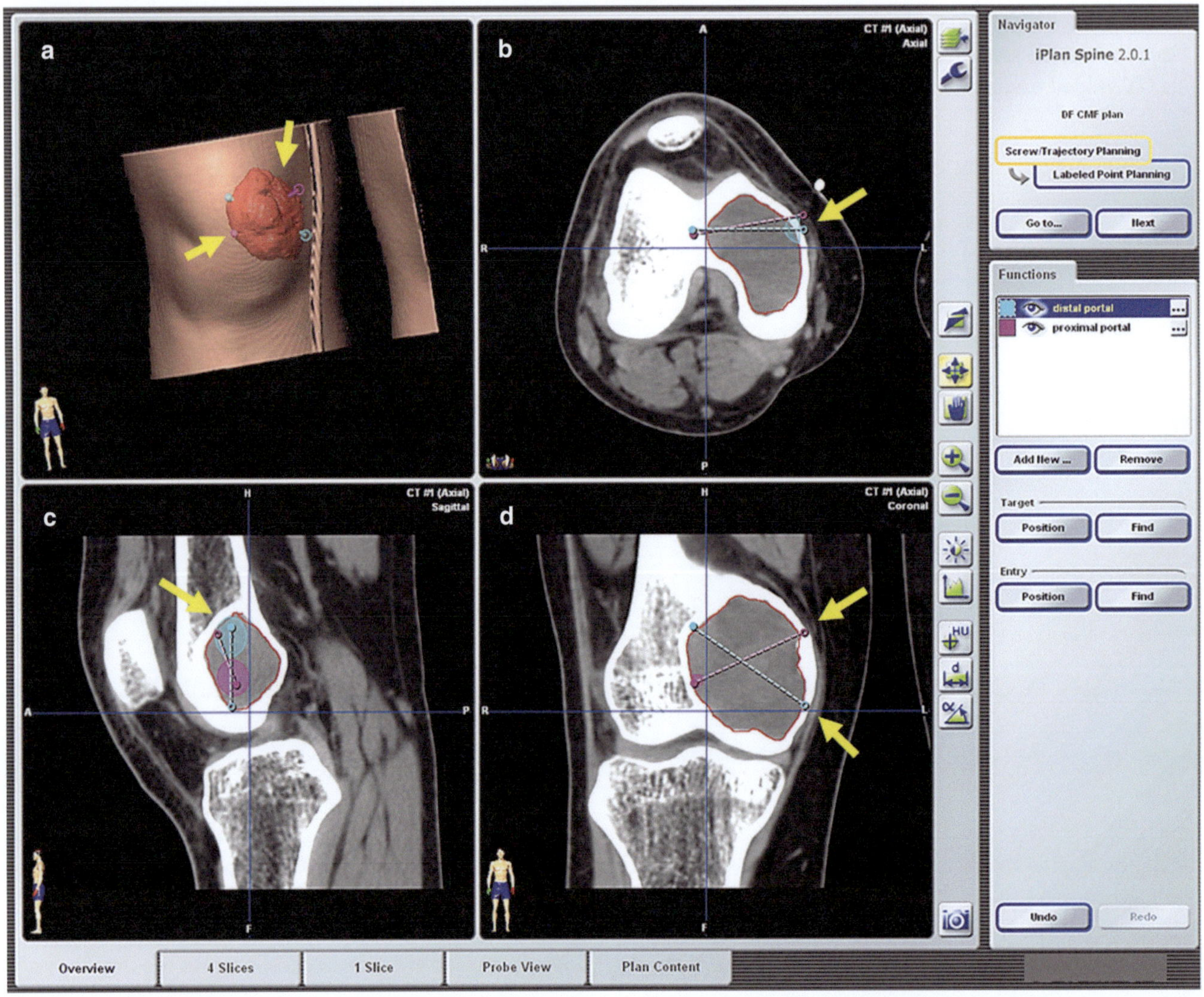

Fig. 13.2 Preoperative CT and MR images were imported and fused in the navigation system. The tumor was mapped (red). The extent of the tumor (arrows) could be examined in the 3D model (**a**), axial (**b**), reformatted sagittal (**c**), and coronal (**d**) images. The volume of the tumor could be calculated to estimate the amount of cement or bone graft needed for filling up the cavity after tumor curettage

13.4.2 Patient Positioning

- The patient was positioned supine on an operating table with a radiolucent board (Fig. 13.3a). An ipsilateral thigh pneumatic tourniquet was applied to provide a bloodless surgical field during the bone curettage. The opposite leg was hanged on leg support to facilitate the intraoperative acquisition of the plain radiograph of the knee (Fig. 13.3b).
- The navigation machine, with its tracking camera, was positioned at the rear end of the operating table (Fig. 13.4).

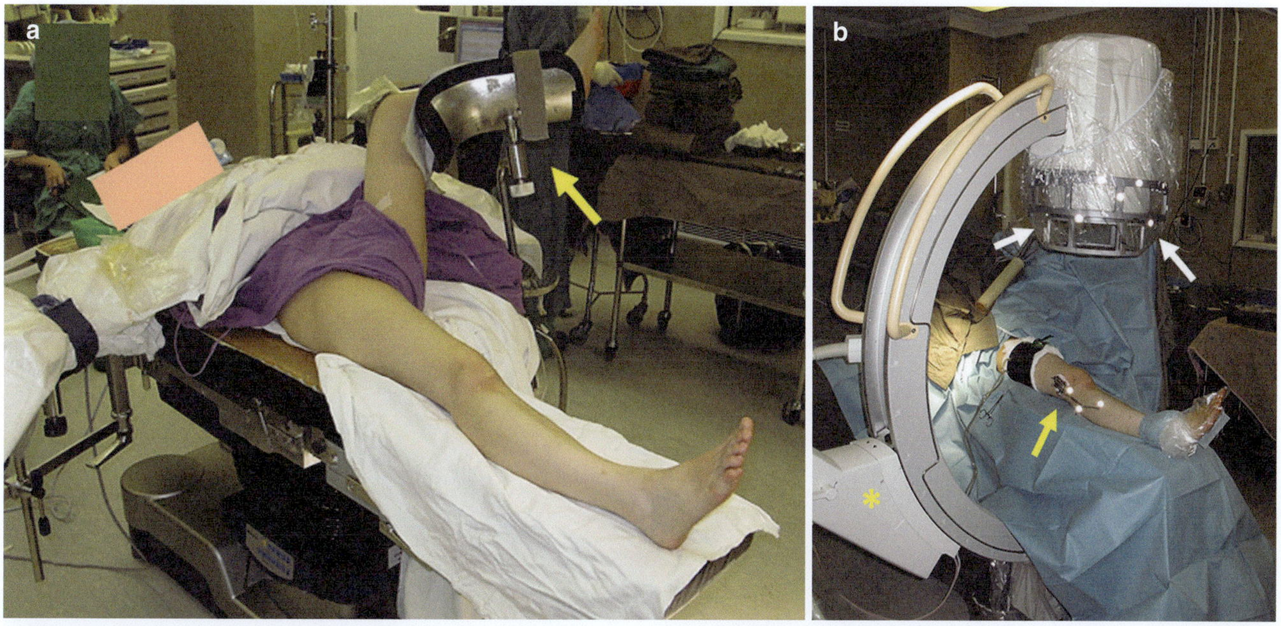

Fig. 13.3 (**a**) The patient was positioned supine with left leg hang on leg support (arrow). (**b**) The patient's position facilitated the C-arm X-ray machine (asterisk) to acquire the anteroposterior and lateral views of the plain radiograph of the right knee for the navigation procedure. A patient tracker (yellow arrow) and a phantom tracker (white arrows) of the C-arm X-ray machine were mounted for the image registration of the plain radiographs

Fig. 13.4 The operative set-up for the NEAT surgery. The navigation system was located at the rear end of the operating table so that no physical objects were blocking between the navigation camera (asterisk) and the patient and instrument trackers (arrows)

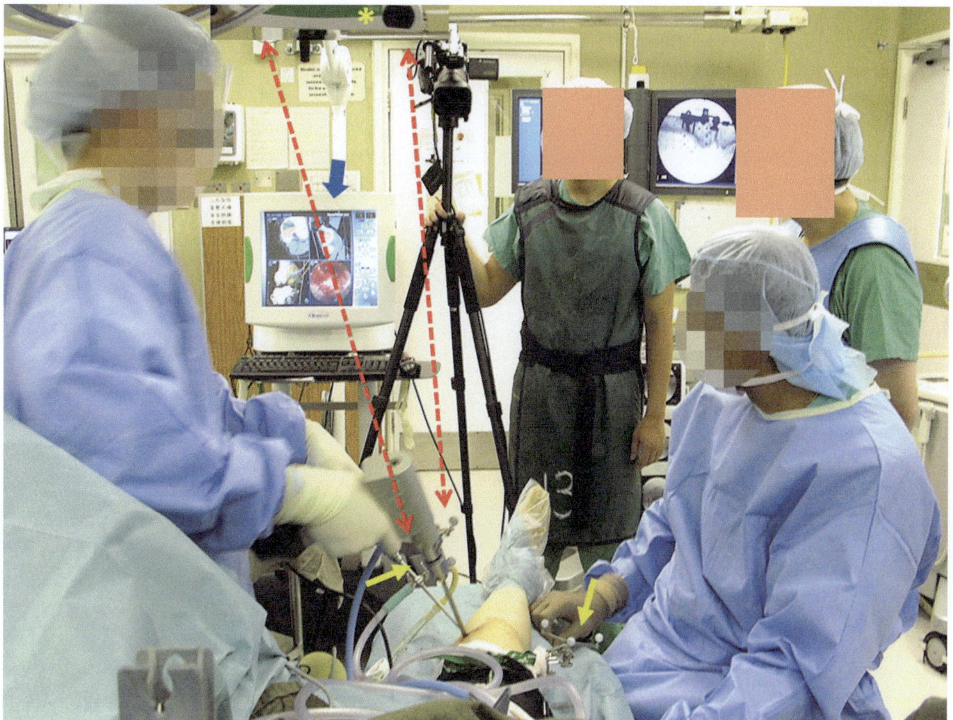

An extra video monitor was located on the right side of the operating table so that the operating surgeon could watch the endoscopic images alone when performing bone curettage without navigation guidance (Fig. 13.5).

- The endoscopic curettage procedure did not require fluid inflow, and the curettage procedure was performed with dry endoscopy.

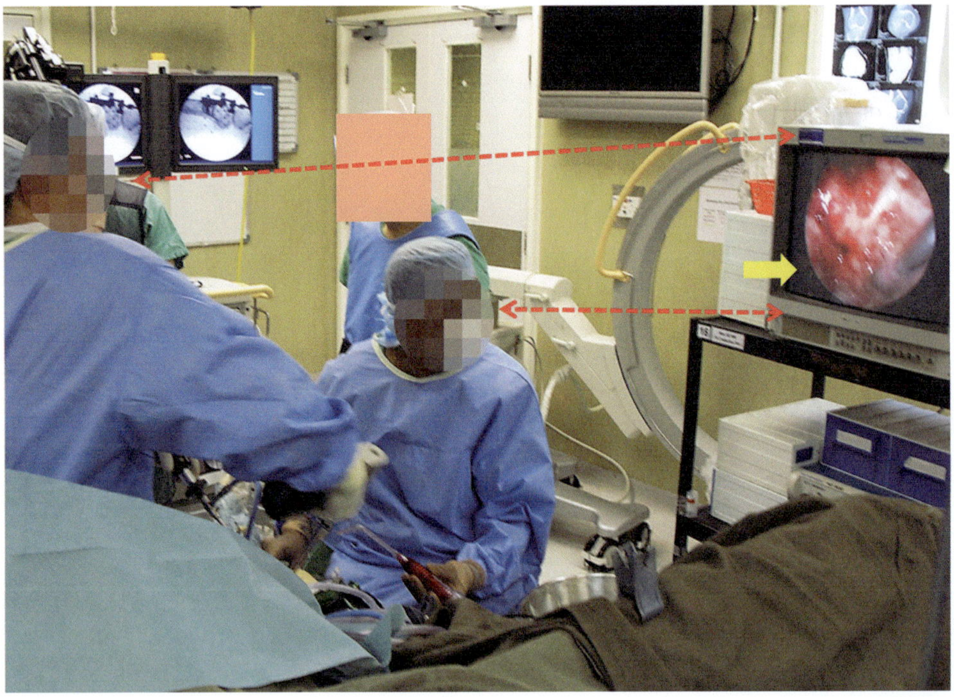

Fig. 13.5 Another arthroscopic monitor (orange arrow) was located on the right side of the patient so that the operating surgeon could concentrate only on endoscopic images when the navigation guidance was not required

13.4.3 Portal Design

- Two portals were used. Two cortical windows of about 1 cm in diameter were planned on the medial and middle aspect of the right distal femoral condyle so that the tumor cavity could be reached during curettage procedure (Fig. 13.6a–c). As the arthroscope, bone curettes, and high-speed burr are straight instruments, the two portals may be connected as one larger portal to facilitate the tumor clearance if necessary.

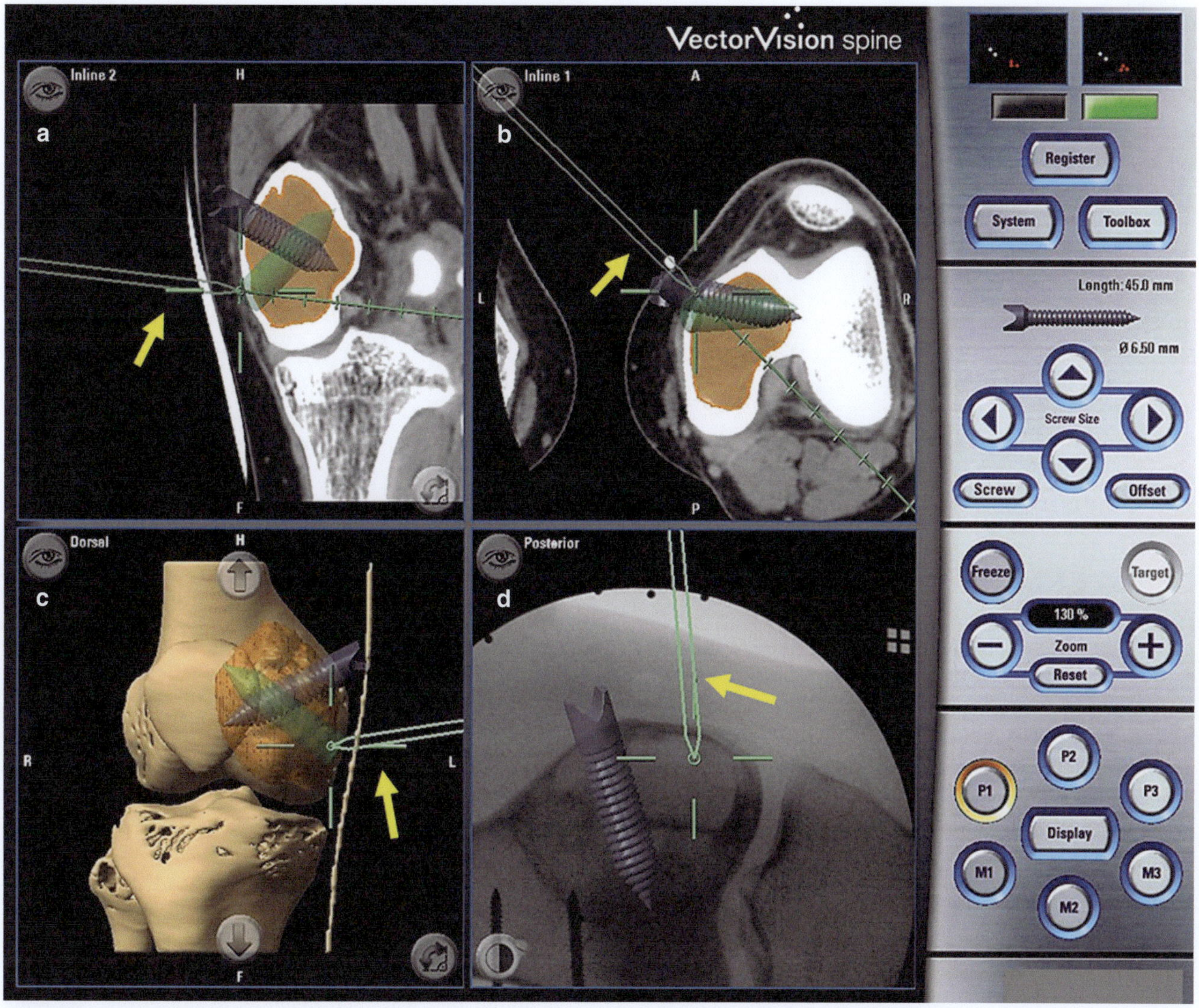

Fig. 13.6 The navigation display shows the locations of the working and viewing portals that were marked as pedicle screws (gray and green) in reformatted coronal (**a**), axial (**b**), 3D bone tumor model (**c**), and intraoperatively acquired plain radiograph (**d**) in the CT navigation spine system. The locations of the portals were planned so that the tumor cavity (orange) could be fully reached. After the image-to-patient registration, the planned location of the distal portal was identified by using the navigation probe (arrows)

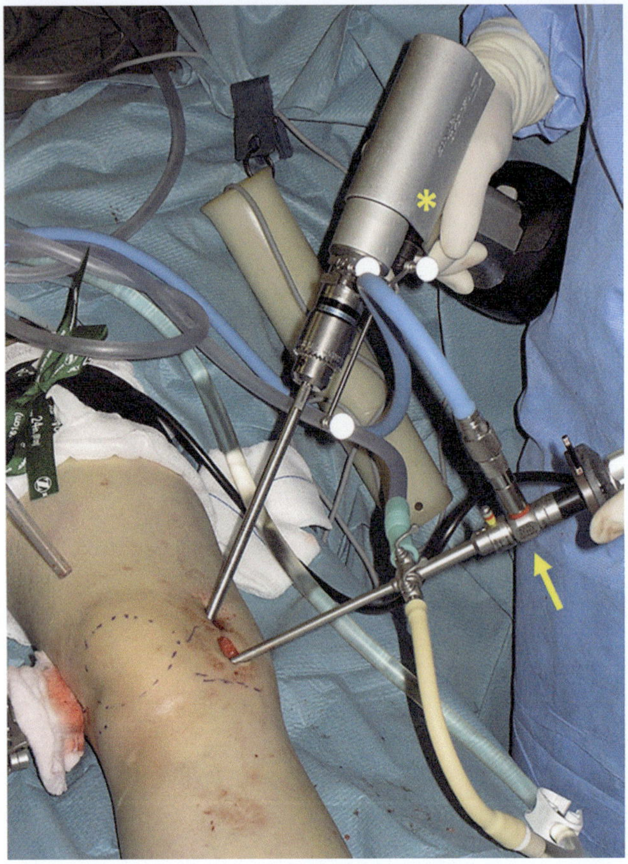

Fig. 13.7 The shoulder arthroscope (arrow) was inserted into the distal viewing portal to visualize the curettage procedure performed by the navigated bone burr (asterisk) at the proximal working portal

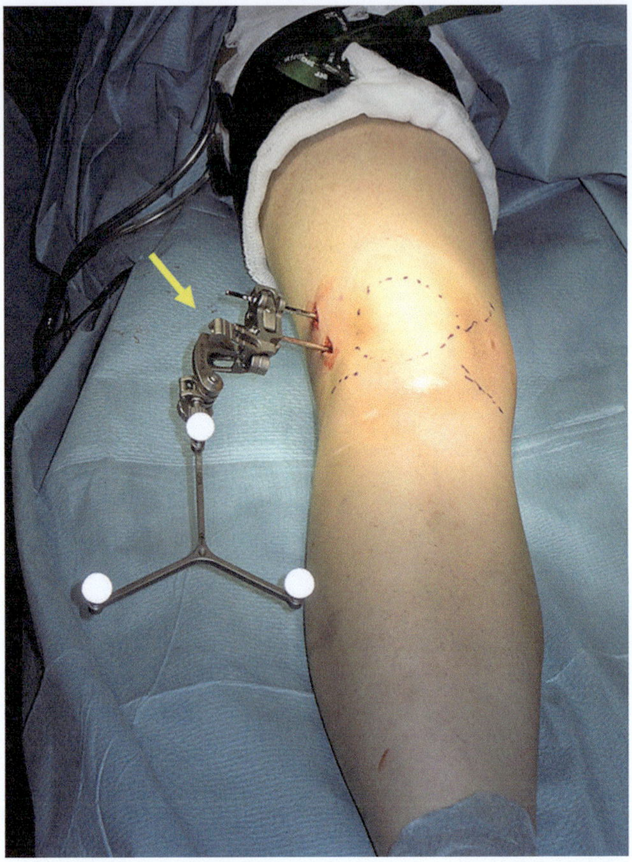

Fig. 13.8 The patient tracker (arrow) was attached to the lateral aspect of the distal femur after inserting two parallel 4.5 mm anchoring pins. The tracker was placed at the lateral side so that it would not be blocking the arthroscope and working instruments on the medial side

- The tumor was removed through one working portal under direct magnified endoscopic visualization at the second viewing portal (Fig. 13.7). The curettage instruments and arthroscope took turns to change the portals for the tumor curettage.

13.4.4 A Detailed Description of the Technique

- A patient's tracker was attached to the lateral femoral condyle by inserting two parallel 4.5 mm pins so that the tracker would not hinder the working and viewing portals at the medial femoral condyle (Fig. 13.8).
- To real-time tracking the operating bone, the navigation surgery requires a registration process in which the operative anatomy matches precisely to the preoperative CT images in the navigation software. A CT-fluoro matching technique was used. An ortho planar (anteroposterior and lateral) fluoroscopic images were intraoperatively acquired that was then matched to the virtual 3D bone

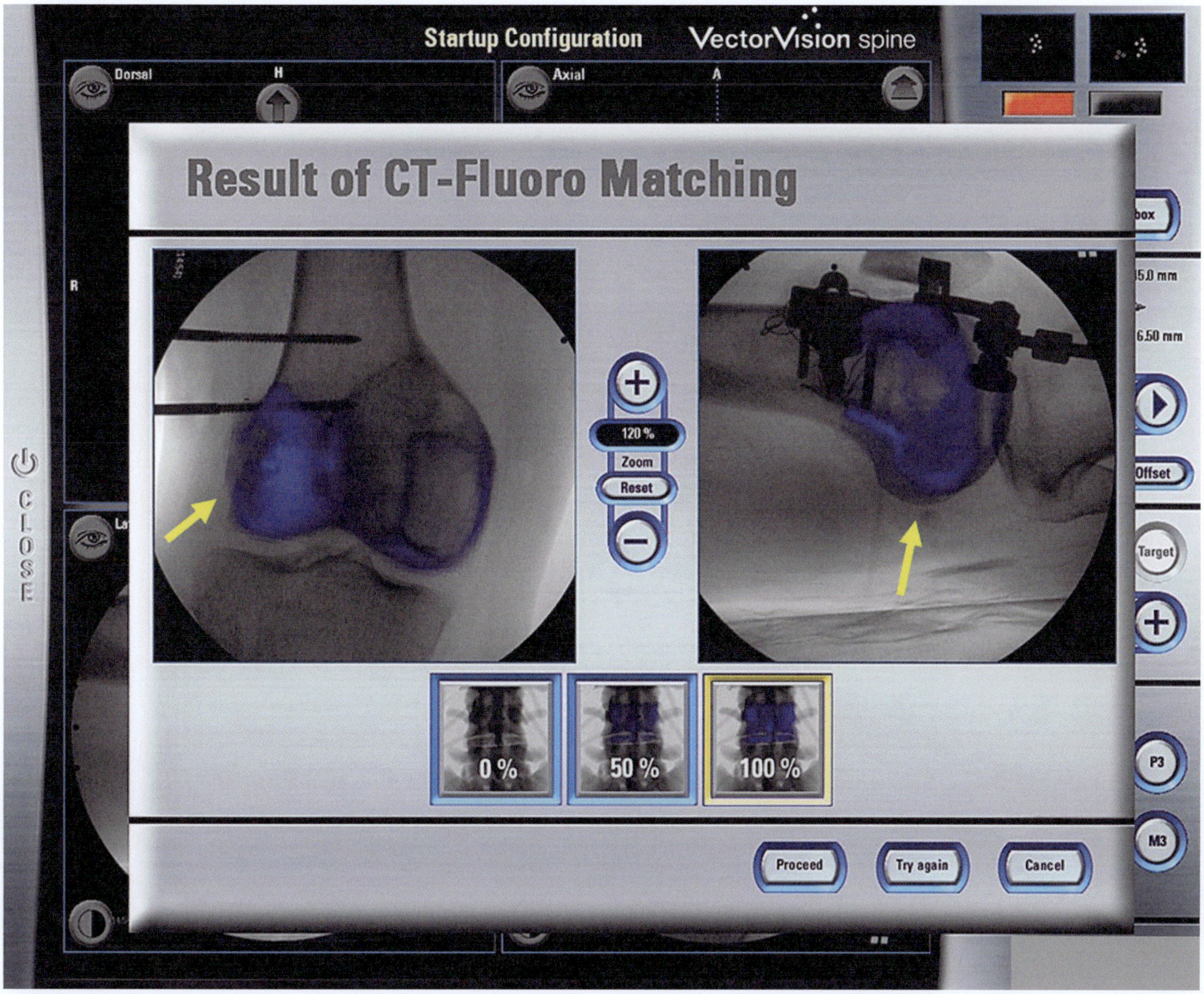

Fig. 13.9 CT-fluoro matching was used for the image-to-patient registration in the navigation procedure. It involved the matching of the 3D model of the distal femur (arrow) generated from the preoperative CT images with intraoperatively acquired anteroposterior and lateral views of fluoroscopic images. The registration was considered accurate when the 3D bone model (blue) was manually moved until its outline overlapped precisely with that of fluoroscopic images

model generated from the preoperative CT images in the navigation system (Fig. 13.9).

- The registration accuracy was further verified by touching the navigation probe on the anatomic landmarks or the

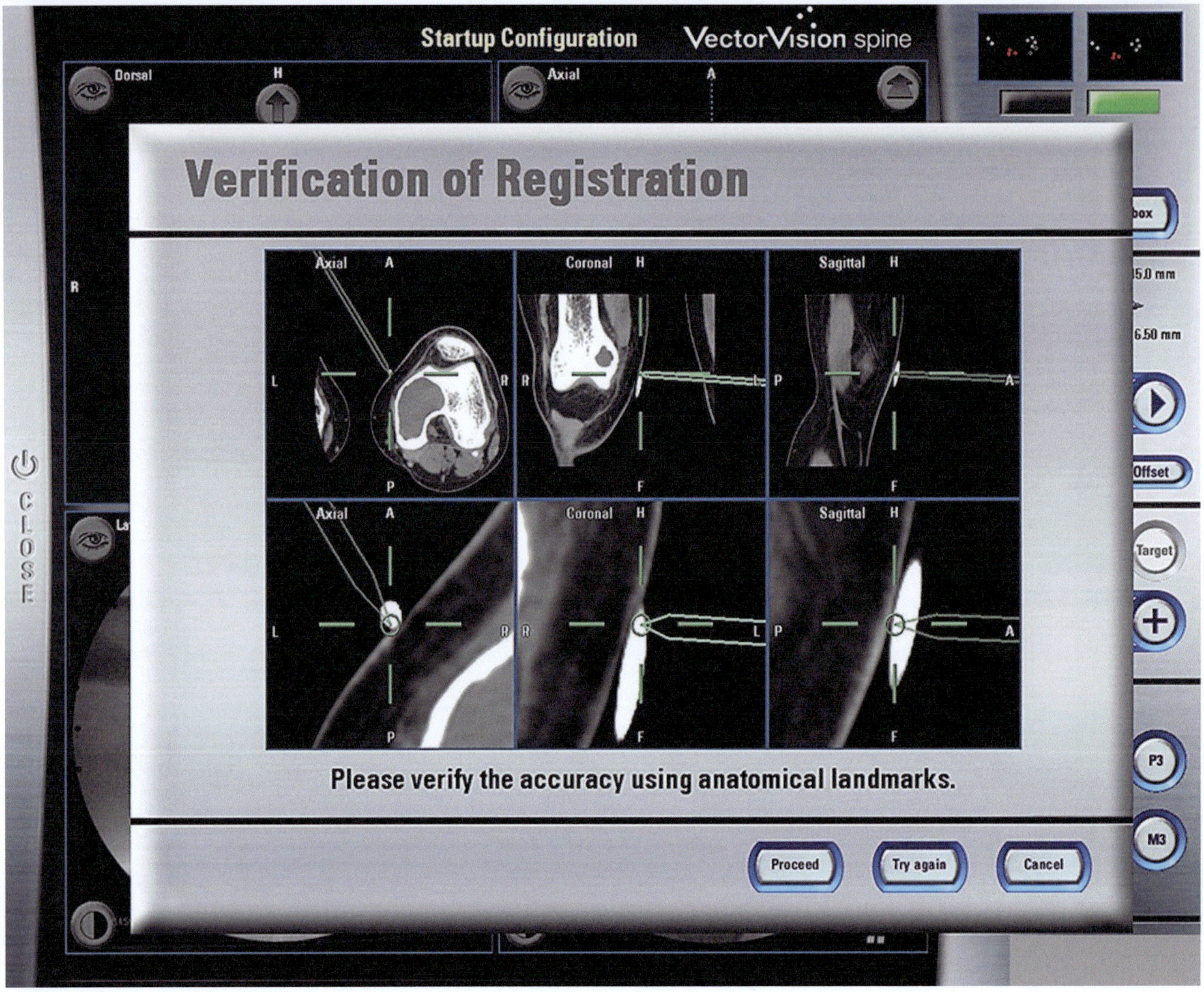

Fig. 13.10 The registration accuracy was verified using the navigation probe (green) touching anatomical landmarks, the skin of the patient, or the bone surface at the portal

bone surface (Fig. 13.10). The navigation system was considered accurate only if there was exact matching between the image on the navigation console and the patient's bone anatomy.

- The skin incision over the planned portals was marked under navigation guidance (Fig. 13.11). A pneumatic tourniquet of the right thigh was put on.
- The sites of the cortical bone window were identified and made as planned under navigation guidance (Fig. 13.6a–d).
- After the central bulk of the tumor was curetted via the two portals (Fig. 13.12), tumor curettage was further performed at the tumor cavity with endoscopic assistance (Fig. 13.13a, b).

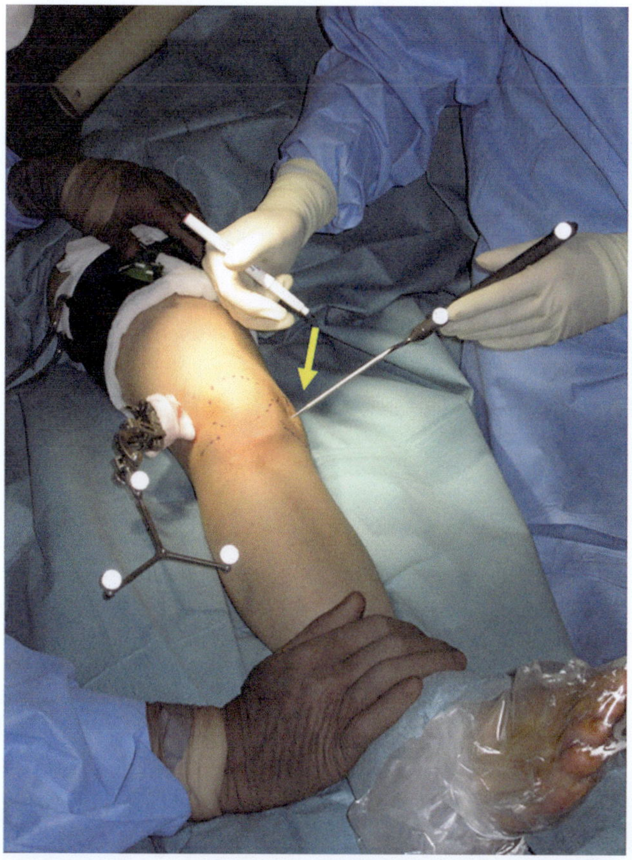

Fig. 13.11 The skin incision (arrow) at the two portals could be precisely marked under navigation guidance with the navigation probe

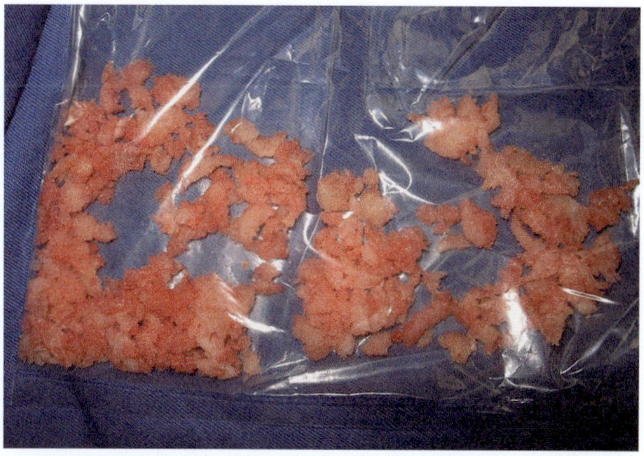

Fig. 13.12 The curetted tumor was sent for the histological examination after the NEAT surgery

Fig. 13.13 (**a**) The tumor was removed by using a curette (asterisk) via the proximal working portal under (**b**) the direct visualization of the arthroscope at the distal viewing portal. The endoscopically assisted procedure then allowed tumor curettage in a minimal access manner with less surgical trauma

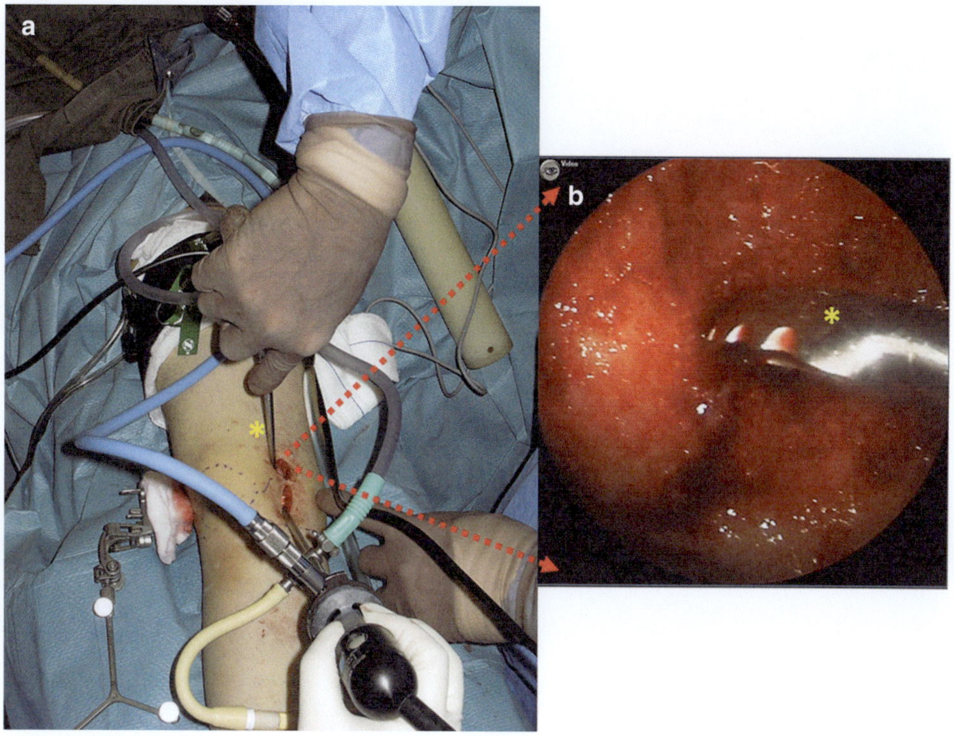

- High-speed bone burr mounted with navigation trackers were calibrated to the navigation system so that the tip of the burr was correctly referenced and spatially visualized regarding the patient's anatomy. The entire intraosseous surface of the tumor cavity was further removed under the navigation guidance and direct endoscopic visualization (Fig. 13.14a–d). The excessive burring of the normal bone could be avoided to minimize fracture or at the subchondral area to reduce the chance of osteoarthritis.
- The endoscopic visualization allowed us to visually identify the residual tumor on the walls of the tumor cavity

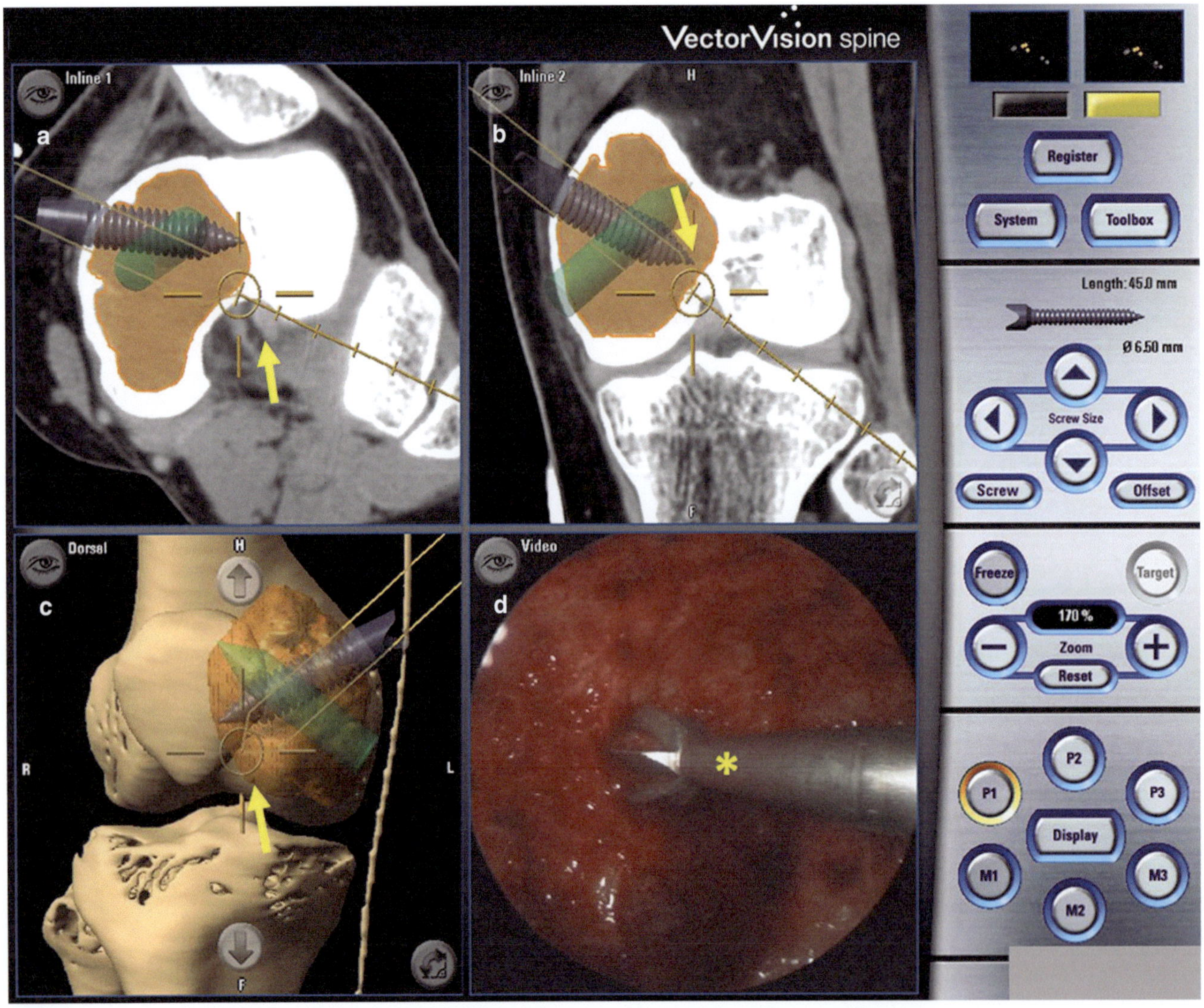

Fig. 13.14 The spatial location of the tip of the navigated bone burr (arrow) could be real-time tracked under the navigation system with reference to the various reformatted CT images, (**a**) axial, (**b**) coronal views, and (**c**) 3D bone tumor model. (**d**) The bone burr (asterisk) could also be visualized with the endoscopic images

while the navigation guidance confirmed the clearance was reaching the peripheral edge of the tumor with reference to preoperative CT images (Fig. 13.15a–d).

- The tumor cavity was irrigated with hydrogen Peroxide and copious normal saline. Cement was injected into the bone cavity using a cement gun via one of the portals

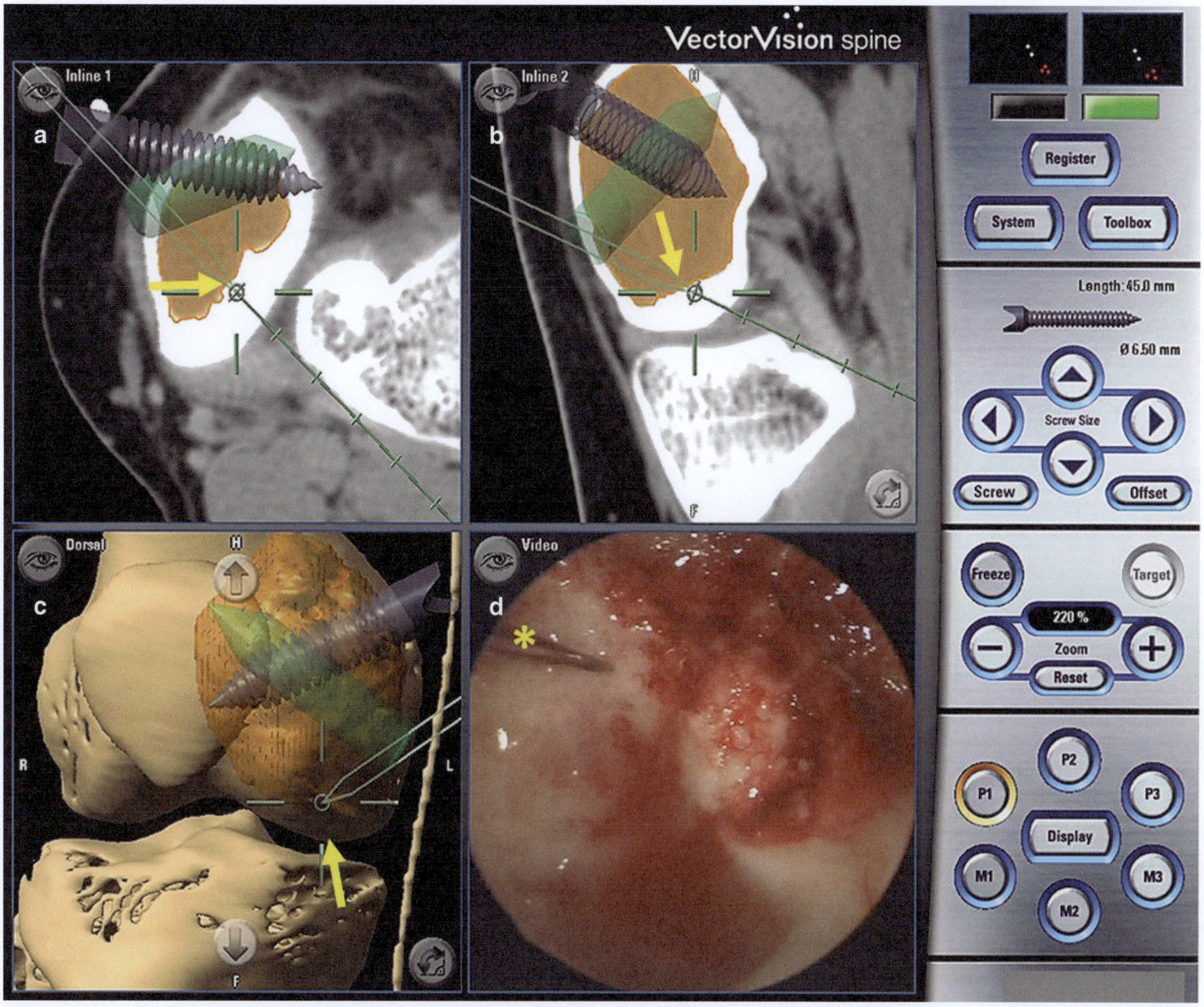

Fig. 13.15 The adequacy of the tumor clearance could be further verified by using the navigation probe touching at the different sites of the curetted tumor cavity. The reformatted coronal (**a**), sagittal views (**b**), and 3D bone model (**c**) show that the tip of the navigation probe (arrows) was just beyond the peripheral edge of the tumor cavity near the subchondral region of the medial femoral condyle. (**d**) The navigation probe (asterisk) could also be visualized with the endoscopic images. The NEAT surgery could facilitate complete tumor clearance while avoiding excessive normal bone removal

(Fig. 13.16a). A suction drain was inserted to prevent wound hematoma due to possible bleeding at the bone-cement junction, and the wound was closed by layers (Fig. 13.16b).

13.4.5 Complications

- Local tumor recurrence depends on the type of benign bone tumors undergoing tumor curettage and the adequacy of local tumor clearance. The technique may facilitate tumor surgeons to achieve better tumor control that may translate into a better clinical outcome.
- Fracture due to the already weakened bone by tumor invasion or excessive bone burring during curettage procedure.
- Late osteoarthritis as a result of the loss of subchondral bone by tumor involvement.

13.4.6 Post-operative Care

- With the minimal access approach in terms of skin incision and cortical bone windows, the patient was allowed to resume full-weight bearing walking and immediate joint mobilization after the suction drain was removed 1 or 2 days after surgery.
- A plain radiograph was taken after the drain was removed and then post-operative 1 month, every 3 months for the first 2 years, every 6 months for 3 years and then annually. Most of the tumor recurrence occurs at 2–3 years after surgery, and an annual plain radiograph was taken to detect late osteoarthritis (Fig. 13.17a, b).

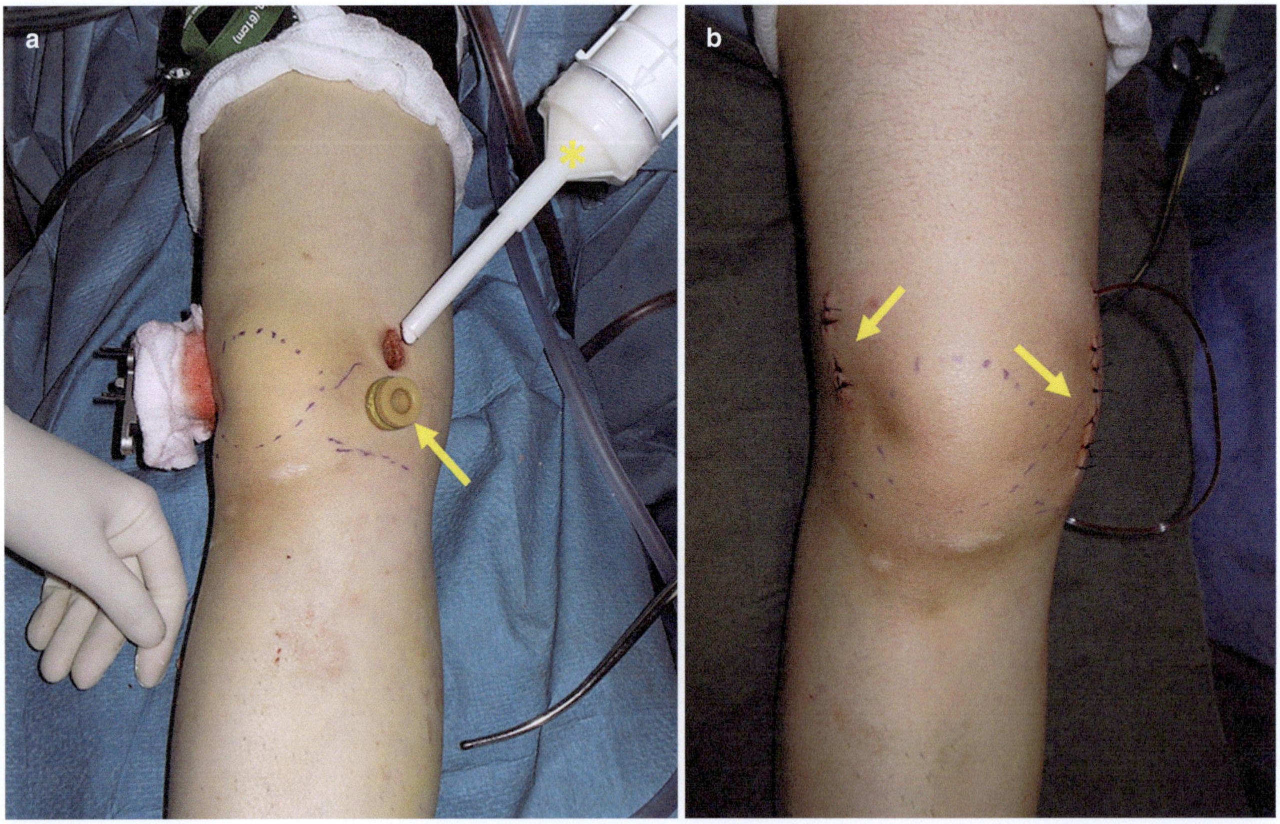

Fig. 13.16 (**a**) The tumor cavity was filled with bone cement by using a cement gun. The cement was pressurized with a plastic stopper at the distal portal; (**b**) shows the final skin closure

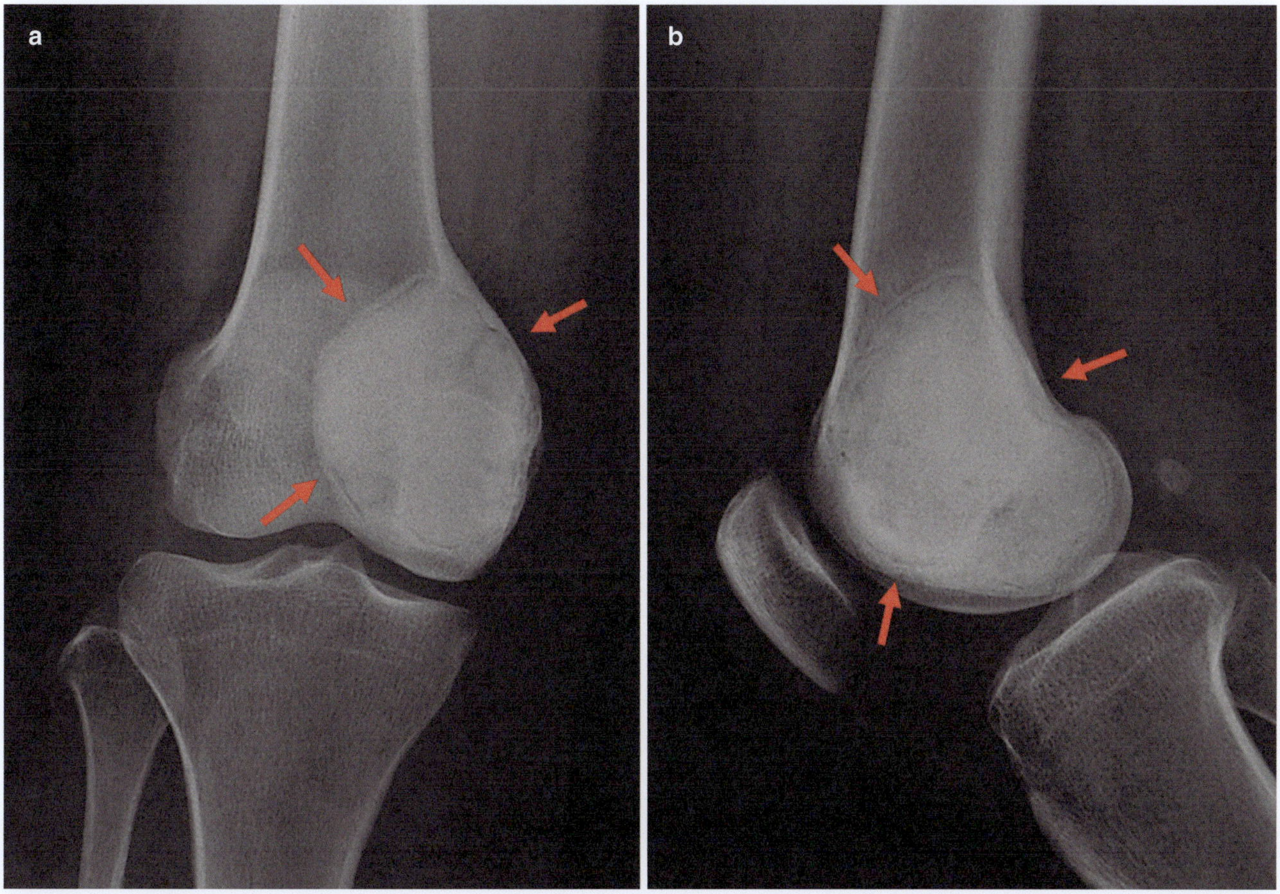

Fig. 13.17 The anteroposterior (**a**) and lateral views (**b**) of the plain radiograph of the knee show no tumor local recurrence nor osteoarthritis at 11 years after the surgery

13.5 Summary

- The NEAT surgery combines the advantages of both bone endoscopy and navigation guidance. It enables surgeons to perform intra-lesional tumor curettage in selected benign bone tumors in minimal access with less surgical trauma. The curettage procedure and the tumor cavity not only can be visualized with an endoscope but also can be assessed for tumor clearance with real-time feedback of navigation information on the preoperative CT images.
- The technique may avoid excessive bone removal to minimize the risk of fracture while preserving limb function. A learning curve is anticipated as it requires both expertise of endoscopic and navigation surgery. There is no long-term result to support the potential benefits that can be translated into a better outcome.
- Currently, there is no commercial system and instruments dedicated to bone endoscopy. It would be helpful to design special curved instruments or protective portal sheath for endoscopic tumor surgery.

References

1. Farfalli GL, Slullitel PA, Muscolo DL, Ayerza MA, Aponte-Tinao LA. What happens to the articular surface after curettage for epiphyseal chondroblastoma? A report on functional results, arthritis, and arthroplasty. Clin Orthop Relat Res. 2017;475(3):760–6.
2. van der Heijden L, van de Sande MA, Heineken AC, Fiocco M, Nelissen RG, Dijkstra PD. Mid-term outcome after curettage with polymethyl methacrylate for giant cell tumor around the knee: higher risk of radiographic osteoarthritis? J Bone Joint Surg Am. 2013;95(21):e159.
3. Ramappa AJ, Lee FY, Tang P, et al. Chondroblastoma of bone. J Bone Joint Surg [Am]. 2000;82-A:1140–5.
4. Turcotte RE, et al. Giant cell tumor of long bone: a Canadian Sarcoma Group study. Clin Onhop Relat Res. 2002;397:248–58.
5. Hu P, Zhao L, Zhang H, et al. Recurrence rates and risk factors for primary giant cell tumors around the knee: a multicentre retrospective study in China. Sci Rep. 2016;6:36332.
6. Stricker SJ. Extraarticular endoscopic excision of femoral head chondroblastoma. J Pediatr Orthop. 1995;15(5):578–81.
7. Otsuka T, Kobayashi M, Yonezawa M, Kamiyama F, Matsushita Y, Matsui N. Treatment of chondroblastoma of the calcaneus with a secondary aneurysmal bone cyst using endoscopic curettage without bone grafting. Arthroscopy. 2002;18(4):430–5.
8. Choi Y, Kwak JM, Chung SH, Jung GH, Kim JD. Tumor treated by endoscopy. Clin Orthoped Surg. 2014;6:72–9.
9. Aiba M, Kobayashi Y, Waguri-Nagaya H, Goto J, Mizutani S, Yamada H, Okamoto M, Nozaki H, Mitsui S, Miwa M, Kobayashi K, Endo S, Saito T, Goto T. Otsuka, treatment of aneurysmal bone cysts using endoscopic curettage. BMC Musculoskelet. Disord. 2018;19(1):268.
10. Dietz JF, Kachar SM, Nagle DJ. Endoscopically assisted excision of digital enchondroma. Arthroscopy. 2007;23:678.e1–4.
11. Wong KC, Kumta SM, Tse LF, Ng WK, Lee KS. Navigation Endoscopic Assisted Tumor (NEAT) surgery for benign bone tumors of the extremities. Comput Aided Surg. 2010;15(1–3):32–9.
12. Wong KC, Kumta SM. Use of computer navigation in orthopedic oncology. Curr Surg Rep. 2014;2(4):47.

MIX
Papier aus verantwortungsvollen Quellen
Paper from responsible sources
FSC® C105338

If you have any concerns about our products,
you can contact us on
ProductSafety@springernature.com

In case Publisher is established outside the EU,
the EU authorized representative is:
Springer Nature Customer Service Center GmbH
Europaplatz 3, 69115 Heidelberg, Germany

Printed by Libri Plureos GmbH
in Hamburg, Germany